The LEARN® Program for Weight Management 2000

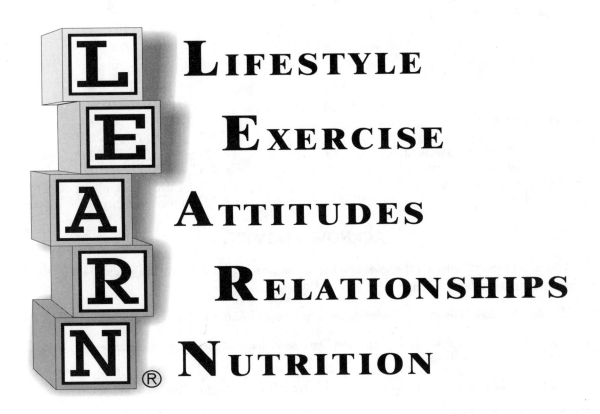

LIFESTYLE

EXERCISE

ATTITUDES

RELATIONSHIPS

NUTRITION

Kelly D. Brownell, Ph.D.
Yale University

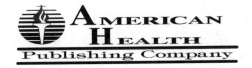

AMERICAN HEALTH
Publishing Company

Written requests for permission to make copies of any part of this publication should be addressed to:

Permissions Department
American Health Publishing Company
P.O. Box 610430, Department 10
Dallas, Texas 75261–0430
Facsimile: 817–545–2211

Library of Congress
ISBN 1–878513–24–9

Address orders to:

The LifeStyle Company™	In Dallas (817) 545–4500
P.O. Box 610430, Department 70	Toll Free 1–888–LEARN–41
Dallas, Texas 75261–0430	Facsimile (817) 545–2211
World Wide Web address	www.TheLifeStyleCompany.com
E-mail address	LEARN@TheLifeStyleCompany.com

ACKNOWLEDGMENTS

I am grateful to several trusted colleagues and friends for providing comments and suggestions for this manual. Their help was invaluable. They are:

Dr. Steven N. Blair, Director of Epidemiology, The Cooper Institute for Aerobics Research, Dallas, Texas.

Dr. John P. Foreyt, Professor of Medicine and Director, Behavioral Medicine Research Center, Baylor College of Medicine, Houston, Texas.

Dr. G. Alan Marlatt, Professor of Psychology, University of Washington, Seattle, Washington.

Dr. Sachiko T. St. Jeor, Associate Professor and Director, Nutrition Education and Research Program, Department of Family and Community Medicine, University of Nevada School of Medicine, Reno, Nevada.

Dr. Thomas A. Wadden, Professor, Department of Psychiatry, University of Pennsylvania School of Medicine, Philadelphia, Pennsylvania.

Permission to reprint cartoons was granted by, Creators Syndicate, Inc., Johnny Hart, King Features Syndicate, North America Syndicate, Tribune Media Services, United Feature Syndicate, Inc., United Media, Universal Press Syndicate, Washington Post Writers Group, Bob Thaves, and Randy Glasbergen.

Finally, I thank my students, colleagues, and especially my clients for providing the challenges and stimulation that encouraged me to undertake this writing.

TABLE OF CONTENTS

Introduction and Orientation Lesson 1
   My Welcome 1
   Watch for the Tape Symbol 2
   What The LEARN Program Is All about 2
   What this Can Mean in Your Life 3
   A Description of The LEARN Program 3
   Format of this Program 4
   Is the Time Right for You? 4
   Weighing the Benefits and Sacrifices 5
   Your Goals and Expectations 6
   Your Quality of Life 8
   Helpful Resources 8
   Congratulations and Good Luck 10

Lesson One 11
   The LEARN Program Cassettes 11
   The LEARN Approach 11
   A Revolution in Thinking about Weight Loss 12
   Diet vs. Lifestyle Change 12
   Building Skills and Confidence 13
   Record Keeping 14
   The Food Diary 15
   Calorie Guides 16
   The Weight Change Record 17
   Getting Started with Physical Activity 19
   A Very Helpful Device 20
   Reasons for Overweight 21
   A Note About Exercise, Relationships, and Nutrition 23
   Your Self-Assessment 23
   My Personal Goals for this Week 23
   My Self-Assessment 24

Lesson Two 29
   About Eating a Sensible Meal 29
   Reviewing Your Food Diary 30
   An Expanded Food Diary 32
   Rating Your Diet 33
   The Role of Exercise 33
   The Benefits of Exercise 34
   Why Losing Weight Is Difficult 35
   On Being a Good Group Member 36
   The Mysterious Calorie 36
   Not All People Are Created Equal 37
   What Makes a Pound 38
   Your Vision of Reasonable Weight Changes 38

My Personal Goals for this Week 39
My Self-Assessment 39

Lesson Three 43
Analyzing Your Expanded Food Diary 43
Determining Your Target Calorie Level. 44
Counting Grams of Fat 46
How Often Should You Weigh Yourself? 48
On the Move 49
Is Exercise Safe for You? 49
Starting Your Walking Program 51
Mall Walking. 52
Cravings vs. Hunger 52
My Personal Goals for this Week 52
My Self-Assessment 53

Lesson Four 55
Barriers to Physical Activity. 55
The 15-Minute Prescription 55
Getting Feedback and Staying Motivated to Be Active. 56
You Can Win a Presidential Sports Award. 57
A Walking Partnership. 58
The ABC's of Behavior 58
Shaping the Right Attitudes 60
Goal Setting. 61
The Principle of Shaping 62
The Mighty Calorie 62
Following a Balanced Diet 63
The Food Guide Pyramid 64
A Graphic Illustration. 65
Selecting an Eating Plan: Calorie Counting vs. Exchange Plan. 66
Introducing a New Monitoring Form 67
Quality of Life 68
My Personal Goals for This Week 69
My Self-Assessment 70

Lesson Five 73
Small Changes in Your Diet 73
More on Quality of Life. 73
Calorie Intake. 74
Taking Control of Your Eating 75
Perfecting Your Walking Program 78
Food and Weight Fantasies 79
Holidays, Parties, and Special Events: A Note 79
Solo and Social Changing 79
Would a Partner Help? 80
Why Social Support Can Be So Important 81
Servings from the Five Food Groups. 82
My Personal Goals for This Week 82
My Self-Assessment 83

Lesson Six. 85
   Slowing Your Eating Rate 85
   More on the Food Guide Pyramid 86
   Your Target Calorie Level. 88
   Choosing a Support Person 89
   Communicating with Your Partner. 90
   Making Physical Activity Count. 91
   The Calorie Values of Physical Activity 93
   The Trap of Negative Self-Talk. 95
   Charting My Progress 96
   My Personal Goals for This Week 97
   My Self-Assessment 97

Lesson Seven 99
   Thinking Your Way to Success 99
   Shopping for Food 101
   The Role of Fat in Your Diet 102
   Planning Healthy Meals 107
   Impressive Reasons to Be Active 108
   Continuing Walking and Lifestyle Activity 110
   Your Body and Your Self-Esteem 110
   My Personal Goals for This Week 113
   My Self-Assessment 114

Lesson Eight 117
   A New Activity Formula for Americans 117
   The Importance of Food 119
   Nutrients Without Energy 119
   Milk, Yogurt, and Cheese in Your Diet. 121
   Storing Foods (Out of Sight, Out of Mouth) 123
   Compulsive Eating and Binge Eating 124
   Selecting and Starting a Programmed Activity. 126
   Cardiovascular Training 128
   Danger! An Exercise Threshold Attitude 130
   Internal Attitude Traps 131
   Quality of Life Self-Assessment 132
   Rating Your Diet 132
   My Personal Goals for This Week 132
   My Self-Assessment 132

Lesson Nine 135
   A Two-Month Review 135
   Serving and Dispensing Food 137
   More on Activity. 139
   The Myth of Spot Reducing 141
   Impossible Dream Thinking 142
   Something for Your Partner to Read 143
   More Facts about Vitamins 144
   Reading Food Labels 145
   The Importance of Protein. 148

The Meat, Poultry, Fish, Dry Beans, Eggs, and Nuts Group 150
A New Weight Change Record 151
My Personal Goals for This Week 152
My Self-Assessment 152

Lesson Ten 155
For You and Your Family to Read 155
Dealing with Pressures to Eat 157
Another Attitude Trap: Imperatives 159
Stress and Eating 160
Let's Consider Jogging and Cycling 162
More about Water Soluble Vitamins 164
Carbohydrates and Your Diet 165
Vegetables in Your Diet 167
How Many Servings? 167
My Personal Goals for This Week 168
My Self-Assessment 169

Lesson Eleven 171
More Good News about Physical Activity 171
Are Aerobics for You? 173
Pleasurable Partner Activities 174
More about Fat Soluble Vitamins 174
Facts, Fantasies, and Fiber 176
Fruit in Your Diet 178
How Much Is a Serving? 180
My Personal Goals for this Week 180
My Self-Assessment 181

Lesson Twelve 183
Eating Away from Home 183
Exercise—The Many Points of Light 187
Using the Stairs 187
Fast Food 189
Breads, Cereals, Rice, and Pasta in Your Diet 190
Breakfast Cereal: The Good, the Bad, the Sugar Coated 192
Reevaluating Your Quality of Life 192
My Personal Goals for This Week 194
My Self-Assessment 195

Lesson Thirteen 197
Taking Stock of Your Progress 197
Bringing it All Together: The Behavior Chain 202
A Pulse Test for Positive Feedback 207
Bracing Yourself Against a Toxic Environment 209
Poultry: Better than Red Meat? 210
Hard Work at the Office 211
My Personal Goals for This Week 211
My Self-Assessment 212

Lesson Fourteen 215
    Preventing Lapse, Relapse, and Collapse 215
    Identifying Urges and High-Risk Situations 217
    Making a List, Checking it Twice 218
    Dichotomous (Light Bulb) Thinking 218
    Cholesterol 221
    Warning: Alcohol and Calories 223
    My Personal Goals for This Week 223
    My Self-Assessment 224

Lesson Fifteen 227
    Coping with Lapse and Preventing Relapse 227
    Becoming a Forest Ranger 229
    Life on Chutes and Ladders 230
    Holidays, Parties, and Special Events 231
    Why Is Nutrition So Important to Me? 233
    More on Minerals 233
    A Note about Breakfast 236
    My Personal Goals for This Week 237
    My Self-Assessment 238

Lesson Sixteen 241
    The Master Monitoring Form 241
    Using the Master List of Techniques 242
    The National Walking Movement 242
    Revisiting Your Eating and Activity Habits 244
    To Record or Not to Record 244
    Weight Loss 245
    Quality of Life Self-Assessment 247
    My Salute to You! 247
    Rate Your Diet 248
    My Personal Goals for This Week 249
    My Self-Assessment 249

Commencement Lesson 251
    Interpreting Your Progress 251
    Remember a Reasonable Weight? 252
    Making Your Habits Permanent 253
    Examining Your Master Monitoring Form 254
    Where to Go from Here 254
    Ending Where We Began 256
    A Final Weight Change Record 256
    Saying Farewell 256

Appendix A—Master List of Techniques 261
    Lifestyle Techniques 261
    Exercise Techniques 261
    Attitude Techniques 262
    Relationship Techniques 262
    Nutrition Techniques 262

Appendix B—Weight Loss Readiness Test 263
    What Is Readiness? 263
    The Consequences of Not Being Ready 263
    Assessing Readiness 264
    The Weight Loss Readiness Test Categories 265

Appendix C—Answers for Self-Assessment Questions 271

Appendix D—Guidelines for Being a Good Group Member 277
    Importance of the Group 277
    Good Chemistry and Teamwork 277
    Guidelines and Responsibilities 278
    In Summary 281

Appendix E—Rate Your Diet Quizzes 283

Index 295

Supplemental Resources and Ordering Information 303
    The LifeStyle Company 303
    The LEARN Institute for LifeStyle Management 303
    The American Association of LifeStyle Counselors 304
    Other Materials 304

Notes 305

About the Author 311

INTRODUCTION AND ORIENTATION LESSON

When I travel in the U.S. and other countries to lecture, I'm often greeted by professionals who use this manual in their work or by individuals who are using the manual to lose weight. Some ask me to autograph their copy of the manual. Some show me their copies of the book, with the pages ragged and bent at the corners and sentences and paragraphs underlined or highlighted with colored markers. I am delighted to see the book used in this way. It shows me that the reader is involved. I urge you to get involved and to give this program your best effort.

I am a great believer in feedback, and I'd very much like yours. If you can suggest changes to improve the program, please let me know. Additions, deletions, alterations—I am open to them all. I can say with sincerity that this manual, now in its tenth edition, has improved dramatically over the years with input from people using it. If you enjoy the manual and it helps you, please let me know. Good news is always gratifying to hear. Also, your words may inspire other people. So, if you contact me, let me know if I can use what you say (without citing names) in future versions of this manual.

To send feedback to me, you may write a letter to my attention and mail it to American Health Publishing Company, P.O. Box 610430, Department 10, Dallas, Texas 75261–0430. You may also fax feedback to me at 1–817–545–2211. If you have access to the Internet, you may e-mail your feedback to me at LEARN@TheLifeStyleCompany.com. I read every word.

I hope this manual and you make a nice pair. Bend the pages, underline liberally, and write notes in the margins. Use this book for all it's worth.

My Welcome

I have put together a program that I hope will make you feel comfortable, is friendly, and will work for you. There will be times you will laugh and other times you will struggle. But, with the right information and your motivation, you'll be surprised by what you can accomplish.

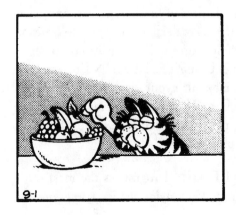
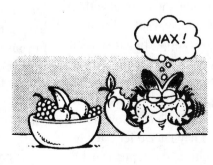
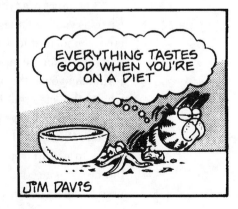

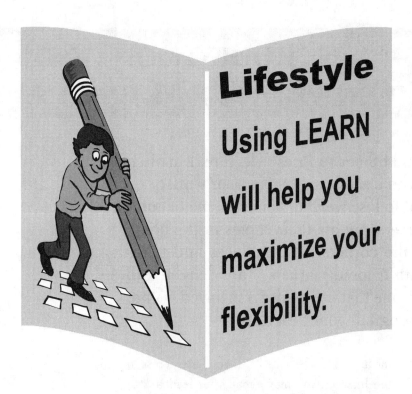

Lifestyle

Using LEARN will help you maximize your flexibility.

Watch for the Tape Symbol

When you see this symbol alongside text in this manual, it means that the topic being discussed in the text is covered on *The LEARN Program Cassettes 2000*. I have recorded a series of four audiotapes to accompany this program. The audiotapes are not a repeat of the program—they are additional material to clarify the program and to lend support to you at critical times. The tapes can provide motivation, inspiration, and education. They offer much helpful information in a friendly tone.

The tapes are typically used in three ways. First, as you read a section in the manual with a tape symbol next to it, you may want to listen to that section on the tape for supporting material. I will refer you to the particular tape and section where the material being discussed can be found. Second, some people just listen straight through the tapes. This gives them an overview of key topics up front. They later refer back to the tapes as needed. Third, the tapes can be used at times of crisis. If you hit a plateau, strug-

gle with cravings, or want to eat in response to difficult moods, the tapes can help. When you find it difficult to get out and walk, the tapes can get you going.

Examples of the topics covered in the tapes include the power of constructive thinking, ways to reward yourself, stress and eating, getting support when you need it, hitting a plateau, compulsive eating, keeping motivated, and much more.

People listen to the tapes in the car, when they are out walking, when they're doing some other form of exercise, when doing things around the house, and in many other ways. The tapes provide me with another way to speak with you.

If you have not ordered the cassette tapes and would like to, see Supplemental Resources and Ordering Information in the back of this manual that begins on page 303. Alternatively, you can order online by visiting us on the Internet at www.TheLifeStyleCompany.com.

What The LEARN Program Is All about

Different people benefit from different approaches to weight management. Some love a structured diet, and others hate the lack of choice; some enjoy being physically active, and others get tired just thinking about exercise; some like support from others, and others are more private. The key is finding the best approach for you.

Your chances of finding the best approach increase if you are flexible. Being flexible means having choices and tailoring your approach to fit your life. Using The LEARN Program will help you maximize your flexibility. The principles of LEARN can help you make long-term changes, no matter what type of nutrition and exercise plan you use.

The LEARN Program is the most thoroughly tested lifestyle change program for weight management available. I wrote the first version about 22 years ago and have revised, updated, and improved it every year or two since then. The object of the program is to help people develop the confidence and learn the skills necessary to lose weight and keep it off. In my work at Brown University, the University of Pennsylvania, and now at Yale, I have used The LEARN Program with thousands of individuals. They have helped me make it better. My hope in creating this new 2000 edition is that it will help you change your lifestyle to manage your weight once and for all.

What this Can Mean in Your Life

TAPE 2
SECTION 1

Living with extra weight can be extremely difficult. The good news is that something can be done. You deserve to feel better and deserve to have the best of what we know about weight management on your side. You deserve to succeed.

Success at weight loss can be wonderful. I can think of many benefits, such as having more energy, being in better health, and looking better. Better yet, think of the boost in self-esteem that comes from dealing with a very difficult problem. Think of how wonderful it feels to receive complements on your progress and for others to be genuinely happy for you. This is all part of well-being—being well as a person. Let's work together to be well.

A Description of The LEARN Program

TAPE 1
SECTION 4

I named this program LEARN for two reasons. The first is that learning implies an educational process in which the learner masters crucial information and applies it to everyday life. Second, the word LEARN is an acronym created from the first letter of the five essential components of the program: Lifestyle, Exercise, Attitudes, Relationships, and Nutrition.

The name LEARN has now been adopted and added to other programs for lifestyle change such as stress management, exercise, etc. When I talk about The LEARN Program, I'm talking about this program. You can refer to the Supplemental Resources and Ordering Information in the back of this manual for a list of programs in the LEARN Life-Style Program Series™.

Each lesson in this program has a self-assessment and a section for setting personal goals for the week. The self-assessment is for *you* to decide whether you have learned the important information in each lesson. This will highlight the key points in each lesson and alert you to areas that may need more work. The section on setting personal goals asks you to experiment with weekly goal setting, so you can learn what works best for you. These sections also remind you about the progress you are making.

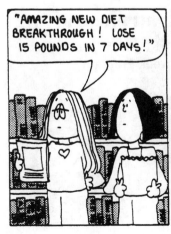
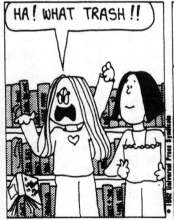
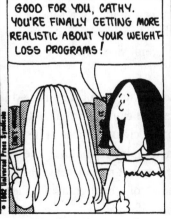
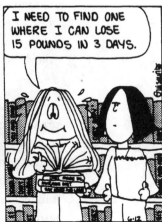

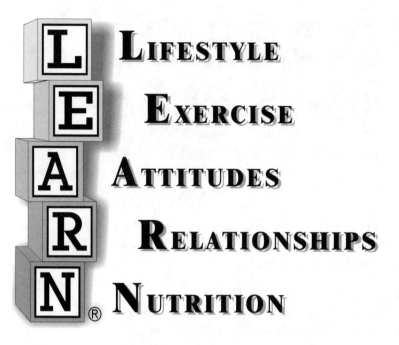

LIFESTYLE
EXERCISE
ATTITUDES
RELATIONSHIPS
NUTRITION

As you go through The LEARN Program, you will become a student of your habits and learn when, how, and why your habits occur and how to change them. You will practice your new techniques so they will become part of your lifestyle. This is what separates the approach of this program from other programs—the focus is on permanent results.

I should mention two other aspects of the program. First, you will not be assigned certain foods; nor are any foods forbidden. I resist the idea of dictating what you can and cannot eat. You will not be asked to rid your life of apple pie or faint with envy when your friends dip into the Haagen-Dazs. Likewise, you will not be running to the fruit stand for papaya and mangoes so you can abide by a senseless series of magic foods. The program is structured around your lifestyle, not vice versa.

The second aspect of The LEARN Program is that you can individualize the program to your unique circumstances. The focus is on learning new habits, whatever the necessary habits are for you. You can weave the principles and techniques of the program into the fabric of *your* life and lifestyle.

Format of this Program

This edition of The LEARN Program is structured to have the Introduction and Orientation Lesson you are reading now, followed by 16 weekly lessons plus a commencement lesson. Each of the 16 lessons contains one week's worth of material. Hence, the program lasts for 16 weeks.

The material you are reading now is part of the Introduction and Orientation Lesson. This lesson introduces The LEARN Program, addresses your readiness to change, and talks about how you can get lifestyle change working for you. This is a quick read—you may be able to pour through this introductory material in a single reading. Lesson One begins the nuts and bolts of the program.

Is the Time Right for You?

I know you want to lose weight. You may marvel at my insight; after all, you are reading a weight management guide! Still, before we begin, let us consider whether the time is right. With some simple guidelines, you can decide whether to move ahead now or to wait for a better time.

Losing weight is much easier than keeping it off. Some people have lost and regained as much as 1000 pounds, in what nutrition expert Jean Mayer labeled "the rhythm method of girth control." Losing and regaining weight is

The LEARN Program Schedule
A 16-week Program

Lessons 1–4 (Month 1)
Lessons 5–8 (Month 2)
Lessons 9–12 (Month 3)
Lessons 13–16 (Month 4)

discouraging, so beginning a program when motivation is high is best.

The first step is to ask whether you are prepared for the rigors of a weight loss program. Despite claims from diet books, most people cannot lose 15 pounds without trying. They do not get addicted to exercise by buying designer jogging shoes and warm-up suits. And, most people do not suddenly yearn for sprouts and tofu when they are used to eating bacon, pork chops, and hot fudge.

Right now you are probably saying, tell me something new! You know that weight management requires effort. Yet, many people start programs when they are only mildly motivated. They may be pressured by family, may be distressed by clothes that don't fit, or may be losing weight to look better for a special event, such as a wedding or reunion. Sometimes these provide sufficient motivation, but not always.

A key decision in any program is deciding whether to begin, but deciding can be tricky. In Appendix B, beginning on page 263, I discuss weight loss readiness and provide a Weight Loss Readiness Test. This test provides guidelines for deciding whether now is the right time for you to begin a program. The guidelines will also help you identify potential problem areas that may need additional effort as you go through The LEARN Program. Take a few minutes now to read through this important material on weight loss readiness.

Weighing the Benefits and Sacrifices

Consider the benefits and sacrifices of starting a weight loss program. Think of the benefits, such as improved health, better figure, self-confidence, better social life, more energy, attractive clothes, and whatever applies to you. The negative aspects should include all the factors like hunger, irritability, explaining your new lifestyle to others, problems eating out, and so forth. Also consider the time you will need to devote to your program to be successful. Each week, you will need to set aside time to read the week's lesson, keep records, and plan for upcoming events. The more time you give to your weight management efforts, the better your chances of success.

Page 7 illustrates examples from two individuals contemplating a weight loss program. Bob wants to lose 40 pounds, and his wife is pressuring him to lose weight. Becky has 27 pounds to lose. She is tired of being heavy. Becky is applying for jobs after taking courses at night and wants to look as good as possible.

Bob and Becky weighed the positives and negatives of beginning a program and came to different conclusions. The positive side of the ledger was stronger for Becky, so she pressed ahead and achieved her goal. Bob was different. He decided against starting a program because it held so many disadvantages for him. He later found himself more motivated and lost his excess weight.

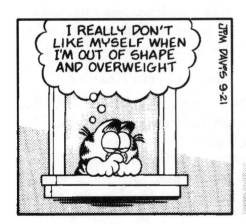
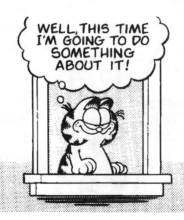
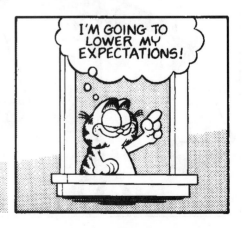

We can learn two morals from Bob's story. First, deciding not to begin a program is sometimes wise. A person who attempts to lose weight and fails can feel bitter and guilty. The decision to wait until later is not a failure—it may prevent a failure.

A second side to Bob's story is also possible, however. A person who decides the time is not right may be looking for a convenient excuse. Such people may deny or avoid the realities of their weight problem or may question their ability to succeed. I recommend that such people take a two-week trial of eating less and exercising more as a test of how they will do later. Difficulty may be a sign that starting a program should be set aside and undertaken later. If they do well, their attitude may continue to improve as they lose weight. Consider this two-week trial if you are uncertain about starting a program now.

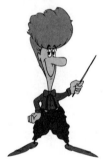

List as many of the benefits and sacrifices you can think of in the figure titled "My List" on page 8. This exercise may help you to see if the balance of benefits and sacrifices leans in the direction of starting a program. If the list of sacrifices outnumber the benefits, you may want

to reconsider whether now is the best time to begin a program.

Your Goals and Expectations

TAPE 1
SECTION 5

This program can help you achieve a "healthier" weight. The LEARN Program produces average weight losses of 20–30 pounds. This has been documented in a number of studies from our research group and from scientists at other centers. This translates into a one- to two-pound weight loss per week for the weeks the program is generally used. What does this mean for you?

Averages can be deceiving. If one person loses 50 pounds and another loses none, their average is 25 pounds. Whether the program is a success depends on which person you consider. Some people lose more than the average, and some lose less, but in general, the program aims for steady weight loss that can be maintained. By the way, you are more likely to achieve the best results by reading and completing each lesson faithfully and by achieving your personal goals each week. A recent study showed that the more weekly goals people accomplish, the greater their weight losses.

If you have 30 pounds or less to lose, this program provides a good opportunity for you to reach your goal weight. If you have more to lose, you can estimate the 20- to 30-pound loss for the initial program and then can continue to lose by applying the techniques you have learned. If you stop losing before reaching your goal, you may go through the program again or add another approach to take you further.

Long-Term Results

The best news about The LEARN Program is the long-term results. Compared with the very high relapse rates from most programs, the maintenance of weight loss for this program is quite good. Again, some people lose even more after the initial 16 weeks while some regain.

Weighing the Benefits and Sacrifices

Benefits

Sacrifices

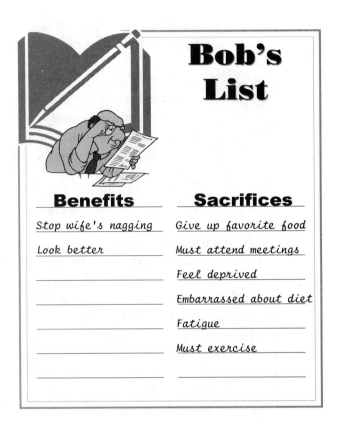

Bob's List

Benefits	Sacrifices
Stop wife's nagging	*Give up favorite food*
Look better	*Must attend meetings*
	Feel deprived
	Embarrassed about diet
	Fatigue
	Must exercise

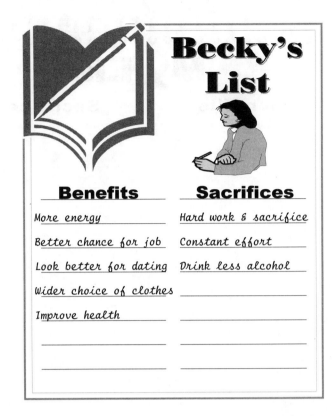

Becky's List

Benefits	Sacrifices
More energy	*Hard work & sacrifice*
Better chance for job	*Constant effort*
Look better for dating	*Drink less alcohol*
Wider choice of clothes	
Improve health	

These numbers have more meaning when compared with the results of other approaches. Dr. Albert Stunkard, from the University of Pennsylvania, once estimated that fewer than 5 percent of people on weight loss programs lose more than 40 pounds and keep it off. Many people (as many as 66 percent) who enter the popular commercial and self-help programs will drop out within six weeks. Techniques like hypnosis, herbal programs, and the best-selling diet books are usually of little use. The key to successful weight management, of course, is stabilization and maintenance.

We will be working on maintenance from the first moment you dive into this program. I want to help you develop a mind-set of *permanent* lifestyle change. You will be changing fundamental behaviors and attitudes that affect your eating and activity. We will work together to make changes that become part of the way you live. Perhaps more than in any other program, I have blended methods to maintain weight loss with ways to lose weight initially. Our vision is focused on both immediate and long-term solutions.

Many programs and books promise quick and easy results, some as much as 10 pounds in the first week. Such diets are drastic measures that may endanger your health. These quick weight losses are more water than fat, because the body rids itself of water when the intake of salt and carbohydrate decreases. The water returns when a person abandons the rigid diet in favor of more normal eating. Losing weight slowly allows your body to adjust to a new weight and will help you look and feel better as you reduce.

The slow and gradual weight loss is not as flashy as fad diets, but may ultimately be more effective. Losing more than three to four pounds per week is physically impossible, even by fasting. So, a one- to two-pound weight loss per week is quite good. Slow and steady are the key words. This represents the most reasonable approach to weight management.

Setting Realistic Goals

You will be most satisfied with your results if you set clear and realistic goals that you have a good chance of attaining. During this pro-

"When Bob and Becky weighed the positives and negatives of beginning a program, they came to different conclusions."

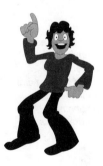

My List

Benefits	Sacrifices

"On the list above, write down as many of the benefits and sacrifices you can think of in beginning a program now."

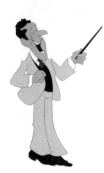

gram, I will speak often about realistic goals, appropriate expectations, and "reasonable weight."

Take a minute now and think about what a 10 percent weight loss would be for you. This is a good starting goal. Whether or not you lose more, the 10 percent loss will be an important achievement. Clinical studies have shown weight loss in this amount improves important factors related to health, such as blood pressure and lipid levels. In the space below, write down what a 10 percent weight loss would be for you today. We'll refer back to this number later in the program.

A 10 percent weight loss for me will be _____ pounds.

Your Quality of Life

TAPE 1
SECTION 7

People begin a weight loss program because of the benefits they hope will occur with weighing less. Looking better, feeling better, having more energy, and having more self-confidence are examples of what we call "quality-of-life" issues. These and other factors shape how you feel every day.

As you progress through this program, you will have a natural tendency to focus on the scale. This can be a problem when the scale shows no change, even when you might be making positive lifestyle strides. Keeping your eye on the many changes that can occur will be helpful. This helps you appreciate the positive effects of your hard work and shows just how many areas of your life can improve by eating better and being more physically active. Focusing on areas other than the scale also gives you more than one means of evaluating your progress.

Please complete the Quality of Life Self-Assessment provided on page 9 to get a feeling about various aspects of your current daily quality of life. I will ask you to complete this assessment several times later in the program to see if the scores have changed.

Helpful Resources

Additional materials have been developed for The LEARN Program that may be helpful to you. Read through the list of additional resources beginning on page 303 and see if these may be helpful to you. If so, you may want to get these resources right away as you begin Lesson One. For more information on ordering these supplemental materials, see Supplemental Resources and Ordering Information on page 303.

The LEARN® Program Cassettes 2000 are a motivational and inspirational supplement to *The LEARN Program for Weight Management 2000.* The tapes do not repeat the pro-

Quality of Life Self-Assessment

Please use the following scale to rate how satisfied you feel now about different aspects of your daily life. Choose any number from this list (1 to 9) and indicate your choice on the questions below.

1 = Extremely Dissatisfied

2 = Very Dissatisfied

3 = Moderately Dissatisfied

4 = Somewhat Dissatisfied

5 = Neutral

6 = Somewhat Satisfied

7 = Moderately Satisfied

8 = Very Satisfied

9 = Extremely Satisfied

1. _____ Mood (feelings of sadness, worry, happiness, etc.)

2. _____ Self-esteem

3. _____ Confidence, self-assurance, and comfort in social situations

4. _____ Energy and feeling healthy

5. _____ Health problems (diabetes, high blood pressure, etc.)

6. _____ General appearance

7. _____ Social life

8. _____ Leisure and recreational activities

9. _____ Physical mobility and physical activity

10. _____ Eating habits

11. _____ Body image

12. _____ Overall quality of life

gram, but provide additional material to clarify and reinforce key principles. The information will help motivate and inspire you as you develop and practice the new skills and principles of weight management.

In addition to *The LEARN Program Cassettes 2000* mentioned earlier, The LEARN Monitoring Forms were developed at the request of many people who had completed The LEARN Program. Although I provide you with daily monitoring forms throughout this manual that you may copy, many individuals find it more convenient to have a pocket-sized form that contains a week's supply of food monitoring.

The LEARN WalkMaster™ is a helpful way for you to monitor your physical activity. This handy little device is a pedometer that keeps track of your steps, how far you walk, and how many calories you use. I will discuss this more in Lesson One, but for now, I would like you to consider ordering one.

The LEARN Healthy Eating and Calorie Guide provides basic information about how to develop a more healthful diet by using the Food Guide Pyramid to plan healthy and nutritious meals. It includes a Calorie Guide for common foods and a special Fast Food Calorie Guide. In addition, the guide has information about vitamins and minerals along with the most recent

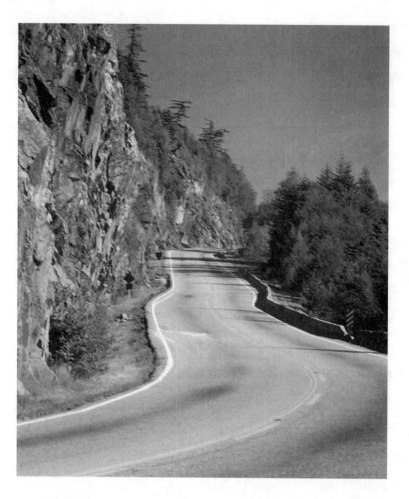

Telephone: 1–817–545–4500
Toll Free: 1–888–LEARN–41
Fax: 1–817–545–2211

E-mail:
LEARN@TheLifeStyleCompany.com
Internet:
www.TheLifeStyleCompany.com

Congratulations and Good Luck

Congratulations on your decision to take control of your weight and health. You can be proud of making an important decision. I wish you every success and look forward to working with you. So, without further delay, let's move on!

"Slow and steady are key strategies in navigating the road to success."

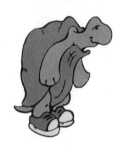

intake recommendations. This guide is a must for individuals wanting to optimize their health through dietary change.

And finally, *The Weight Control Digest®* was developed as a newsletter for both professionals and nonprofessionals to keep abreast of the latest developments in the field, as well as keeping up-to-date on the latest methods and techniques that help individuals maintain their weight.

All of these materials and others are more fully described in the Supplemental Resources and Ordering Information in the back of this manual on page 303. Information on other materials can be obtained by calling or writing to the address shown below.

The LifeStyle Company
P.O. Box 610430, Department 70
Dallas, Texas 75261–0430

Today you begin Lesson One of The LEARN Program. This program contains the best of what science and clinical practice have to offer. In writing this manual, my intention is for us to form a partnership. Together we can make it work.

When you lose weight on this program, only one person deserves credit. I would be happy to claim credit, but I deserve no more than Rand McNally does when you use their atlas to drive from one city to the next. The atlas supplies the possible routes, and may even suggest the best. Yet, you choose the route and you determine whether you reach your destination. Most important, you do the driving. With that in mind, let's go!

The LEARN Program Cassettes

TAPE 1
SECTION 2

As I mentioned in the Introduction and Orientation Lesson, when you see the symbol of the tape cassette, it indicates that the topic is covered in detail in *The LEARN Program Cassettes 2000*. The set has four cassettes with me speaking to you about topics such as motivation, commitment, dealing with plateaus, compulsive eating, dealing with food cravings, rewarding yourself, crisis intervention, body image, and stress and eating.

The tapes are designed to be educational, inspirational, friendly, and supportive and will help me share with you my experiences gained over my years in the field of weight management. The cassettes can be ordered by calling toll-free 1–888–LEARN–41 or by using the Internet (www.TheLifeStyleCompany.com).

The LEARN Approach

The word "LEARN" represents the five components of this program: Lifestyle, Exercise, Attitudes, Relationships, and Nutrition. The lessons in this program contain information in each area. In some weeks the information in one area is particularly important, so it will receive the greatest emphasis.

Appendix A on page 261 has a detailed master list of techniques that you will be learning as you go through The LEARN Program. The techniques are referenced by page number in this manual to easily guide you to where I discuss each topic. Refer to this appendix often when you find yourself having difficult with a particular lifestyle-change technique.

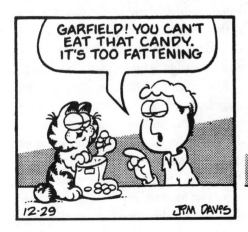
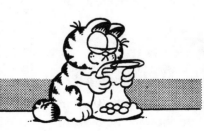
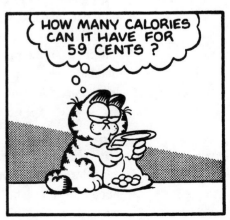

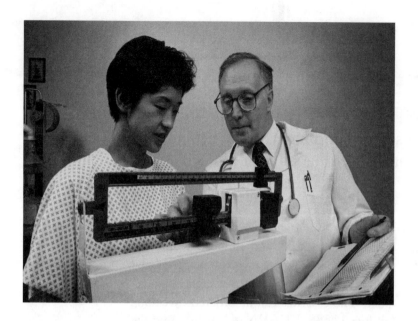

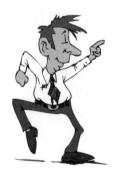

given a goal weight based on the ideals from these tables. The message is that you must lose to a magic level to benefit from weight loss. Far from being "ideal," these weight tables are a source of enormous frustration given their unrealistic view that "one size fits all." Say goodbye to this way of thinking.

A large collection of scientific evidence now converges on an important conclusion—that even a modest weight loss can have important health benefits. High blood pressure, diabetes, elevated cholesterol, sleep disturbances, and a variety of other common medical problems are often improved, if not controlled, by modest weight loss. This changes everything.

The new weight loss goals are designed to help people achieve a *healthier* weight, and to push aside the notion of *ideal* weight. Virtually everyone can achieve a healthier weight at which they will feel better, have more energy, and reduce their risk of health complications.

Diet vs. Lifestyle Change

TAPE 1
SECTION 4

The LEARN Program is not a diet; it is a system for lifestyle change. This is more than just a matter of words—it is a fundamental difference in philosophy that affects nearly every aspect of the LEARN approach.

I designed this program to teach you new skills, skills to challenge today's bad environment that promotes weight gain in just about every way imaginable. Many of the skills you will learn in this program weren't needed 20–30 years ago. Back then our environment didn't contribute to weight gain as much as today's world. Think back over the past 20–30 years. How many high-calorie, high-fat, fast-food restaurants have entered our world during this time? How many labor-saving devices have been introduced and are now part of your daily life? Thousands! In fact, technology has introduced more fast-food restaurants and labor-saving devices during this time than in the entire

"Even modest weight loss can have important health benefits."

Because we are partners in The LEARN Program, your role will be an active one. You will have forms to fill out and homework assignments. Upcoming weeks will be filled with experimentation because you will be trying many new approaches to eating and physical activity. The program is both exciting and challenging.

In some cases, this manual will be used in conjunction with classes or with some degree of professional assistance. The LEARN Program is also used as a companion or guide in many other weight loss and weight management programs. I developed this program for you to use as a self-help program or in a group setting. Remember that group sessions do not replace the manual. They simply cannot cover the details of a program like a manual can. The manual permits you to examine the information at *your* pace and at a time when *you* can pay attention. Also, you can refer to the manual at different points in the program. Be sure to read the manual each week, and use it as a reference after the program ends.

A Revolution in Thinking about Weight Loss

Most of us have had years of worrying about "ideal weight." Height-weight tables are everywhere, and in many programs, people are history of humans. I don't have to tell you the impact these environmental changes have had on our health and weight. As you go though this program, you will learn important skills to help you overcome today's environmental challenges. This is what I mean by lifestyle change; changing the way you interact with your environment.

The word diet conjures up a number of images. To many, it implies deprivation and suffering, but most of all, it is something that you go on or off. Whether someone is "on a diet" or "off a diet" is part of our modern language. This is a problem, of course, because changing habits is not something that happens while a person is on a diet and then stops later when the diet ends. This implies a temporary solution, a quick patch job that only requires minor effort over the short term.

We are seeking a permanent solution. Instead of a quick but temporary fix, we want lifestyle change. This involves establishing new habits and working hard to make these part of day-to-day life. Most people who struggle with weight have a chronic problem. Chronic problems require attention over the long term.

Reflect for a moment on the difference between going on a diet and changing your lifestyle. The lifestyle approach, which emphasizes gradual, sustainable, and permanent changes in eating, exercise, thinking, and feeling, is the hallmark of this program. As you go through the program you will learn important skills that will help you build confidence to succeed and make lifestyle changes that are permanent.

Building Skills and Confidence

TAPE 1
SECTION 1

A highly respected psychologist at Stanford University, Albert Bandura, developed a concept known as self-efficacy. His thought includes two parts. First, the notion states that an individual's chance of accomplishing some goal depends on

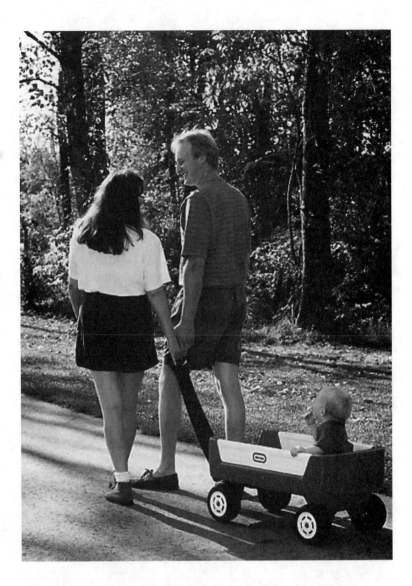

having the skills to make the change. The second part includes the individual having the confidence that the change can occur. This idea applies beautifully to weight management.

"Establishing new habits that will become a part of your day-to-day life is the hallmark of this program."

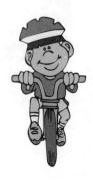

As I said earlier, skills are what this program is all about. I will suggest many approaches to developing important weight management skills. You'll take each for a test drive and find the ones that work best for you. The skills will deal with what you eat, whether you are active, and perhaps most important, the thoughts, feelings, and attitudes you have about many important factors. Thinking helpful thoughts and looking at the world in a constructive way involve skills that you can cultivate.

Confidence is the second part of the picture. If you are confident that you can handle high-risk situations, bounce back when you falter, and keep your motivation high, you'll have the strength to hang in there when things get tough. You'll approach situations with a new sense of control. I will be speaking often about confidence.

Sometimes these discussions of confidence will sound like a pep talk, but pep talks can be really helpful. One of the most important things you can do is to have your own internal pep talks. What you say to yourself when you do well can have an important impact on your success. Moreover, what you tell yourself when you slip or when you are pondering how best to continue will be central to your success. The number of times I talk about the discussions you have with yourself may surprise you.

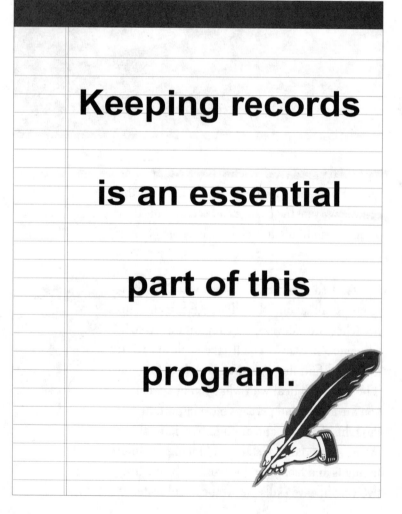

Keeping records is an essential part of this program.

TAPE 1
SECTION 8

Record Keeping

The first and perhaps most important lifestyle behavior you will learn is to keep records. You will be keeping records of your eating, exercise, and weight. You'll have more records than an accountant! Don't worry. I'll explain the reasons for this.

Purpose and Importance

This lesson introduces two records. The first is the Food Diary, which is a daily record of the food you eat. The second is the Weight Change Record, which is a weekly graph of your weight. Both will increase your awareness of eating and how it affects your weight.

Awareness is a key step in changing habits. You may already know a great deal about your habits and your weight patterns, particularly if you have kept records for an earlier program. You will be surprised by how much more there is to learn. The awareness you gain from record keeping has several benefits. These will become clear within a few weeks. Here is a sampling of what you will learn from keeping good records.

⇨ *You learn about calories*. Calories are lurking where you least suspect. One cup of fruit yogurt can have more calories than an ice cream cone. Ten innocent potato chips contain 110 calories, more than five cups of plain popcorn. Becoming a calorie expert insures you won't be derailed by calorie surprises.

⇨ *You become aware of what you eat*. You might be thinking, "Of course, I know what I eat." However, one does not always recall the exact number of Doritos consumed at happy hour or the ounces of milk poured into the bowl of Wheaties. These are forgotten calories, sometimes because we want to forget them!

⇨ *You increase control over eating*. Knowing exactly where you stand with the day's calorie count is important. This helps you to judge whether you can afford certain foods. You may have the calories banked to have that snack you are considering. Your choices are much easier with this information.

⇨ *Your eating patterns become clear*. You may discover that most of your eating takes place between dinner and bedtime. Some people eat when they have certain feelings (anger, anxiety, etc.), and others find they eat when doing something else, like watching TV. Knowing your patterns is a big help in changing habits.

⇨ *You learn how to bank calories*. Your body is like a bank account in which you make calorie deposits and withdrawals. If you eat less, you have some calories to bank for a special occasion. If you have a party to attend on the weekend, you can cut back during the week. With this knowledge, you can afford to indulge with some special dessert. Calorie records give you the information to make informed food choices.

⇨ *You learn not to despair*. You may experience one or more weeks during this program when you fail to lose weight, or even worse, gain weight! Many reasons exist for this. I will discuss them later. Such a discouraging bout with the scale can make life difficult. Reviewing your change in weight over many weeks can prevent this despair.

A slight gain is easier to tolerate when your records remind you that you have been losing weight in a steady manner.

The Food Diary

The Food Diary is your holy book during this program. You will use it to record amounts and calories of the foods you eat. You may resist this part of the program. Recording everything you eat and estimating calories may be hard to do initially. When it becomes easy, you may find it repetitive. Conquering this resistance and keeping the records is important. Research has shown this to be one of the most, if not the most important part of lifestyle change.

A blank Food Diary is provided on page 27, along with a sample that has a typical person's eating records filled in on page 26. I will provide blank food diaries (later called Monitoring Forms) for each lesson in The LEARN Program. You may make photocopies of the blank records for your own use. Many people using this program find it difficult to make copies of the diaries and monitoring forms. To help with this difficulty, The LEARN Program Monitoring Forms (described on page 303 in the back of this manual) can be ordered by calling toll-free 1–888–LEARN–41 or on the Internet at www.TheLifeStyleCompany.com. Each of these forms contains a week's worth or monitoring and can easily be carried in a pocket or purse. Following are the instructions for completing your Food Diary in this lesson.

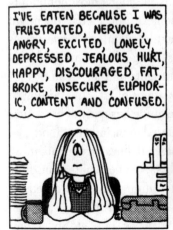
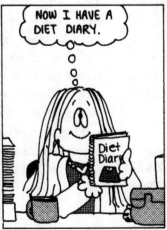
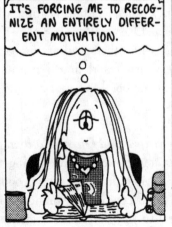
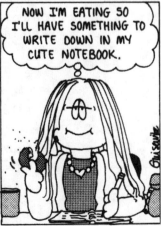

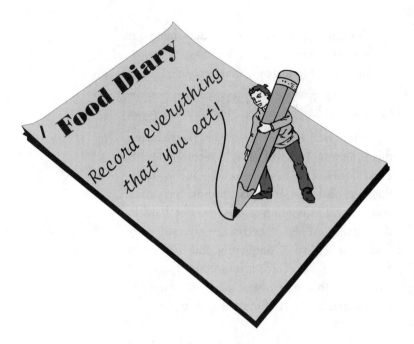

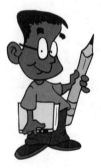

⇨ ***Record everything, forget nothing.*** Every morsel of food goes in the Food Diary. If you eat pretzels, count how many. You must enter every ounce of food and beverage. Don't forget to count the foods you taste when you are cooking.

⇨ ***Record the food, the amount, the calories.*** Record the type of food you eat, how it is prepared (baked, fried, etc.), how much, and the number of calories.

⇨ ***Record immediately after eating.*** Do not wait until you are ready for bed, until the next morning, or even later! You will have trouble remembering how many peanuts you ate at the cocktail party or how much juice you had for breakfast if you wait too long. When you finish eating, whip out the Food Diary and make your entries. If you are with others and are embarrassed, excuse yourself and find a private place, like a phone booth. Clark Kent did it, and so can you!

⇨ ***Carry your Food Diary always.*** Food is lurking about everywhere waiting to leap into your mouth. Keep your Food Diary with you (except when swimming or in the shower) so you won't be caught off guard.

Some people use a pocket notebook or small notepad during the day and then transfer the information to their Food Diary later.

Calorie Guides

To record the number of calories in foods, you'll need a calorie guide. For some foods, you can probably look at the food label on the package and find the calories in foods. Other foods, like fruits and vegetables, do not come in packages. Many times you may eat out and be served foods from friends or family, or otherwise be in a position where there will be no indication of the calories in the foods you eat.

How Do I Get a Good Calorie Guide?

Calorie guides are readily available. I can make two suggestions. The first is to go to a bookstore and look in the section on diet and nutrition. Easier yet, ask someone who works there to help you find a book with the calorie and nutrition values of foods. The guides may vary a bit in the calories and nutrition listed for given foods, but this is nothing to worry about.

The second option is *The LEARN Healthy Eating and Calorie Guide* (described on page 303 in the back of this manual). This guide has been designed to be used with The LEARN Program and the other programs in the LEARN LifeStyle Program Series™. This guide contains the foods most commonly eaten, and even some exotic foods you might try. The guide includes standard serving sizes and calories per serving. Also, the guide includes all of the nutrients that have calories for each food (such as grams of fat). In addition to common foods, the guide has a list of beverages and has been expanded to include fast foods, vitamin and mineral guidelines, menu planning strategies, and will help you estimate your daily calorie needs. This guide can be ordered by calling toll-free 1–888– LEARN–41, by using the Internet site (www.TheLifeStyleCompany.com), or by writing to the address listed at the back of this manual.

Using the Calorie Guide

You will need to do some arithmetic to calculate calories. For instance, the guide may list a pat of margarine as having 36 calories. If you have two pats on a roll, the contribution from margarine will be 72 (36 x 2) calories. If you have only half the pat, you will record 18 calories.

Your judgment is important when estimating calories because a calorie guide provides only estimates and may not apply to the food you are actually eating. For instance, a calorie guide may show that a roast beef sandwich has 347 calories. This refers to a regular sandwich with about 2 oz of meat with no mustard, mayonnaise, or whatever else you use. If your deli sandwich has two inches (rather than 2 oz) of roast beef, the calories could be three or four times what the guide lists.

The challenge is to estimate the portion sizes and composition of the foods you eat. This can be difficult, especially when you eat out. At home, using a food scale can simplify the job. Many people feel they do not need a scale, especially the veterans of weight loss programs who have been keeping calorie records for years. Some colleagues and I did a study on this. We had individuals in our program estimate the quantities and calories in common foods and beverages, such as milk, green beans, meat, and soda. Some estimated high and some low, but the average error was 60 percent too low! This means they were eating 60 percent more calories than they thought. Food scales are available and are not expensive.

Finding the hidden calories in foods is also important. Examples are butter on vegetables, whipped cream on desserts, dressings on salad, and sugar used as a sweetener. Be painfully honest since these are sources of extra pounds. Did you know that one extra pat of margarine

per day, which has only 36 calories, can add up to four pounds of weight in one year?

As you progress through the program, you will be able to estimate food portions, the composition of foods, and calories more easily and accurately. The Food Diary will be easier to keep and the exact calories will become less important.

The Weight Change Record

TAPE 1
SECTION 8

You can track your progress by using the Weight Change Record. Once each week, record the date and your weight change from the previous week. I have provided a sample on page 19.

Keeping the Weight Change Record has several advantages. First, it is a reminder of how you are faring with the program. Second, it shows the relationship between your eating and your weight. The record can help you estimate how many calories you need to lose weight. Take the average daily calorie values from several weeks of your Food Diary and compare with your weight changes from your Weight Change Record. Third, the graph puts your weight change in perspective. If you gain a pound during your eighth week, you can take heart from the steady loss in earlier weeks.

You will notice that the Weight Change Record is a graph of change, not of weight per se. This is done so people can place the graph

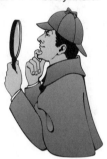

"Count everything you eat, and be on the lookout for those hidden calories lurking about everywhere."

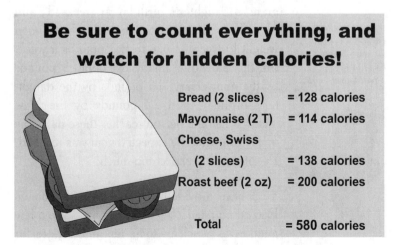

Be sure to count everything, and watch for hidden calories!

Bread (2 slices)	= 128 calories
Mayonnaise (2 T)	= 114 calories
Cheese, Swiss	
(2 slices)	= 138 calories
Roast beef (2 oz)	= 200 calories
Total	**= 580 calories**

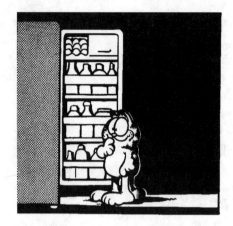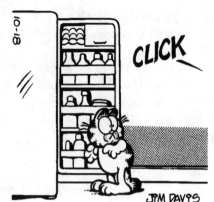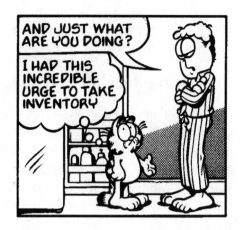

in a public spot, like on the refrigerator door, if they wish. Your weight does not appear on the graph, just your progress. Many people like to have the graph posted in a place where they see it frequently, so it can act as a source of encouragement. The sample on page 19 shows how this could happen.

On the sample graph provided on page 19, you will see a straight line. This represents what weight would look like if a person lost the same amount of weight each week. Of course, life does not occur in a straight line. The realistic line on the graph shows some weeks where weight stays stable and even weeks when weight increases.

A terrific help in setting reasonable goals is to think ahead to how much weight you are likely to lose by landmark dates. Let's use the sample graph on page 19 as an example. A person's anniversary might be at week 6 of the program, a daughter's birthday at week 11, and New Year's celebration at week 15. A good weight loss goal is one to two pounds a week. So, this individual might lose about 9 pounds by the anniversary, 16 pounds by the daughter's birthday, and 22 pounds by the New Year. When the person reaches these dates, he or she can see if the expected goal was reached. People usually expect too much!

I have provided a blank Weight Change Record on page 25 for you to use. Take a few minutes to pencil in some landmark dates for

"Keeping your own personal Weight Change Record has many advantages."

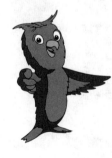

this graph for the next eight weeks. Use holidays, birthdays, or other special dates as target dates. When those dates roll around, compare your weight loss with the graph. A weight loss that seems disappointing may look good when compared with a reasonable standard.

You should know right now to expect some weeks when your graph looks more like the realistic line than the straight line. What matters in a given week is where you are compared with where you started. This is far more important that what you weighed the week before. Gaining a pound is a small setback in the scheme of your total program, but your *reaction* to the pound can be devastating. Therefore, think of this sample graph often, and remember that you are a real person and that the realistic line may best reflect your experience.

Sample Weight Change Record

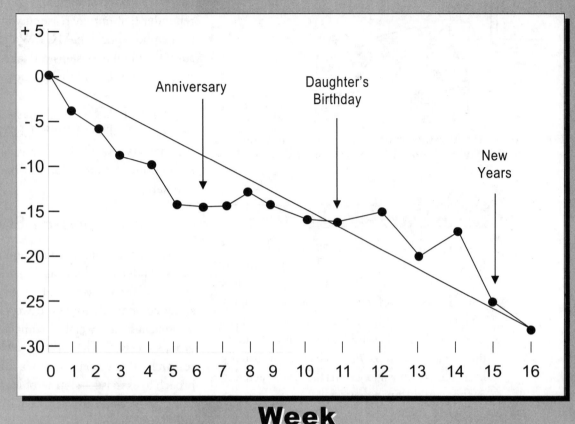

Weight Change (in pounds)

+ 5
0
- 5
-10
-15
-20
-25
-30

0 1 2 3 4 5 6 7 8 9 10 11 12 13 14 15 16

Anniversary

Daughter's Birthday

New Years

Week

 TAPE 1
SECTION 9

Getting Started with Physical Activity

You'll read a lot about being physically active in the lessons that follow. Physical activity is really, really important, even if you only do a little. In fact, physical activity is one of the best predictors of long-term success. The best news of all is that you don't have to knock yourself out doing it. Even in modest amounts, exercise can be good for your health, good for your weight loss, and good for your self-image.

One issue I will discuss several times is just how much exercise you should do. Contrary to old notions that you have to exercise a certain number of minutes and get your heart rate into a target zone, anything will help. The task is to increase your movement and activity beyond what you do now. Work your way into a pattern of regular, healthy physical activity. *Anything you do to increase your activity will be helpful and "counts."*

A great way to start is to do two things. The first is to use every chance you get to be a bit more active. Try walking places, using stairs when possible—just making an effort to move around will help. Every time you're active it is a reminder you are making progress. The second thing is to do some regular walking—even in small amounts. Begin with walking that is comfortable for you, and work your way up. Doing a series of short walks is as good as taking one long walk.

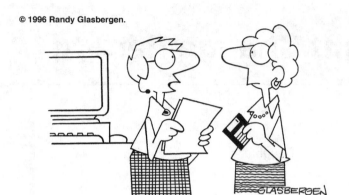

"I'm trying to fit 30 minutes of daily exercise into my busy schedule. Today I took 120 fifteen-second walks."

A Very Helpful Device

I would like you to consider purchasing a handy and helpful device called a pedometer. The more advanced versions of the pedometers not only track how far you walk but other important factors as well, such as calories burned. These devices measure motion and calculate the number of steps you take. People usually keep a log of how many steps they take each day or the total distance they walk.

The LEARN WalkMaster™ is one of those devices—one that my colleagues and I use ourselves and is used by people with whom we work. It gives you credit whether you are in Boston running the Marathon or are meandering through the house. The LEARN WalkMaster can detect increases in your activity even when you don't notice. This feedback can be highly rewarding and can be a constant reminder that *any* increase in your activity can be helpful. The LEARN WalkMaster measures the number of steps you take, the total distance you move, and the calories you burn.

The LEARN WalkMaster can be ordered by calling 1–888–LEARN–41, by Internet (www.TheLifeStyleCompany.com), or by using the order form at the back of this manual.

An Impressive Study

Let me mention a study conducted by Drs. Ross Andersen, Thomas Wadden, and colleagues at the University of Pennsylvania. This study compared people on two quite different approaches to weight management. Both groups received The LEARN Program. The researchers gave one group a traditional approach to exercise—step aerobics at a fitness facility, three times a week, requiring about 60 minutes each time.

The other group was encouraged instead to increase "lifestyle activity." This group was asked to increase their activity by 30 minutes most days of the week by adding short bouts of activity throughout the day, by walking rather than driving short distances, etc. To help these people keep track of their increased activity and to boost motivation, a device like The LEARN WalkMaster was provided.

At a one-year follow-up after the initial program ended, both groups had lost the same amount of weight. In addition, both groups showed the same changes in important medical factors, such as blood pressure. This shows that reasonable, attainable amounts of activity can be valuable, even if it's not strenuous. The LEARN WalkMaster can help with this. It can show even small changes in your activity and will help you realize that these changes

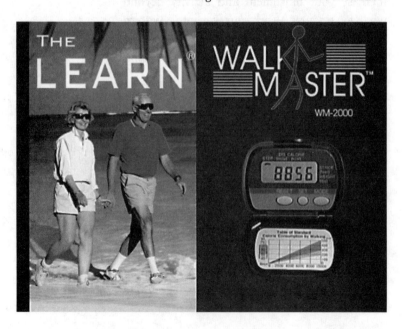

make a difference. I suggest you use one of these devices.

Reasons for Overweight

TAPE 1
SECTION 11

Why people are overweight is still somewhat of a mystery, although scientists from many countries have been working on the problem for years. Exciting discoveries occur frequently, yet we still have a long road to travel before we can unravel the complex causes and consequences of weight problems. Meanwhile, it is helpful to examine the popular reasons people use to explain overweight.

I cover this information here because the reasons people use to explain weight problems create attitudes that can help or hinder efforts to lose weight. A person who feels genetics has determined his or her weight may be discouraged from attempting to lose weight. The information that follows may counter some misconceptions.

⇨ *Glands*. An underactive thyroid used to be a popular reason to explain weight problems. The truth is, most overweight people have no gland problems. If they do, the problems are not serious enough to account for much of their excess weight. If you suspect gland problems, don't hesitate to see your doctor, but remember that fewer than 5 percent of overweight persons have these difficulties.

⇨ *Metabolism*. The issue of metabolism will be covered later in our discussion of exercise. Metabolic rate, which is the energy (calories) your body uses for living, varies widely among people. This influences the way they gain or lose weight. Some women will lose weight rapidly on 1600 calories per day while there are rare individuals who lose slowly on only 800 calories per day. A thrifty metabolism that conserves energy and promotes weight gain curses these people. Determining your exact metabolic

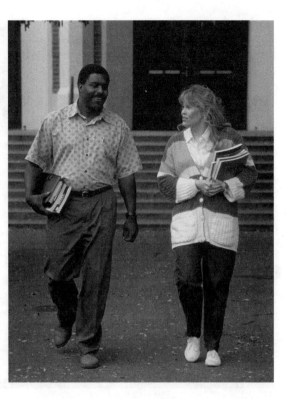

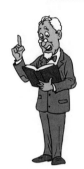

"Individuals become overweight for a variety of complex reasons."

needs is more costly than it is worth, because you approach weight loss in the same way regardless of your metabolism. If you have a thrifty metabolism, exercise is especially important.

⇨ *Genetics*. Overweight runs in families. A child with no overweight parents has less than a 10 percent chance of being overweight. If one parent is overweight, the chances increase to 40 percent. With two overweight parents, the odds are 70 percent. This could, of course, reflect the tendency of families to pass along their eating and exercise habits to children.

We have known for years that people can breed animals to be fat. The meat you buy at the supermarket comes from an animal bred to have a certain percentage of body fat. But, what do we know about humans?

The past 20 years have brought an explosion of research on the genetics of body-weight regulation. Among the ways to study genetics is to examine identical twins. Studies have compared body

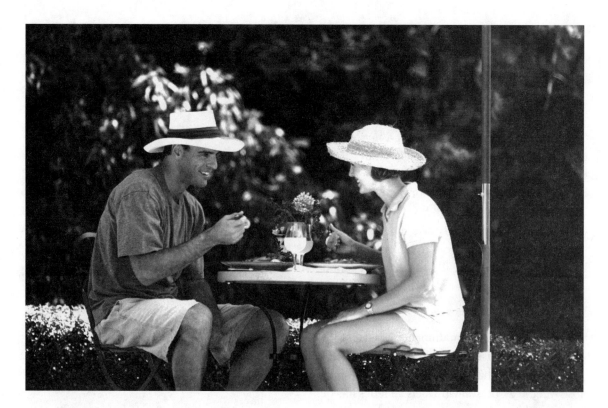

weights of twins who were reared together to weights in twins reared apart. If genes are important, we would expect the weights within twin pairs to be similar despite whether they were reared together. If the twins reared apart are more dissimilar than twins reared together, the environment would seem to exert an important influence. The studies show that the similarity in body weights within twin pairs is nearly the same whether twins are reared apart or reared together. This suggests that genes are important.

This does not mean that genetics completely controls weight. How we eat and exercise will determine whether our genetic predisposition to be heavy or thin is expressed. One virtue of this research is that it relieves some of the blame people place on themselves for being overweight. One danger is that people overstate the importance of genetics. They may come to feel they are destined to be heavy and nothing can be done.

⇨ **Fat cells**. The body accumulates and stores fat in fat cells, also called adipose tissue. Some people have too many fat cells (hyperplastic obesity) while others have the normal number but their fat cells are too large (hypertrophic obesity). Still others have both types. People who were overweight in childhood or are very heavy tend to have an excessive number of fat cells as well as enlarged cells. Early researchers in this area speculated that people with too many fat cells would have difficulty losing weight. Researchers have not tested this sufficiently to know whether it is true.

⇨ **Family upbringing**. Some families foster overeating for emotional or even cultural reasons. Some people may eat for psychological reasons related to their family upbringing. A program aimed at behavior change is the right approach for these people. Behavior change helps to separate emotions from eating and helps to identify other sources of gratification.

⇨ **Psychological factors**. Many overweight people have trouble controlling their eating in response to stress, depression, loneliness, anger, and other emotions. Does this mean that being overweight is a symptom of deep psychological distress? If so, the remedy would be to root out the underlying psychological problems in hopes that the symptom (overeating) would disappear.

This theory rings true intuitively for many people, but does not have much support among experts. Many normal-weight persons have psychological problems but cope without overeating. In people who undergo intensive psychotherapy, weight problems generally remain after their psychological difficulties have been resolved. If you feel that psychological problems are at the root of your weight problem, deal with either the weight (through this program) or the psychological problems (with therapy). Do not labor under the notion that you must remedy the psychological problems before you can lose weight.

When all is said and done, and all the reasons for overweight are debated, the fact remains that people gain weight because they consume more calories than their bodies use. Becoming overweight is usually a gradual process and may result from small errors in what we eat. One business executive gained five pounds each year for 20 years. He did not notice the five pounds each year, but he was unhappy with the 100 pounds he accumulated over time. This could have occurred from nothing more than two to three drinks per week. The solution

to such a problem is a gradual change in eating and exercise habits so that long-term weight loss can occur.

A Note About Exercise, Relationships, and Nutrition

The emphasis this week is on lifestyle (record keeping) and attitudes (causes for overweight). Exercise, relationships, and nutrition will be covered in detail later. They will receive much attention as we progress through The LEARN Program.

Your Self-Assessment

You may recall that in the Introduction and Orientation Lesson I discussed the self-assessments that are included at the end of each lesson. These self-assessments are simple true/false quizzes to help you decide whether you have learned the important points of each lesson. If you answer all the questions correctly, pat yourself on the back. You can boast about being a weight loss whiz! When you answer a question incorrectly, review the material in the lesson again.

My Personal Goals for this Week

TAPE 2
SECTION 2

Each lesson of The LEARN Program will end with a section on setting personal goals. This section will include specific issues for your attention, based on the material in the lesson. In some ways, this is an assignment to practice the new activities you read about. This will also offer

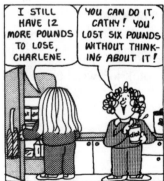

I STILL HAVE 12 MORE POUNDS TO LOSE, CHARLENE.

YOU CAN DO IT, CATHY! YOU LOST SIX POUNDS WITHOUT THINKING ABOUT IT!

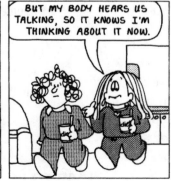

BUT MY BODY HEARS US TALKING, SO IT KNOWS I'M THINKING ABOUT IT NOW.

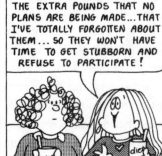

I HAVE TO SOMEHOW CONVINCE THE EXTRA POUNDS THAT NO PLANS ARE BEING MADE...THAT I'VE TOTALLY FORGOTTEN ABOUT THEM...SO THEY WON'T HAVE TIME TO GET STUBBORN AND REFUSE TO PARTICIPATE!

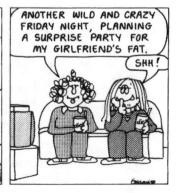

ANOTHER WILD AND CRAZY FRIDAY NIGHT, PLANNING A SURPRISE PARTY FOR MY GIRLFRIEND'S FAT.

SHH!

you a chance to reflect on what you want to accomplish before moving on to the next lesson. Sometimes the goals will be broad, like being more aware of temptations to eat, but others will be more specific. An example is being physically active for a certain number of minutes each day.

Goal setting is important. This process gives you something to strive for, a standard against which to measure your progress. As you establish your personal goals each week, remember several things. The first is to set goals that are reasonable. The tendency for many people is to set goals too high. This makes good progress seem trivial. I will discuss this issue of setting realistic goals in greater detail as the program moves ahead.

TAPE 3
SECTION 8

The second thing to remember is to reward yourself, even with a few kind words. Too often people dismiss important changes they make and focus instead on how far they have to go. People are notoriously reluctant to reward themselves, perhaps because it seems like bragging. Yet, you can be your biggest fan—you know how much time and effort you have invested in making important changes. Most people would not dream of praising themselves for something they would routinely praise a friend for doing. Getting in the habit of praising yourself is a good habit indeed!

The primary goal this week is not to start a diet but to learn about your eating and weight habits. The Food Diary and the Weight Change Record are an important first step in this learning process. I will discuss specific calorie levels in Lesson Three. Set a personal goal this week to make copies of the Food Diary provided on page 27 of this lesson. If you have ordered the pocket-sized forms discussed on page 9, that's terrific; you won't need to make copies. Complete your Food Diary each day of the week and begin to chart your weight change on the Weight Change Record on page 25.

Setting personal goals to complete these forms is critical, for three reasons. First, it is a good test of your motivation. Difficulty in keeping the records may reflect inadequate motivation. If this is the case, you may want to think about beginning the program later when motivation is higher. Second, the information will teach you about your habits. Third, the information will be valuable to a group leader or professional who may be working with you.

My Self-Assessment

Lesson One

(Circle either T for true or F for false.)

T F 1. Discovering the psychological roots of your weight problem is the most important factor in weight reduction.

T F 2. All overweight people have an excessive number of fat cells.

T F 3. There is no such thing as a slow or underactive metabolism.

T F 4. Very few people can accurately estimate the quantity and calories of foods.

T F 5. Record keeping may be the most important aspect of a weight management program.

T F 6. Using a tool like a pedometer is not very helpful for weight management.

(Answers in Appendix C, page 271)

My Weight Change Record
(Weeks 1–8)

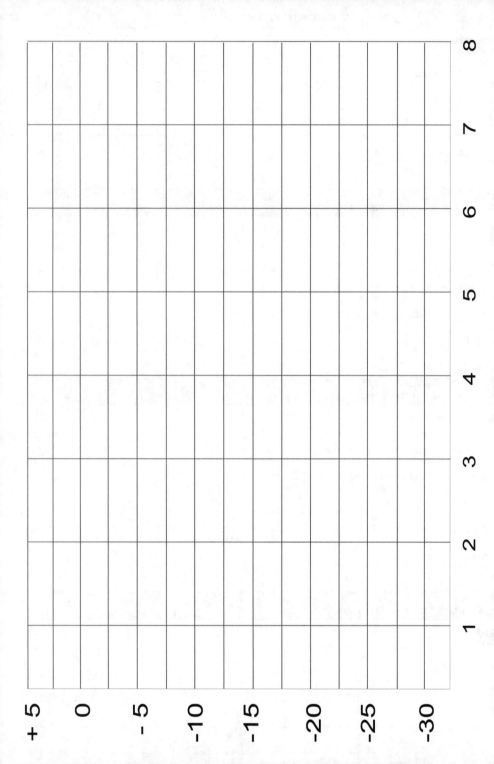

Weight Change (in pounds)							
+ 5							
0							
- 5							
-10							
-15							
-20							
-25							
-30							
1	2	3	4	5	6	7	8

Week

Food Diary—Lesson One *(Sample)*

Today's Date:_____

DESCRIPTION	CALORIES
BREAKFAST	
Orange juice, ½ cup	60
Cheerios, 1 cup	89
Skim milk, 1 cup	86
White toast, dry, 1 slice	64
TOTAL CALORIES FOR THIS MEAL	299
LUNCH	
Apple, 1 medium	81
Vegetable soup, 2 cups	144
Chicken salad sandwich, 2 oz, with 2T mayonnaise	332
Ritz crackers, 5	70
Diet Pepsi, 12 oz	1
TOTAL CALORIES FOR THIS MEAL	628
DINNER	
Garden salad, 1 cup, fat-free dressing	160
Chicken breast (roasted), skinless, 3.5 oz	173
Green beans, 1 cup	26
Cauliflower, 2 cups	60
Wheat bread, 1 slice	61
TOTAL CALORIES FOR THIS MEAL	480
SNACKS	
Yogurt, low-fat, 8 oz	144
Apple, 1 medium	81
TOTAL CALORIES FOR SNACKS	225
TOTAL CALORIES FOR THE DAY	1,632

Food Diary—Lesson One

Today's Date:_____

DESCRIPTION	CALORIES
BREAKFAST	
TOTAL CALORIES FOR THIS MEAL	
LUNCH	
TOTAL CALORIES FOR THIS MEAL	
DINNER	
TOTAL CALORIES FOR THIS MEAL	
SNACKS	
TOTAL CALORIES FOR SNACKS	
TOTAL CALORIES FOR THE DAY	

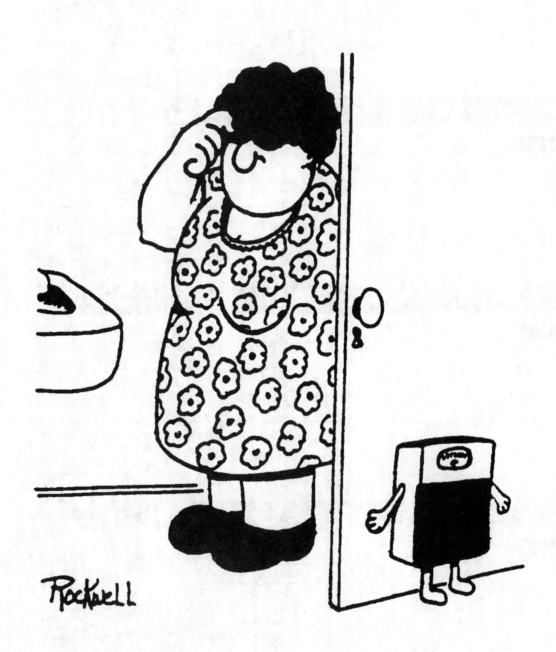

W elcome back after your first lesson! I hope you did well and are on your way to permanent weight loss. Many people think of weight management as "going on a diet." If you follow this way of thinking, banish these thoughts from your mind. Think of weight management as making better food and activity choices. This new way of thinking leaves the door open for enjoying your food and eating sensible meals that are filling. Let me show you how.

About Eating a Sensible Meal

Making the meals count that you do eat is important. By this, I mean you want your meals to be satisfying, good tasting, pleasing to the eye, nutritious, and have a texture that is pleasing to your palate. Otherwise, you'll feel deprived when there is no need to, and you will keep your body from getting good nutrients. You don't have to eat a sparse and boring "diet meal." Your meals can be filling and nutritious, include much variety, taste delicious, and be low in calories and fat. You may have to do some planning in advance and make good food choices.

Eating Great Meals

You will hear me talk a lot about eating "sensible" meals throughout The LEARN

Program. I am a firm believer that you should enjoy every bit of food you eat. The object is for you to eat delicious, filling, and nutritious meals—not a plate with one stalk of asparagus and a beet. Keeping your calories low while accomplishing your dietary goals and being satisfied is quite possible—if you make good choices. Let's examine such a meal.

The Baked Italian Chicken dinner is shown in the picture on page 30 and described in the box below the photo. This is a fine meal from a nutritional standpoint with less that 9 grams of fat, more than 14 grams of fiber, and only 540 calories. Just look at the picture—there's a lot of food to eat. Think of having three vegetables, plus a potato and salad, not to mention the chicken and fruit. The meal has great variety, a pleasing mix of foods, and a fine nutrient breakdown.

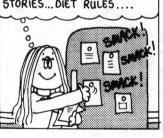
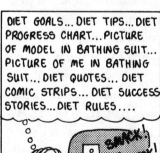
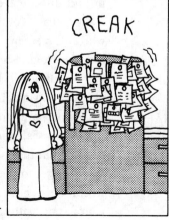
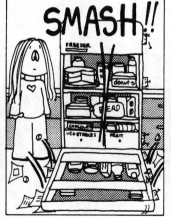
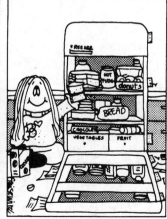

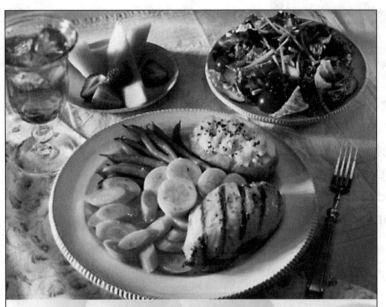

Baked Italian Chicken Dinner

Yield: 1 Serving*

Per Serving: 540 calories; 8.7 gm fat

Ingredients:

4 oz	Chicken breast, skinned
1 t	Italian seasoning
	Nonstick cooking spray
1 medium	Potato, baked
1 t	Butter replacement (Butter Buds)
½ cup	Squash, steamed
1 t	Butter replacement (Butter Buds)
½ cup	Carrots, sliced, steamed
1 t	Butter replacement (Butter Buds)
1 cup	Lettuce, red leaf, chopped
1 cup	Lettuce, romaine, chopped
3 slices	Cucumber
2 medium	Radishes
4	Cherry tomatoes
2 T	Salad dressing (low-fat lite)
½ cup	Melon
½ cup	Strawberries
	Ice Tea

Directions:

Spray coat chicken breast with nonstick cooking spray and sprinkle with Italian seasoning. Broil for approximately 15 minutes (7–8 minutes on each side). Serve with baked potato and steamed vegetables seasoned with butter replacement such as Butter Buds; salad of fresh lettuce, cucumber, radishes, and tomato topped with a non-fat lite salad dressing. Beverage of ice tea with artificial sweetener and lemon. Dessert of melon and strawberries.

*May be multiplied to provide for entire family.

Some people like to feel really full when they eat. If this sounds like you, a meal like this will probably do the job. The meal contains a large quantity of food, and the foods that are in the meal tend to be filling. Eating a sensible meal can mean eating a fun meal, a delicious meal, and a meal that makes you feel virtuous.

You can substitute soup for the salad or replace vegetables and the fruit with others you might like more. You may have turkey or fish instead of the chicken, and still come in around the same low-calorie levels as the chicken dinner (540 calories). So, when you hear "sensible" meal, think of good food, plenty to eat, and a boost for your body.

You can find many good ways to put together healthy, low-calorie meals. In Lesson Seven under the section on Planning Health Meals that begins on page 107, you will find a list of cookbooks and healthy eating books loaded with ideas.

Reviewing Your Food Diary

TAPE 2
SECTION 8

Your Food Diary contains information about very important issues—your eating patterns. The better you understand these patterns, the easier it will be to establish new ones. After a week of recording, you should have a better idea of how many meals you typically eat each day and the types of food you enjoy. You should also be more aware of when you are hungriest and the places in and outside the home where you are most likely to eat. Your job is to become a detective who analyzes your eating habits and tries to correct the troublesome ones. Sometimes this requires only small changes such as taking a piece of fruit or a small bag of pretzels to work so you will be prepared for the three o'clock munchies. In other cases, you may have to take more time to plan your meals. You may need to make sure that you get to the supermarket at least once a week. Let's now search to see what some of your eating patterns might be.

Searching for Patterns

One purpose of completing the Food Diary is to examine your eating patterns. Much of our eating is automatic and occurs with little thought or appreciation. We miss much of the pleasure in food and eat more than we need. Think of munching from a large bag of potato chips. Would you remember how many you ate? Would you taste each bite of each chip? Would you have just the right amount to satisfy yourself?

A good example of automatic eating is from a client of mine named Ginny. She loved ice cream and would have a bowl every night. With instruction, she began counting her bites and noting the pleasure in each one. She averaged 16 bites. She found that the first four bites were delicious, then there were about 10 bites where she paid little attention to what she was eating (automatic eating). The final few bites were good because she was nearly finished. With her increased awareness, Ginny decided that the middle 10 bites were needless calories.

Examine your Food Diaries for the past week and look for patterns. The patterns you find will be the foundation for later parts of the program. This is where I work with you. I will give you guidelines for tailoring techniques to your specific eating and exercise patterns. On page 32 is the "My Eating Patterns Worksheet" to help you identify your unique

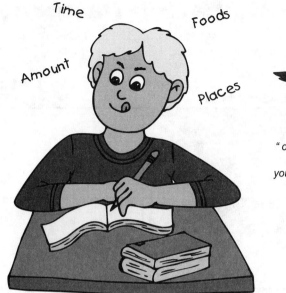

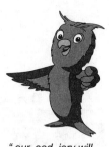

" our ood iary will help you discover your eating patterns."

eating patterns. As you review your Food Diaries for the last week and complete this worksheet, pay careful attention to the following topics as you search for *your* eating patterns.

⇨ **Time**. Look for times of the day when you are likely to eat. A typical pattern shows little eating at breakfast and lunch, but much eating and snacking at dinner and after. Do you crave a snack just before bed? Do you always have something in mid-afternoon? Are your meals irregular? Do you skip meals?

⇨ **Amount**. Look over the quantities and calories of the food you eat. One key is to enjoy the food you eat so that you do not

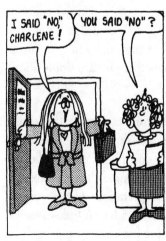

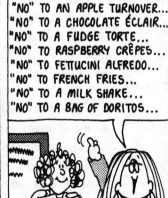

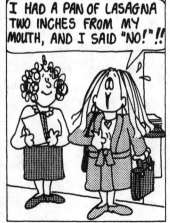

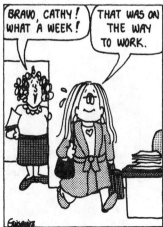

My Eating Patterns Worksheet

week of: _____

Description	My Eating Patterns	Eating Patterns to Change
TIME		
AMOUNT		
FOODS		
PLACES		
OTHER		

"The better you understand your eating patterns the easier it will be to establish new ones."

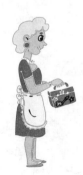

waste calories. Are there foods you could eat less of or avoid completely? Do you eat specific amounts each time without thinking about how much you need and want?

⇨ *Foods*. Pay close attention to the foods you eat. Can you find patterns in the foods you choose? Which foods contribute most to your calories? Can you think of substitutes for high-calorie foods?

⇨ *Places*. Are there certain places where you eat? Do you frequently eat in places other than your kitchen or dining room? Some likely candidates are the den, the office, and the car.

An Expanded Food Diary

This week you will find several categories added to your new Expanded Food Diary. These categories are Time, Feelings, and Activity. In addition to the food and calories, you will be able to record the time you are eating, how you feel, and whether you are doing something else.

These are important factors in the eating habits of many overweight people. Therefore, use the Expanded Food Diary as you did the Food Diary for Lesson One. In the next lesson, I will discuss the interpretations of the new diary. A blank diary is provided in this lesson on page 41, and a sample from one of my clients is shown on page 40 to show you how the diary might be completed. Be sure to make copies of the blank diary to use between now and the next lesson.

Rating Your Diet

Nutrition is one key to successful weight management. What you eat affects how you feel, whether you are healthy, and how you look. Much information on nutrition awaits you in this program. To start the process, let's evaluate your diet.

I have provided on page 283, the "Rate Your Diet Quiz" for Lesson Two. This quiz was developed by the Center for Science in the Public Interest and published in the *Nutrition Action Healthletter*. Take a few minutes to complete the quiz and to score your answers. You have probably changed your diet since beginning the program. Complete the quiz as you would have *before starting the program*, so you will see how you would score ordinarily. In Lessons Eight and Sixteen I will have you take the quiz again to see how your eating habits have changed.

Better diets will receive higher scores on this quiz. You will see which choices for each question contribute to or subtract from the total score. Taking the quiz can be educational because it may help provide new ideas for healthy food choices. Later in the program you will be asked to take the quiz again and compare your scores.

The Role of Exercise

TAPE 1
SECTION 9

Throughout this program, I will speak about ways to eat a balanced diet. Keeping calories low is one good way to help your body create an energy deficit. However, there is much, much more you can do. Now it is time to talk about the other side of the weight loss equation—increasing the num-

ber of calories you expend by increasing your physical activity. Are you ready?

I cannot overstate the importance of increasing physical activity. Theoretically, you can eat less, exercise more, or do both to alter your energy balance and your weight. I feel strongly that doing both is the best approach. This comes from experience with hundreds of clients and from research showing that people who exercise are most likely to achieve long-term weight loss.

The Importance of Being Active

Don't get nervous! Increasing your activity does not have to involve calisthenics, weight lifting, or marathon running. Many overweight people avoid exercise because it hurts, it takes time, they are embarrassed, and they are not skilled at athletic activities. Solutions exist to these problems. I will discuss these in upcoming

"Increasing your activity does not have to involve calisthenics, weight lifting, or marathon running."

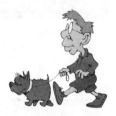

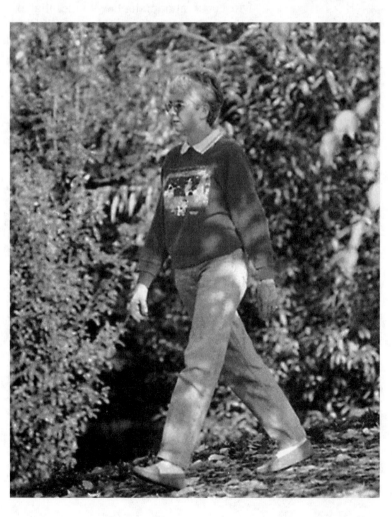

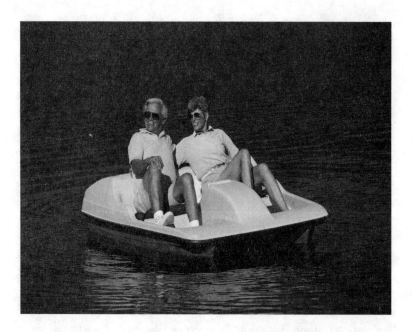

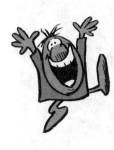

"Physical activity is central to weight management, and the key to staying active is to do things you enjoy doing."

lessons. For now, I want you to be aware of the importance and benefits of being active.

A New View of Exercise

Most of us labor under the old idea that exercise has to be taxing to be beneficial. In fact, this is what most of the experts preached for years and years. Much to the delight of people struggling with their weight, the view of exercise has changed entirely in the last several years. What we know now, and what prestigious groups like the American College of Sports Medicine and the Centers for Disease Control and Prevention have emphasized, is that low levels of activity can be beneficial for health. We also know that low levels can be helpful for weight management.

This turns everything upside down. It means that making small increases in physical activity counts as exercise. Even with modest changes, you may improve your health. It also means that we can set aside the biggest barrier to exercise—the thought that high levels are the only acceptable amounts. I hope you don't tire of me saying that any amount of exercise is beneficial. I raise this issue often in the program.

The Benefits of Exercise

Physical activity is central to weight management for seven reasons. Most people know

only the first—that it burns calories. Let's explore the other six.

⇨ **Burns calories**. Exercise does burn calories, but this may be its least important benefit. Be careful to avoid feeling that a modest amount of exercise entitles you to more calories at the table. You will probably eat more calories than the exercise expended.

⇨ **Counteracts the ills of overweight**. Exercise can help change the physical and psychological problems associated with being overweight. It can lower blood pressure and cholesterol and improve the metabolism of carbohydrates.

⇨ **Helps control appetite**. Studies with both animals and humans suggest that exercise can help control appetite. It certainly does not stimulate appetite when people exercise in moderate amounts. If you exercise and feel increased hunger, your mind is at work rather than your body.

⇨ **Preserves the body's muscle**. Your body looses both muscle and fat when you lose weight. The aim is to maximize fat loss. Combining exercise with diet does this more effectively than using diet alone.

⇨ **Increases metabolic rate**. When you are eating less and are losing weight, your metabolism slows. This is bad news because your body then uses less energy (calories) for basic functioning at a time when you want to burn more calories. Exercise speeds up your metabolism, although the degree and duration of this increase are subject to debate. Exercising while eating less may help offset this drop in your metabolic rate.

⇨ **Improves confidence and psychological factors**. Exercise makes people feel good. Each time you are active is a symbol that you are making positive changes. This improves confidence and gives you a boost that can carry over to your eating plan. In addition, many people exercise to relieve stress. If you are a person who eats to relieve stress, exercise may accomplish the same thing but will burn rather than add calories.

⇨ **Correlates with long-term success**. Exercise is the factor that best predicts who will lose weight and keep it off. If people are followed a year or more after a weight loss program, those who are exercising tend to be the ones who keep the weight off. Furthermore, those individuals who are prescribed a structured exercise program during weight loss do better than those who just diet.

As you can see, the evidence in favor of exercise is clear and powerful. In the next lesson I will begin with specific suggestions for increasing activity. Walking will be the first step, so if you are walking now, keep up the good work! If not, don't hesitate to begin—but don't overdo it.

Throughout this program, I discuss the importance of exercise and physical activity. I also provide many helpful ways to help you become more active and to stay active. However, there is much more to be learned than I can present in this program. In this program, I simply help you get started. Dr. Steven Blair, of The Cooper Institute for Aerobics Research in Dallas, has written an excellent book for those individuals who find it difficult to find time to exercise. *Living with Exercise 2000*, part of the LEARN LifeStyle Program Series™, is a step-by-step guide designed to help people incorporate increased physical activity into their daily lifestyle. For more information on this guide, contact The LifeStyle Company toll free at 1–888–LEARN–41.

Why Losing Weight Is Difficult

Let's face it—losing weight is hard work. Most overweight people really want to lose weight, but often find it difficult. Many factors are at work here. I will discuss several here. Appreciating the complexities of weight management, so you don't get demoralized when you encounter tough times, is important.

Eating is a complex activity. When you face temptation from food, say a piece of cake after dinner, many factors combine to determine whether you will eat it. Physiology is at work because seeing the cake might stimulate hunger. Your family upbringing can enter the picture because you may have learned that foods (especially desserts) are associated with love. Culture plays a part, particularly if you are dining with someone else and you feel obliged to eat everything, including dessert. Psychology might take part if you are feeling depressed or lonely and want food for gratification. A single reason cannot be pinpointed. To keep your attitude on the

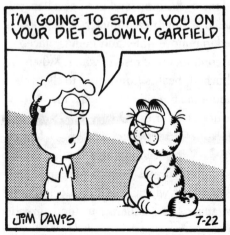
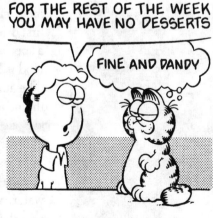
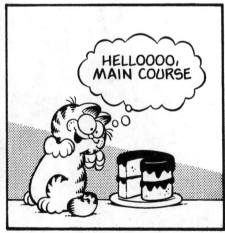

right track, remind yourself that getting the actual eating and exercise habits under control is the best course to weight loss. Instead of feeling guilty about what you eat, or resentful about what you cannot eat, you can learn about food and calories and enjoy yourself!

On Being a Good Group Member

Many people who use this program do so on their own. Others are part of a group program. If you are part of a group and are with others who struggle with problems like yours, there are several important matters to consider.

Being in a group can be a wonderful experience, with support, encouragement, and good ideas flowing from one member of the group to another. This is why groups can be so beneficial. To make the group a positive experience, each member must realize that working in a cooperative way and with a team spirit will allow the group to reach its potential. Each member in the group has the opportunity, the *responsibility*, to follow certain guidelines. Some effort will be required, but the payoff will make it worthwhile.

Detailed guidelines for being a good group member are presented in Appendix D, beginning on page 277. If you are participating in a group program, I urge you to read these over, and to take the advice seriously. Being a contributing and constructive member of the group will support the other group members, who in turn will support you. This can go a long way toward motivating you when times are tough and giving you fresh ideas for specific problems.

The Mysterious Calorie

In Lesson Four, I discuss your option of counting calories or using food exchanges. No matter which option you choose, you need to know more about calories.

The word "calorie" is on the lips of millions of Americans. Food products boast about being "low calorie" and diet soft drinks sell because they have "no calories." Just what is this thing we call a calorie?

A Calorie Is

The calorie is a measure of energy available to the body. This is much like a gallon is a measure of volume, the inch a measure of length, and the pound a measure of weight. When you eat something, the number of calories it contains is the number of energy units it provides to the body for its needs. The calorie is also a measure of energy your body uses, so it is a measure of both intake and expenditure. That is why I talk about the number of calories burned during exercise.

How do we measure the calories in foods? This is done by burning food in a special instrument called a bomb calorimeter. The food is first dried to remove water and then is placed in a special container that rests in water. When the food is burned, heat is transferred to the water. The amount the burning food heats the water is the measure of calories. One calorie is the energy needed to raise the temperature of 1 gram of water 1 degree centigrade. Foods contain proteins, carbohydrates (sugars and starches), and fats, each of which provide calories. The water, vitamins, and minerals in food provide no calories.

Most foods are measured in kilocalories, which is 1000 times the energy in a small calorie. In common usage, as in diet books and calorie guides, the word calorie actually refers to kilocalorie.

This may sound technical, but you need only know the calorie values of foods. A piece of apple pie has 400 calories, and a fresh apple has 100. The pie gives you four times the energy (calories) as the apple. This would be fine if you were starving, but when your basic energy requirements are met, the body stores the excess as fat. The pie contributes four times as many calories to your fat stockpile.

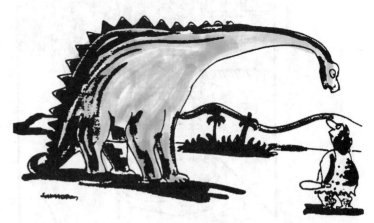

"How many calories are you?"

Not All People Are Created Equal

People differ greatly in how their bodies use calories. We all know people who eat like crazy and gain very little. These fortunate folks are well served in a society where food is abundant and thin is in. In a famine, however, they would be the first to go. Their bodies are not efficient at converting ingested calories to precious energy stores (fat).

The unfortunate ones among us are those who are food efficient. Their bodies make good use of calories, so they are prone to gain weight. This is adaptive if food is scarce, but promotes weight gain when food supplies are adequate. To lose weight, such a person must cut his or her intake to very low levels.

This is one reason that some heavy people have a more difficult time losing weight than others. Let's consider two individuals (Sheri and Bonnie) who fight different battles. Both weigh 180 pounds. Sheri eats 2500 calories each day to maintain that weight and will lose about one pound each week by cutting to 2000 calories. Bonnie, on the other hand, maintains the 180 pounds on only 1800 calories each day, and must reduce to 1300 calories to lose the one pound each week. Is it surprising, then, that Bonnie will have a more difficult time losing weight than will Sheri? Because of these individual differences, prescribing the same calorie goal to these two different people would not be fruitful.

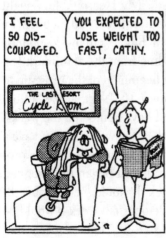
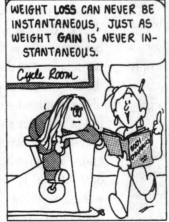
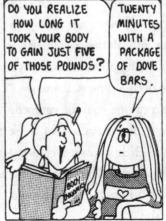
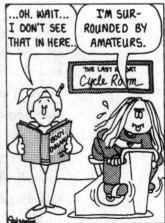

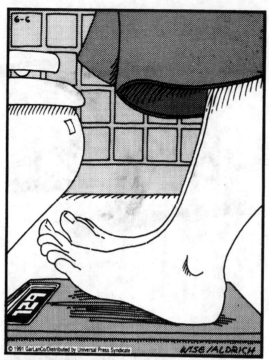

If you stand on the scale just so, you weigh less.

What Makes a Pound

In a related matter, we often hear that 3500 calories equals a pound (it takes 3500 extra calories to gain one pound). If we decrease intake by 3500, one less pound will adorn our bodies. The typical arithmetic is as follows. If you eat 500 fewer calories each day than your ordinary intake, you will create a 3500 calorie deficit in a week and will lose one pound. These numbers are helpful to show how we can translate calories into pounds, but again, the numbers are rough averages. People are highly variable in the number of calories necessary to lose a pound, so these numbers may or may not apply to you. The key question is, therefore, "How do you choose a calorie goal for yourself?" Think about this question over the next week. In Lesson Three, I'll help you set a calorie target for yourself. As you consider this important question, think about weight changes that are reasonable for you.

Your Vision of Reasonable Weight Changes

People begin weight loss programs with differing ideas about how much weight they will lose and how fast they will lose it. A common story might be of Sally, with 50 pounds to lose. She may begin a program in March in anticipation of the upcoming swimsuit season. Sally may not consider how much weight might *reasonably* be lost in the few months ahead. Instead, she focuses on how she will look when she hits the beach.

Having unreasonable expectations of how fast weight will drop can be a problem. When this happens, people with perfectly respectable or even enviable weight losses can feel disappointed. Let's return to Sally's example. She might lose 20 pounds in three months. This is terrific progress, but when she steps on the beach, Sally might feel like a failure knowing that she is still 30 pounds heavier than she wants to be. This feeling could translate into self-doubt, anger, hurt, resignation, and the feeling that it was not worth trying in the first place.

You can avoid this trap and allow yourself to have the good feelings you deserve when you do well. First, having a clear idea of how much weight you might lose is important. I'll give you a suggestion for accomplishing this.

On page 42, I have provided another blank weight graph called "My Reasonable Weight Loss." Assume you will lose 20 pounds by Week 16. This is slightly less than 1½ pounds per week. Draw a line from the zero mark (no pounds lost) at the beginning of the program to the 20 pounds at week 16. Next, at the bottom of the graph where I have numbered the weeks, put in dates for each of the weeks so you have a specific date recorded for each week of the program. For instance, if you began the program on October 1, week 1 would be October 8, week 3 would be October 22, week 6 would be November 12, and so forth. Then, make a special mark on weeks in which some important date occurs (your birthday, your parent's or child's birthday, July 4th, Thanksgiving, Halloween, Valentine's Day, etc.).

When a specific week rolls around, like when your birthday arrives, you can look at your graph and evaluate your progress. This gives you a reasonable standard against which to do so. A person beginning a program on October 1, could pull out this graph on Halloween, see that a reasonable loss is about five to six pounds, and then feel great about a nine-pound loss.

Completing this exercise is important. Referring to it could make the difference between feeling good (as you should) or bad (as is possible) later in the program. Feeling bad is a good state to avoid, and you don't want bad!

My Personal Goals for this Week

You have several program goals for this week. First, you need to make copies of the new Expanded Food Diary on page 41 and complete it each day. Record the types and amounts of food you eat, times, places, and activities associated with eating. Remember that you can order blank week-at-a-time diaries by calling The LifeStyle Company toll-free at 1–888–LEARN–41 or visiting the web site at www.TheLifeStyleCompany. Second, make the meals that you eat count and work on making them enjoyable, delicious, and nutritious. Review your food diary from Lesson One and search carefully for patterns. Using the Rate Your Diet Quiz beginning on page 283, rate your diet. Be sure to rate your diet as it was before you started this program.

Finally, think about your attitudes toward physical activity as you prepare to increase your activity this week. Can you exercise in a more positive light after reading this lesson? Increased activity brings many rewards, one of which is long-term weight management. Remember, even small increases can help. Don't forget to record you weight change on your Weight Change Record on page 25. Good luck achieving your personal goals for this week!

My Self-Assessment

Lesson Two

T F 7. Being on a weight management program means that you can't enjoy good meals.

T F 8. Automatic eating is common in overweight people and distracts them from the taste of food.

T F 9. The Food Diary helps uncover patterns in your eating habits.

T F 10. Exercise isn't of much use for weight loss because it burns relatively few calories.

T F 11. Exercise can help prevent the loss of muscle tissue during weight loss.

T F 12. It is possible to change dietary habits to lose weight and still eat meals that are satisfying, good tasting, and nutritious.

T F 13. The calorie is the measure of the amount of fat in food.

T F 14. The calorie level necessary to lose weight is the same for all people.

(Answers in Appendix C, page 271)

Expanded Food Diary—Lesson Two *(Sample)* Today's Date:_____

DESCRIPTION	TIME	FEELINGS	ACTIVITY	CALORIES
BREAKFAST				
Coffee, 6 oz	7:30	Tired	Reading paper	0
Poached egg, 1 medium				79
Bagel, ½ medium				92
Orange juice, 1 cup				111
TOTAL CALORIES FOR THIS MEAL				282
LUNCH				
Roast beef sandwich, 2 oz, with 2T mayo	12:30	Hurried	Working at desk	442
Water, 1 glass				0
Raspberry yogurt, 8 oz				90
TOTAL CALORIES FOR THIS MEAL				532
DINNER				
Chicken breast-grilled, 3.5 oz	7:30	Relaxed	Watching TV	193
Green beans, 1 cup				44
Carrots, 1 cup, cooked				70
Wheat bread, 1 slice, dry				61
Skim milk, 1 cup				86
TOTAL CALORIES FOR THIS MEAL				454
SNACKS				
Celery, 4 stalks				24
Apple, 1 medium				81
TOTAL CALORIES FOR SNACKS				105
TOTAL CALORIES FOR THE DAY				1,373

Expanded Food Diary—Lesson Two

Today's Date:_____

DESCRIPTION	TIME	FEELINGS	ACTIVITY	CALORIES
BREAKFAST				
TOTAL CALORIES FOR THIS MEAL				
LUNCH				
TOTAL CALORIES FOR THIS MEAL				
DINNER				
TOTAL CALORIES FOR THIS MEAL				
SNACKS				
TOTAL CALORIES FOR SNACKS				
TOTAL CALORIES FOR THE DAY				

My Reasonable Weight Loss

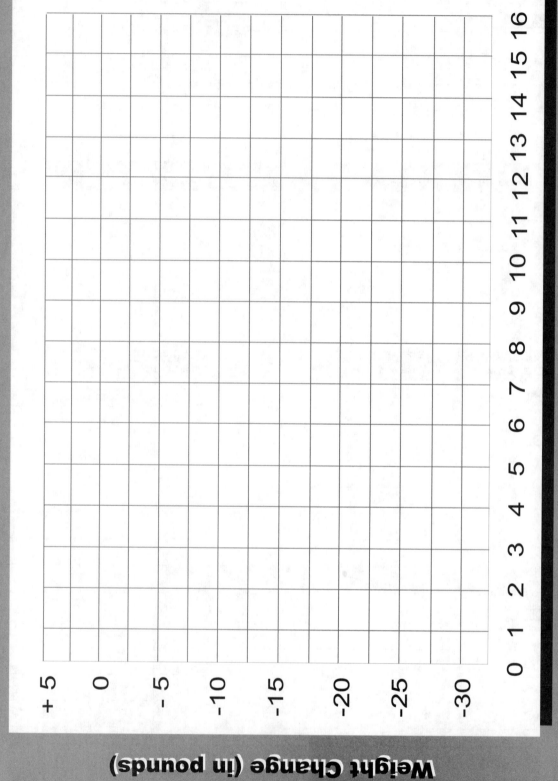

Weight Change (in pounds)

+ 5
0
- 5
-10
-15
-20
-25
-30

0 1 2 3 4 5 6 7 8 9 10 11 12 13 14 15 16

Week

We are ready to move on to new and exciting things. The emphasis in this lesson will be on Lifestyle, Nutrition, and Exercise, with information also on the other parts of The LEARN Program.

Your interpretation of the Expanded Food Diary (Lifestyle) will teach you to be aware of when you are eating from hunger or habit. You will begin to see how the areas of the LEARN model complement each other. For example, I will discuss the all important calorie and help you to determine your individual target calorie level (Nutrition). You will begin a structured walking program (Exercise) and I end the lesson with a discussion about cravings versus hunger (Attitudes). I hope you can see how I have woven the different aspects of the program together.

Analyzing Your Expanded Food Diary

Now that you have experience with the Expanded Food Diary, let's discuss what the information means. You are looking for several things. The first involve eating patterns that tell us whether your eating follows a reliable course from day-to-day. The second are triggers—the circumstances that provoke overeating. Let's see if you can find some patterns and high-risk situations.

The Search for Patterns and High-Risk Situations

The Expanded Food Diary includes spaces for the time of eating, feelings, and other activities. Did you find any patterns?

⇨ **Time**. Did your eating cluster in certain parts of the day? Your eating times may vary depending on the day of the week. Some people keep a strict schedule on weekdays and then have less control on weekends. If you find times when control is difficult, think about scheduling alternative activities (like exercise).

⇨ **Feelings**. Did you eat when you were bored, depressed, anxious, angry, or lonely? Other feelings may also be involved, like resentment, hostility, jealousy, or even joy. Seeing a pattern is a sure sign that you can learn more adaptive ways to cope with difficult feelings.

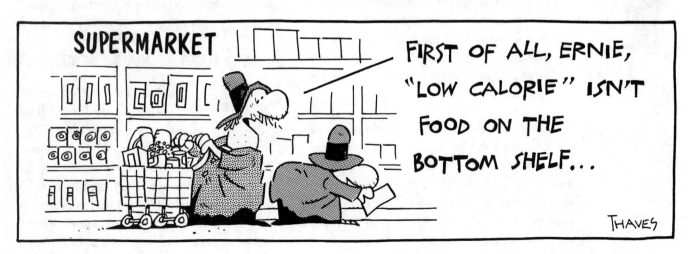

SUPERMARKET

FIRST OF ALL, ERNIE, "LOW CALORIE" ISN'T FOOD ON THE BOTTOM SHELF...

THAVES

TIME
What are the times you eat during the day?

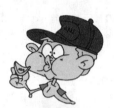

FEELINGS
Do you eat when you are bored, depressed, anxious, angry, or lonely?

ACTIVITY
Do you do other things while you are eating?

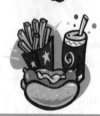

FOODS
What type of foods do you eat? Do you eat some foods because they are fast and convenient?

"Reviewing your food diaries will help you uncover important eating patterns and behaviors."

⇨ ***Activity***. What do you do while eating? Watching television is the main culprit, but reading a newspaper, listening to a radio, or browsing through magazines also can be a problem. Doing two things at once insures that neither gets full attention. Eating already gets less attention than it deserves. Later I will discuss how eating can be separated from other activities.

⇨ ***Foods***. What types of foods do you eat? Do you crave carbohydrates at certain times? Do you eat foods because they are available or do you seek out the foods you love? Are some foods very difficult to eat in moderation?

I have provided you with a worksheet titled "My Eating Patterns" on page 45. You may find this worksheet helpful in uncovering your unique eating patterns. After you have reviewed your Expanded Food Diaries for eating patterns, let's now focus on triggers that may cause you to begin eating.

High-Risk Situations— Triggers for Eating

What are your triggers for eating? Talking to your mother-in-law may do it, being bored at home, or having your spouse eat ice cream in front of you. It could be a trying day at work, a fight with someone, or fear about money matters. Most people have well-defined triggers. What are yours?

This is where the notion of ***high-risk situations*** becomes so important. Throughout this program, you will learn methods for avoiding or coping with situations that spell trouble. Identifying these situations, or triggers, is the first step. What you learn from the Food Diaries and from your own study of yourself will provide valuable information for later stages of the program. You can learn to predict the situations that increase your risk and plot your course accordingly.

Triggers are typically a mix of the factors included in your Expanded Food Diaries. Given the right time, feelings, and other circumstances, eating can be hard to resist. You may encounter positive pressure, like offers of food from friends, or negative pressure, like feeling upset. Once the trigger loosens your control, stopping can be difficult.

List your four main triggers in the "My Eating Triggers" worksheet on page 46. Remember these; I will make many suggestions later about how to counter your eating triggers.

Determining Your Target Calorie Level

TAPE 2
SECTION 5

In Lesson Two I discussed the calorie and asked you to think about what a reasonable calorie level is for you. We now come to the point in the program when it is time to identify your target calorie level. As you explore your body's calorie requirements, you will soon learn (if you do not know already) whether you are more like Sheri or Bonnie, the

My Eating Patterns Worksheet

week of: _____

Description	My Eating Patterns	Eating Patterns to Change
TIME		
FEELINGS		
ACTIVITY		
FOODS		
OTHER		

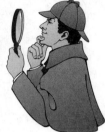

two people mentioned on page 37 in Lesson Two.

The guidelines are simple. You want to find the calorie level at which you can lose one to two pounds each week. Faster loss can be a clue that you are making drastic changes that can be difficult to maintain. You can probably make a good guess about what this level might be. Start there, and experiment to see whether you need to increase or decrease the calories. If you are uncertain, I have three suggestions.

First, if you ordered a copy of *The LEARN Healthy Eating and Calorie Guide*, you will notice that it includes several simple methods for estimating your body's daily calorie requirements. If you have access to the Internet,

you can log onto The LifeStyle Company's website at www. TheLifeStyleCompany.com and go to "Self- Assessments You Can Do." From there, go to the "Find Your Daily Calorie Needs." You will need to answer a few simple questions then the calculator will give you an estimate of your daily calorie needs to maintain your current weight.

Finally, if you are uncertain about the calorie level, consider using 1200 calories per day for women and 1500 for men. These are commonly used figures that represent calorie levels at which many people will lose weight. As you know, however, this is just an average, which means that some people will need fewer calories and some can afford more. In the space below,

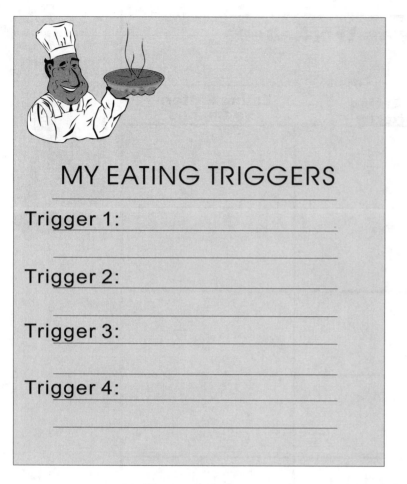

MY EATING TRIGGERS

Trigger 1: _____

_____

Trigger 2: _____

_____

Trigger 3: _____

_____

Trigger 4: _____

_____

write in the calorie level you will use as the first step in identifying your long-term target.

Over the next few lessons, you will have time to experiment with this beginning calorie level and to arrive at your target number. This number is important. I will ask you to enter your

Your Calorie Target

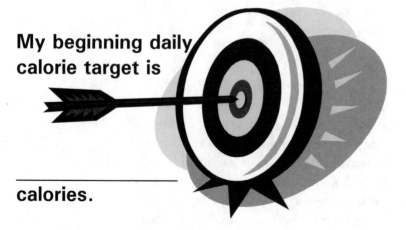

My beginning daily calorie target is

_____

calories.

daily calorie target onto your Monitoring Forms for each week in future lessons. You will note your daily calorie target number on each daily monitoring form. You will then have a record of whether you attained the goal each day of the program. The space for the precise calorie level in the Monitoring Form is left blank, so you can write in your personal number.

Dropping your calorie level below 1000 calories per day is not advisable. By eating fewer than 1000 calories, you may be losing weight at the expense of good nutrition. Diets of less than 1000 calories per day should be supervised by a physician.

Diets that fall below this level are labeled very-low-calorie diets (VLCD). Again, these are to be used only under medical supervision, preferably in a program where a registered dietitian is available to provide expert nutritional input. The body goes through complicated changes when it is on such diets. If a person is not screened and monitored adequately, a potential for danger exists if the food or supplement to be eaten does not contain the right mix of nutrients.

Counting Grams of Fat

As I discuss later in this program, there are many reasons why dietary fat is a central issue in a weight management program. For instance, fat has many calories. Also, research has related fat intake to risks of heart disease and some cancers. For these reasons, some nutrition experts recommend that individuals keep a record of their fat gram intake—in addition to or in lieu of counting calories.

Your primary dietary objective will help you decide whether to count calories or fat grams. If your objective to making dietary changes is to reduce the risk for chronic disease, counting fat grams would be sensible. If weight management is the issue, counting calories is the reasonable choice. A diet high in fat is typically high in calories, and vice-versa, but exceptions exist. For instance, you could drink 25

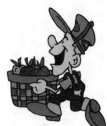

"Be careful. Low fat does not mean low calories."

cans of Coca Cola each day and take in little fat. Yet, you could still gain weight because of the high sugar (calorie) content.

Some individuals who use this program choose to record grams of fat and calories. Because fat intake is so important, I have provided the grams of fat as well as calorie values in many tables throughout this book and in *The LEARN Healthy Eating and Calorie Guide* (see page 303 for information). Feel free to record fat grams if you wish, but remember that keeping an accurate record of your calorie intake is essential.

Reduced-Fat Foods

The food companies have been working hard to develop products with less fat. The enormous popularity of reduced-sugar items such as diet soft drinks has led to a frantic search for ways to preserve the taste of foods while lowering the amount of nutrients that may contribute to health problems.

Today, we see more and more food items that have reduced fat, in some cases because they include fat substitutes. For the most part, I believe these are positive developments as they will allow people to enjoy some of the foods they like but with fewer calories and grams of fat. One risk lies in the way people interpret and then make use of terms like "low fat."

Low fat does not mean low calories. In fact, some low-fat cookies now on the market have nearly as many calories as the cookies they hope

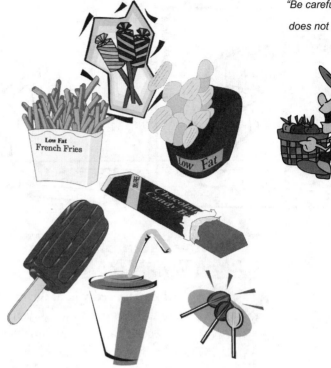

to replace. True, if one is destined to eat a certain number of cookies, then it would be better to have the reduced-fat versions. Still, we cannot assume this will cut calories. Some people feel that because a food seems healthy that they can eat more. So, if you encounter cookies, crackers, and other foods that are low in fat, be certain to check the calories. For some people, the marketing of these products has had a paradoxical effect—people feel they can eat more and thus **increase** their calorie intake.

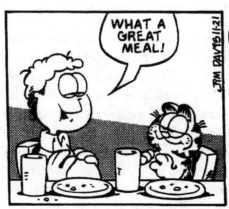

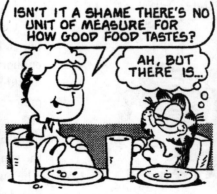

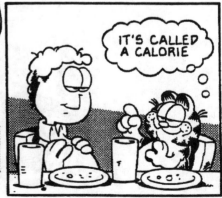

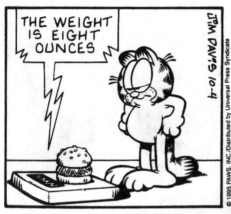

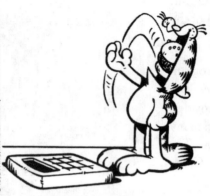

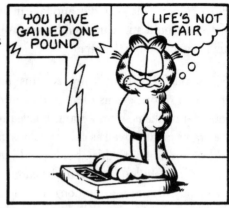

How Often Should You Weigh Yourself?

TAPE 2
SECTION 9

I encouraged you at the outset of the program to weigh yourself weekly and to record the results on your Weight Change Record (on page 25). Many people wonder how frequently they should weigh themselves. One popular self-help group, Overeaters Anonymous, does not have its members weigh themselves at all. The theory is that more frequent weighing gives "too much power to the scale." Other programs recommend that participants weigh regularly to get feedback on their progress. Some people weigh themselves many times each day. The average for people who enter weight loss programs is about once per day.

Feedback from the scale can be a kind incentive for some individuals. It reminds them of the progress they have made and spurs their efforts. Others despair when the scale shows no change, and they look with horror at how much weight they have to lose to reach their goal. Since the scale represents various things to different people, it can be either friend or foe. Please remember that it can be a *powerful* friend or foe, so think seriously about how often you and the scale should communicate.

This is where *your* judgment must prevail. Weigh yourself as often as you see fit. I recommend no less than once each week and no more than once each day. If you are a frequent weigher, you may get discouraged by weight gains beyond your control. Fluid shifts alone can lead to gains or losses of several pounds. However, if you feel the scale can be a motivating factor, try weighing more often.

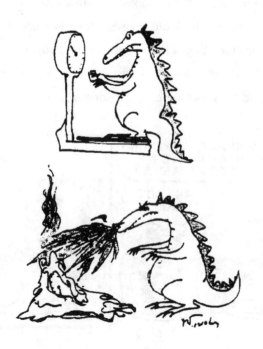

One problem with paying too much attention to the scale is that it can lead to undeserved euphoria or disappointment. An example would be a person who does not do well on his or her eating plan. The scale may show a weight loss anyway, perhaps due to water loss from a menstrual cycle. This person may think he or she can stray from the plan and still lose weight. The opposite side of the coin is the person who does well on the program and gains weight anyway. Again, this can happen for several reasons, including fluid shifts. The danger lies in the person assuming that his or her efforts are fruitless.

The scale should be a general guide about progress, not a day-to-day index of whether your program is working. This is why the Food Diaries (later called Monitoring Forms) at the end of each lesson ask you to record your calorie intake, your behavior changes, and your exercise. If these change, you *will* lose weight. Paying attention to *all* the lifestyle changes you are making will make you less vulnerable to the vagaries of the scale.

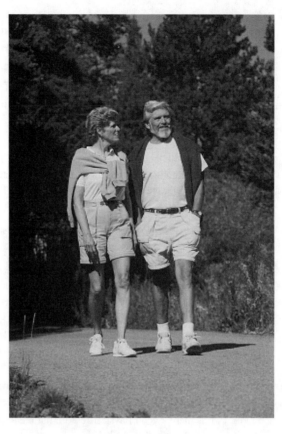

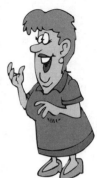

"Walking has many advantages and is a terrific way to begin to increase your activity level."

On the Move

TAPE 3
SECTION 3

Much has been said about the glories of exercise. Some joggers boast of a runner's high, and others feel that sweating and panting are the path to heaven. Some overweight people react to this hysteria by giving up on exercise. However, the LEARN concept of physical activity is not your usual exercise program. The object of the LEARN program is to make exercise fun and to increase the number of activities you consider to be *exercise*. The first example is walking. Other activities will follow later in the program.

Is Exercise Safe for You?

Today you can begin a walking program. If you are doing more vigorous activity, keep it up if you feel comfortable and have medical clearance. If you are not exercising regularly, the walking program may be for you. Walking has many virtues. It is healthy and helps you lose weight. Walking is easy and poses little physical risk (depending on where you walk!). But before you begin, we must ask if exercise is safe for you.

Moderate activity, including the walking discussed here, is safe for most people. Some people with physical problems, however, should not begin an exercise program without

being checked carefully by a physician. This should extend beyond a simple checkup. The physician should be alerted that the person is being checked to decide whether regular exercise is advisable.

The Physical Activity Readiness Questionnaire (PAR-Q) on page 50, provides a simple questionnaire you can complete to see if it is safe for you to increase your physical activity. Read and answer each question carefully. If any factor applies to you, see your physician before doing any exercise. This is serious and goes beyond the usual warning to *see your doctor* that is found in every diet book. If you are uncertain about what the terms mean or about whether you qualify, play it safe, and consult your physician. The list is adapted from the Canadian questionnaire by Dr. Steven Blair of The Cooper Institute for Aerobics Research.

The Physical Activity
Readiness Questionnaire (PAR-Q)

The PAR-Q is designed to help you help yourself. Many health benefits are associated with regular exercise, and the completion of the PAR-Q is a sensible first-step to take if you are planning to increase the amount of physical activity in your life.

For most people, physical activity should not pose any problem or hazard. The PAR-Q has been designed to identify the small number of adults for whom physical activity might be inappropriate or those who should have medical advice concerning the type of activity most suitable for them.

Common sense is your best guide in answering these few questions. Please read them carefully, and circle the YES or NO for each question as it applies to you.

1. Yes No Has your doctor ever said you have heart trouble?

2. Yes No Do you frequently have pains in your heart and chest?

3. Yes No Do you often feel faint or have spells of severe dizziness?

4. Yes No Has a doctor ever said your blood pressure was too high?

5. Yes No Has your doctor ever told you that you have a bone or joint problem, such as arthritis, that has been aggravated by exercise, or might be made worse with exercise?

6. Yes No Is there a good physical reason, not mentioned here, why you should not follow any activity program, even if you wanted to?

7. Yes No Are you over age 65 and not accustomed to vigorous exercise?

If you answered YES to one or more questions:

If you have not recently done so, consult with your personal physician by telephone or in person BEFORE increasing your physical activity and/or taking a fitness test. Tell him or her what questions you answered YES.

After a medical evaluation, seek advice from your physician as to your suitability for:

Unrestricted physical activity, probably on a gradually increasing basis, or

Restricted and supervised activity to meet your specific needs, at least on an initial basis. Check for special programs or services in your community.

If you answered NO to all questions:

If you answered the questions on the PAR-Q accurately, you have reasonable assurance to your present suitability for:

A graduated exercise program. A gradual increase in proper exercise promotes good fitness development while minimizing or eliminating discomfort.

An exercise test. Simple tests of fitness may be undertaken if you so desire.

Postpone exercise or exercise testing:

If you have a temporary minor illness, such as a common cold.

Adapted with permission from Blair SN. (1991). *Living With Exercise*. Dallas, TX: American Health Publishing Company.

Starting Your Walking Program

Walking has many advantages. Below are a few:

⇨ *It can be done by almost anyone*. Compared with many activities like swimming, basketball, or horseback riding, walking is an activity available to most people.

⇨ *It can be done at any pace*. You can walk fast or walk slow, and you can do it anywhere you choose—not just when the health club is open.

⇨ *It is easy*. You need not strain with exertion when you walk. Even low levels are helpful.

⇨ *It is enjoyable*. Think of all you can see while walking. You can enjoy the sights, listen to a portable tape player, or walk with friends.

⇨ *It is inexpensive*. You do not need a health club membership or expensive equipment.

⇨ *It can be a social event*. You may like company while you walk. It is a delightful time to be with someone you enjoy.

This may surprise you, but walking burns almost the same number of calories as running the same distance. How far you go is more important than how fast you go. It needn't knock you out for it to help.

Clothes, Shoes, and Weather

Before you begin, consider clothes, shoes, and weather. Wear clothes that make you feel comfortable. Expensive jogging suits have nothing special about them. Walking will help just as much if you are adorned with an old sweatshirt and jeans.

Shoes are important and may be worth the money for a good pair. Go to a sporting goods store and try on several brands. Pick one that feels good. Good shoes can help your feet, keep you from tiring, and reduce the chance of orthopedic injury.

Weather can be tricky. Avoiding exercise when it is too hot or too cold is wise. If the temperature is above 90 degrees or is below zero, getting your exercise inside is best. This still leaves most days of the year available. Most people manage to do their walking in nearly any weather.

Wear layers of clothing in cold weather. When it gets quite cold you might wear a cotton T-shirt, several sweatshirts, and a windbreaker. The cotton will absorb the perspiration. You may feel cold for the first few minutes, but you will warm up rapidly. If you get too hot, you can remove a layer. Wear a hat because much of the body's heat loss occurs through the head (especially if you are a hot head!). Mittens will keep hands warmer than gloves.

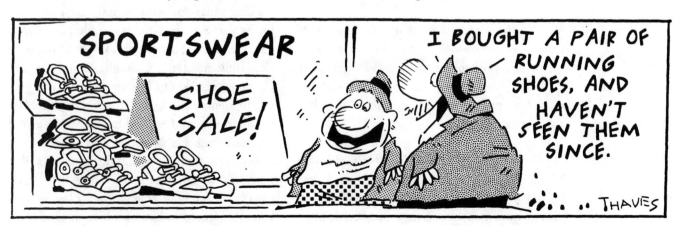

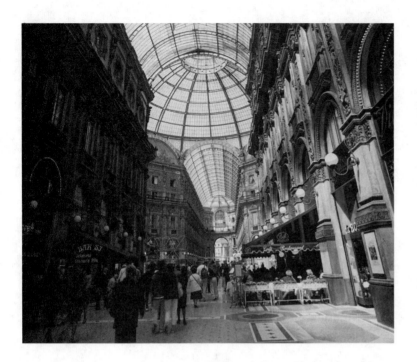

device takes the guess work out of physical activity. I'll talk more about walking in the next lesson.

Cravings vs. Hunger

Here is the place where your mind and body deceive each other, and where the "A" (Attitudes) part of The LEARN Program comes to the fore. When you eat, are you responding to physical hunger or to psychological cravings? Take the Cravings vs. Hunger Quiz on page 53 to find out which is the mind and which is the body.

Situations 1, 3, and 5 usually indicate psychological cravings. Situations 2 and 4 signal physical hunger. Situation 6 could be either. Distinguishing cravings from hunger is important. Once you can distinguish the cravings, we will work on special anti-craving techniques.

You can identify cravings by paying careful attention to when you want to eat. Does something stimulate the urge beside actual hunger? Does someone offer you food? Does something make you think about food? Do you have bad feelings that food would help satisfy? You can note these cravings on your Food Diary. This will remind you of the situations in which food will be hard to resist. Information on conquering the cravings is in the next lesson.

"Shopping malls are excellent places to walk."

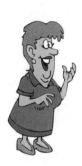

Being careful in hot weather is also important. Walking in the morning or evening may help avoid the hottest parts of the day. Wear as few clothes as possible, and never wear rubber suits or other clothes designed to make you sweat. You will regain whatever weight you lose in sweating. Also, trapping the body's heat in hot weather can be dangerous. Drink plenty of water. Drinking water before, during, and after exercise is safe.

Mall Walking

Shopping malls are a good place to walk in inclement weather or even when the weather is nice. In many parts of the country, *mall walkers* go to malls early in the morning and walk alone or in groups. This is a terrific idea.

The walkers who go with friends or who make new friends find the social contacts helpful in adhering to a regular schedule. Also, walking by the stores each morning leaves you poised for action the minute a new "SALE" sign is posted!

If you ordered The LEARN WalkMaster (discussed on page 20, in Lesson One), keeping track of your steps, distance, and calories burned from walking is a snap. This handy little

My Personal Goals for this Week

The main goal for this week is to begin your walking program. Walk as many days as possible by using the guidelines included in this lesson. Be sure to take it easy if you have not been exercising regularly. Continue to use the Expanded Food Diary this week. This will help you to identify eating patterns and triggers. Remember what you learned from reviewing your previous week's food diaries. See if you can develop even more insight into situations that place you at high risk for overeating. Finally, record your weight change on The Weight Change Record in Lesson One, on page 25.

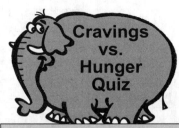

**Cravings
vs.
Hunger
Quiz**

*Answer each question below
by circling either T for true or F for false.*

T F 1. Even after a large meal, I still want dessert.

T F 2. I often have a gnawing feeling in my stomach.

T T 3. When someone mentions a food I love, I feel like eating.

T F 4. I feel light-headed after not eating for hours.

T F 5. When I drive by a fast-food restaurant, I want to eat.

T F 6. There is a time every day when I feel hungry.

My Self-Assessment

Lesson Three

T F 15. You can identify your triggers and high-risk situations for overeating by keeping a food diary and examining it carefully.

T F 16. You should weigh yourself every morning.

T F 17. Walking one mile burns almost as many calories as running the mile.

T F 18. Expensive exercise suits are worth the money because the special materials help the body.

T F 19. The amount of low-fat food you eat is not important.

T F 20. Walking is a good way to begin increasing your physical activity.

T F 21. Overweight people do not experience hunger, only psychological cravings for food.

(Answers in Appendix C, page 271)

Expanded Food Diary—Lesson Three

Today's Date:_____

DESCRIPTION	TIME	FEELINGS	ACTIVITY	CALORIES
BREAKFAST				
TOTAL CALORIES FOR THIS MEAL				
LUNCH				
TOTAL CALORIES FOR THIS MEAL				
DINNER				
TOTAL CALORIES FOR THIS MEAL				
SNACKS				
TOTAL CALORIES FOR SNACKS				
TOTAL CALORIES FOR THE DAY				

LESSON FOUR

In this lesson, I continue with the discussion of physical activity. I'll discuss the typical barriers to exercise and cover ways to make walking fun and enjoyable. I will also introduce you to a new approach to lifestyle change—the ABC's of behavior. This discussion is followed with techniques to conquer food cravings and to set realistic goals. The possibility of a walking partnership will be raised. Finally, I will introduce the Food Guide Pyramid and describe methods of following a balanced diet. You have many interesting topics to look forward to in this lesson. Let's begin this lesson with a brief discussion about barriers to exercise.

Barriers to Physical Activity

Many overweight people are reluctant to exercise because they are embarrassed. This occurs for several reasons. The extra weight can make exercise physically difficult. People who have been overweight all their lives may have unpleasant experiences with exercise. Most important, however, is the fear of what others will think when a heavy person jogs by or cruises past on a bike.

Put aside these feelings right now! You have nothing to be ashamed of. Your weight loss program is more important than being shy or embarrassed. Losing weight is a long process as it is and will be even longer if you wait to trim down before starting to exercise. Don't worry

about what others think. In fact, most normal-weight people give heavy people much credit for making positive changes.

The 15-Minute Prescription

After all the information discussed in the last lesson on walking, it is time to begin. Begin gradually and work your way up. Starting with less than you can tolerate is not dangerous, but starting with more can be painful and discouraging.

Begin walking for 15 minutes each day. If you have difficulty doing this all in one bout, try three 5-minute walks. When you can do this with ease, increase by 5 minutes each day to the point you feel some exertion. If the 15-minute

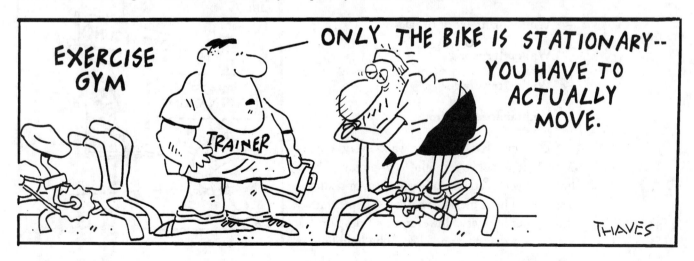

55

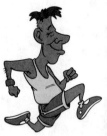

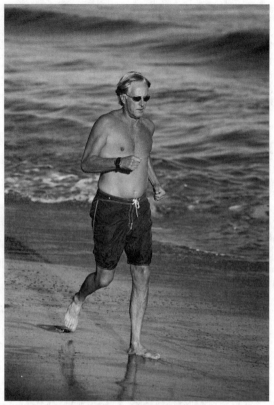

walk is too difficult, subtract time until you feel comfortable. *The goal is to walk 30 minutes to one hour each day.* Try to gradually increase your walking to this level, so as not to make it difficult or unpleasant.

You know best when your schedule can adapt to your walking. Below are six suggestions:

⇨ **Get up 30 minutes early to walk**

⇨ **Walk at lunch**

⇨ **Walk during work breaks**

⇨ **Walk after work**

⇨ **Walk after dinner**

⇨ **Walk before bedtime**

Do your level best to walk every day. Making it part of your routine is important, like brushing your teeth, making your bed, or taking a shower. This is the only way you will integrate it into your lifestyle. However, don't despair if you miss a day now and then. The long-term

picture is more important than if you occasionally miss a day. I will discuss your attitudes about exercise later in the program.

Experiment with walking different places, at different times, and with different people (or try it alone). Find the way you like it best. In Lesson Five, I will present specific ideas about making walking fun.

Getting Feedback and Staying Motivated to Be Active

You may remember that in Lesson One I mentioned The LEARN WalkMaster, a device that counts steps, the distance you move, and the calories you burn. This device has a simple but very important purpose—to keep you motivated and to give you positive feedback about increases in physical activity.

The LEARN WalkMaster, because it can detect small changes in your activity, provides a nice way to see if you're getting more activity. This handy device shows that even small changes do count. You can really help yourself by doing things that you may not have considered helpful before, like walking a little extra distance. Research shows how helpful this "lifestyle" approach to exercise can be, so I suggest you use a pedometer like the LEARN WalkMaster. You can order one by calling

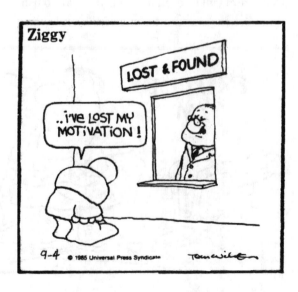

toll-free 1–888–LEARN–41 or by using the Internet (www.TheLifeStyleCompany.com).

You Can Win a Presidential Sports Award

A program of the President's Council on Physical Fitness and Sports, administered by the Amateur Athletic Union, now makes awards available to adults for participation in several activities. The award, called the *Presidential Sports Award*, can be earned by participation in one or more of 68 qualifying sports. Examples of these sports are backpacking, bicycling, bowling, fitness walking, golf, jogging, racquetball, rowing, running, sailing, swimming, tennis, and general types of exercise. Most of these activities can be done at a spa, aerobics class, a gym, or even at home. Chances are, whatever activities you like and can do are on the list.

These awards are for regular people doing regular exercise—you do not have to be an Olympic athlete. You simply write to the address below and receive a sheet called the Personal Fitness Log. The sheet explains which activities are included and what you must do to be granted the award. You fill out the sheet as you exercise and send in the completed signed fitness log along with $8 to receive the award. You will then receive a handsome Personalized Certificate of Achievement with your name and qualifying sport, suitable for framing. You also can receive an attractive lapel pin. You can win as many awards in as many sports as you would like. To receive the information on the award, just send a stamped, self-addressed envelope to:

Presidential Sports Award/AAU
c/o Walt Disney World Resort
P.O. Box 10,000
Lake Buena Vista, FL 32830–1000
Telephone (407) 934–7200
(www.aausports.org)

To show how these awards are truly achievable, we will list the criteria for earning awards

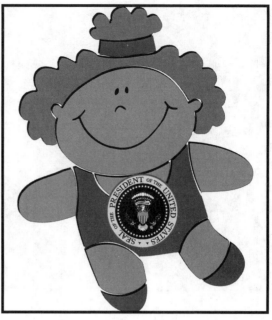

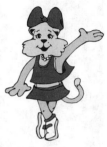

"Even you can win the Presidential Sports Award."

in the "Fitness Walking" and "Tennis" categories.

For fitness walking, a person must do the following within a four-month period:

❶ **Walk a minimum of 125 miles,**

Each walk must be continuous, without pauses for rest, and the pace must be at least four m.p.h. (15 minutes per mile), and

❷ **No more than two and one-half miles in any one day may be credited to the total.**

For tennis, one must:

❶ **Play tennis a minimum of 50 hours,**

❷ **No more than one and one-half hours in any one day may be credited to the total, and**

❸ **The total must include at least 25 sets of singles and/or doubles.**

These examples show that you can win the awards, even if you are struggling with your weight. Winning will require some effort, but then effort is just what we want, right? This program can be very motivating. You may or

"You can win the Presidential Sports Award for playing tennis."

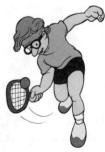

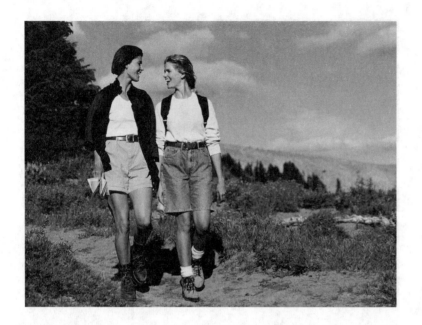

may not be up to the required amount of exercise now, but you probably will be before long. So, write now! You may win the award before you know it.

A Walking Partnership

This is a good time to introduce the "R" (Relationships) part of the LEARN approach. Since we are focusing on walking, we can discuss its social aspects. Some people like to walk with others, while some like to go solo. You are the best judge of what is right for you.

Walking with another person can be a powerful way to make it more enjoyable. The company is a nice distraction because you can talk about politics, speculate about the stock market, bet on ball games, or best of all, gossip! A part-

ner also can help by establishing a regular time for walking. You may be tempted to stay home on some days, but knowing that a partner is waiting may be just the stimulus you need to get out and get going.

Having a partner is not for everyone. Walking can be a delightful time to enjoy yourself, to reflect, and to think about important matters. Don't feel pressured to have a partner, because going it alone may be best for you. Think about the advantages of walking with a partner or walking alone. You might try it both ways to see which you like.

The ABC's of Behavior

As we progress through the program, you will learn ways to change your behavior. We will use the ABC approach. The letters stand for Antecedents, Behavior, and Consequences.

Antecedents

Antecedents are the events, feelings, and situations that occur *before* eating. These usually occur together in a series of steps called the Behavior Chain, which I will discuss in Lesson Thirteen.

Behavior

Behavior refers to eating itself and to the related events and feelings. The relevant factors are the speed of eating, rate of chewing, taste of food, and the events that take place *during* eating.

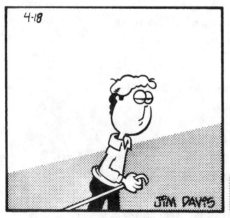
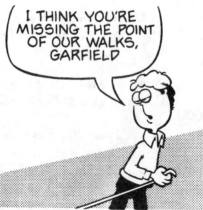
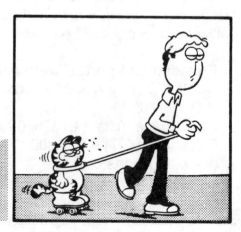

Consequences

Consequences are the events, feelings, and attitudes that follow eating. These factors happen *after* eating and can determine whether the eating will occur again.

You can see each aspect of the ABC approach in the case of Steve. He was home on the weekend watching a football game. The game excited Steve because he bet $20 with his neighbor. He went to the kitchen to get his favorite TV snack, cheese curls. Steve ate the cheese curls rapidly and did not taste each one. He ate until he was very full and then felt guilty about eating so much.

The antecedents were being at home, watching the football game, being excited, and having the cheese curls available. The behavior was eating rapidly until very full. Steve did not taste all the cheese curls. The consequences were an unpleasant, full feeling in his stomach and guilt about overeating.

This analysis gives us many ideas about reducing Steve's chances for overeating. Steve could alter the antecedents by doing something other than watching the game. This activity is a high-risk situation for Steve. He could also alter the antecedents by not having the cheese curls in the house. The behavior could be changed by eating slowly and savoring every bite. The consequences could change if he had different attitudes and could prevent the guilt and self-doubt that might stimulate more eating.

The ABCs of Behavior Change

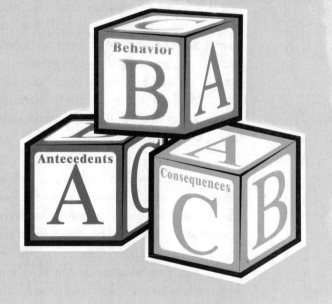

We will use the ABC approach in upcoming lessons. You can prepare yourself by thinking about the antecedents, behaviors, and consequences related to your eating. One way to do this is to review your Food Diaries from the past weeks and raise your level of analysis a notch or two. You have been thinking about events that trigger eating (the antecedents), but think of the eating itself and the consequences. If you think ahead to situations that may be risky for you, you can predict in advance what

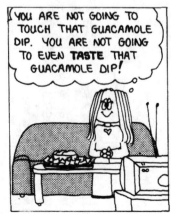
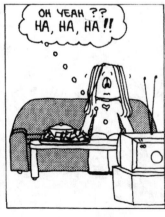
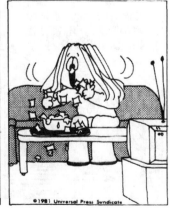
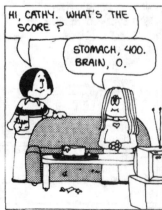

the A, B, and C parts are likely to be. This puts you in a good position to cope with even the greatest challenges.

Let's now look at the example of Sandy. Her greatest risk is after work when she is driving home. She is happy her day is over, and she is tired. Sandy is used to stopping at the convenience store or a fast-food place for something to help her unwind. When she gets home, she feels guilty and loses more of her control, and then bingo, she has a bad night. Because she has done this so often, the pattern may seem impossible to control.

What can Sandy do? She can look at the antecedents, the behavior, and consequences. Sandy can change this sequence of events in several ways. She could have something healthy to eat (like an apple) just before she leaves work. Sandy could take a few minutes to relax before leaving work. She could drive a different way home or react differently by not falling apart when she arrives home. These are only a *few* ways to use the ABC approach. See if you can apply it to events that happen in your life.

Shaping the Right Attitudes

In Lesson Three, we learned to separate food cravings from physical hunger. Once you can spot the cravings, there are two ways to deal with them: distraction and confrontation.

Conquering the Cravings

The *distraction* approach involves ignoring the cravings. When you know a craving is about to engulf you, do something else. Think about something wonderful, plan a dream vacation, or do anything to take your attention away from the urge to eat. The craving will usually pass.

The distraction method works best for people who have a good imagination or can change activities or thoughts at an instant's notice. You only have to do these things for a few moments, because cravings generally pass within minutes or even seconds. If you are bombarded by cravings throughout the day, confronting the cravings may be most effective.

The *confrontation* approach pits you against the craving. Let's say you want to raid the refrigerator for ice cream. You could pretend the urge is another person trying to convince you to eat the ice cream. Argue with this person and say why you will not give in to the urge. Another approach is to visualize the ice cream container beckoning to you and tempting you with promises of fulfillment. Imagine how silly it is to let the ice cream get the best of you.

A typical confrontation scene might be as follows. You get the urge to stop for a snack while driving home from work. You recognize

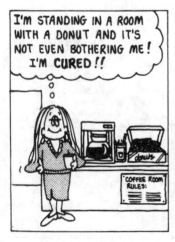

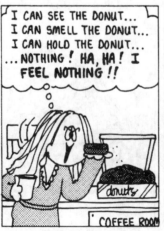

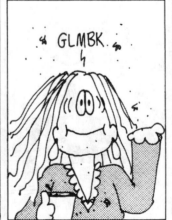

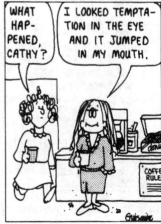

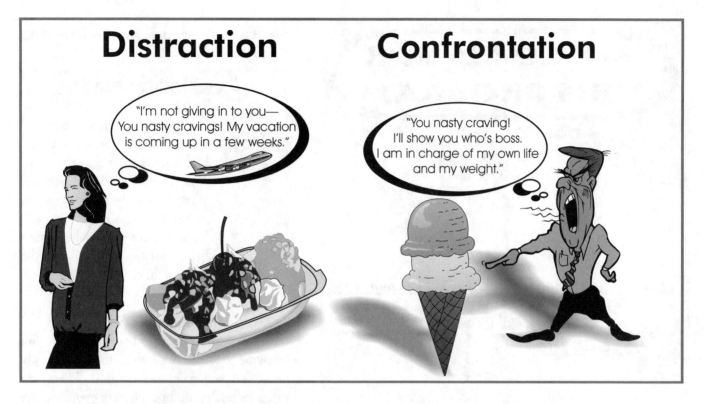

the craving and decide to get the best of it. You say, "You nasty craving! You want me to stop for peanut butter cups when I'm not really hungry. I'll show you who's boss. I am in charge of my own life and my weight."

Think of these two approaches now and decide which will work for you. If you are in doubt, experiment with both. Try to arrive at a strategy as soon as possible, be it distraction or confrontation. This will prepare you in advance for the inevitable cravings you will face. Do your best not to give in.

Goal Setting

TAPE 2
SECTION 4

I have talked about setting reasonable goals in earlier lessons and will bring up this topic often in the lessons that follow. One common attitude problem is having unrealistic goals. Some individuals do not recognize they are setting unattainable goals, but they do so nonetheless. Examples of this are starting a program in May for swimsuit season when you have 50 pounds to lose. Having fantasies of being thin and having life improve immediately is another example. These things may happen, but not right away.

Think about your goals for the program. Think of specific answers to these four questions:

⇨ **How much weight do you expect to lose each week?**

⇨ **How soon do you expect to be thin?**

⇨ **Will your life be different when you lose weight?**

⇨ **Do you expect losing weight to be easy and quick?**

These are just examples of some tricky areas. You are a sensible person and can formulate reasonable goals. Do you think your hidden or unconscious goals are unrealistic? If so, remind yourself time and time again that setting unrealistic goals is a setup for trouble.

In the space on page 62, list your four major goals for this program and decide whether they are realistic. The goals may be specific weight loss accomplishments (to lose one pound each week, or to lose 25 pounds total) or other changes (clothes will fit better, look better for daughter's wedding).

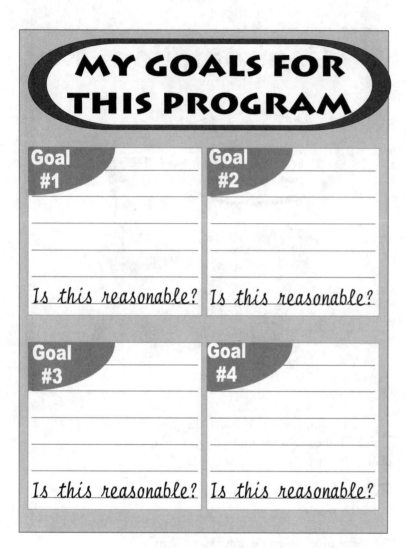

MY GOALS FOR THIS PROGRAM

Goal #1

Is this reasonable?

Goal #2

Is this reasonable?

Goal #3

Is this reasonable?

Goal #4

Is this reasonable?

The Principle of Shaping

Shaping refers to making gradual, step-by-step changes in your behavior. Two examples can highlight how this works. If your weakness is donuts and you begin every day with three of your favorite kind, dropping them completely may be difficult. You could start by cutting down to two donuts, then one, and finally to none. The approach to exercise is another example of shaping. You began with comfortable levels of walking with the goal of increasing in a gradual way to a final level.

You can see how the shaping principle applies to goal setting. Setting realistic goals means starting from a point you can master and then working up gradually to the level you de-

sire. This will come through many times in the lessons that follow.

The Mighty Calorie

In Lesson Three, I explained what a calorie is. We eat at least a half-million calories each year. You might wonder, therefore, what difference a few calories can make. They can make a big difference. Even the smallest number of calories add up over the course of a week, month, or year.

As I mentioned earlier, 3500 calories will translate into a pound of body weight. If you consume 7000 calories more than your body uses, you will gain two pounds. These are rough estimates, and people vary greatly in the precise number of calories needed to gain or lose weight. What is clear is that calories do count. Let's examine the effects of adding an innocent 10 calories per day to your total.

If you add 10 calories per day to what you ordinarily eat, you will gain an extra pound in a year. Added over a decade or two, this is 10–20 pounds; and all from 10 crummy calories per day! If the difference each day were 100 calories, this would be 10 pounds per year and 100 pounds for 10 years! Let's look at the 10-calorie difference for the moment. The chart on page 63 shows you how little you have to eat to get 10 extra calories.

Think how easy it is to have an extra teaspoon of ketchup, one bite of an orange, or less than 1 oz of Pepsi. This shows the need for careful calculation of calories on your Monitoring Form and a vigilant attitude about foods. You also can take a positive outlook on this calorie equation. Cutting out 10 calories each day will save you a pound each year. You certainly won't miss the 10 calories, but you can easily do without the pound.

Following a Balanced Diet

TAPE 1
SECTION 10

Recording what you eat and the times, places, and activities associated with eating will make you more conscious of your food choices. Some people can use this information to craft a healthy meal plan, but many like to learn more about the components of a nutritious, well-balanced diet.

There is no end to advice on nutrition. When I visit bookstores or listen to the radio, I am amazed at the half-baked schemes concocted by "experts." One day it is apricot pits for cancer or papaya juice for arthritis. The next day it is mega doses of vitamins for stress and prune pulp for bad breath.

It is inviting to believe some of these nutty plans because they provide hope for difficult problems. But think back over the years. There was the Scarsdale Diet, The Rotation Diet, The Beverly Hills Diet, The Carbohydrate Addicts Diet, The Zone Diet, among many, many others. Each promised breakthroughs, grand solutions, and results that seemed guaranteed. Do you know anyone who lost weight and kept it off on one of those programs? Where are the programs now? How much would you bet that the miracle book that comes along next week, next month, or next year will be different than the rest—that it will deliver on what it promises and offer a final solution?

When it comes to nutrition, there is no magic, just common sense and rational eating. The key word to remember is balance. This means eating a variety of foods from the different food groups. This may sound like what you learned in the sixth grade, but the message is just as important today.

The body needs a balance of nutrients. It does not function well with too little or too much of any nutrient. If your body needs a certain amount of vitamin E each day, you will be worse off with one-half that amount or with 100 times more. This is similar to making your fa-

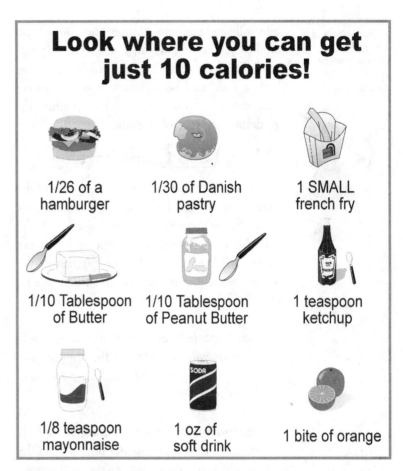

Look where you can get just 10 calories!

1/26 of a hamburger	1/30 of Danish pastry	1 SMALL french fry
1/10 Tablespoon of Butter	1/10 Tablespoon of Peanut Butter	1 teaspoon ketchup
1/8 teaspoon mayonnaise	1 oz of soft drink	1 bite of orange

vorite cake. Each ingredient is important. One ingredient may give the cake a very good taste, but too much will ruin it.

Some clients in my clinic ask why nutrition is so important. The answer is simple. What you eat helps determine how healthy you are, which in turn influences how you cope with life both physically and psychologically. You could lose weight by eating nothing but grapefruit, but your body would suffer greatly from deficiencies in the nutrients grapefruit does not provide. How much you eat (calories) is only part of the answer. How well you eat must also be considered.

You will notice that I say not a word about forbidden foods. I do not believe in prohibition for people losing weight. Such an approach is doomed to fail. If you like cheesecake, but feel it is illegal, you will eventually eat it and feel guilty. This will weaken your restraint even more. If you have the expectation that the first

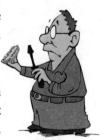

"Ten little innocent calories can add up to many unwanted pounds over the year."

63

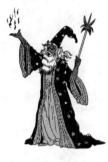

bite will send you into a frenzy and you will eat all the cheesecake in sight, you are setting yourself up to fall apart when you might otherwise have a little and be satisfied. It is fine to eat cheesecake, as long as it occurs within the guidelines for sensible nutrition.

The Food Guide Pyramid

The pyramid is a graphic illustration of the research-based food plan developed jointly by the U.S. Department of Agriculture (USDA) and the Department of Health and Human Services (HHS). The following represent the dietary guidelines developed for Americans by the USDA and the HHS:

⇨ **Eat a variety of foods**. Eating a variety of foods will help you get the energy, protein, vitamins, minerals, and fiber you need for good health.

⇨ **Maintain a healthy weight**. Many studies show that maintaining a healthy weight can reduce your chances of having high blood pressure, heart disease, certain cancers, a stroke, and the most common kind of diabetes.

⇨ **Choose a diet low in fat, saturated fat, and cholesterol**. Diets that are low in fat, saturated fat, and cholesterol may reduce your risk of heart attack and certain types of cancer. Fat contains more than twice the calories of an equal amount of carbohydrates or protein, so a diet low in fat can help you maintain a healthy weight.

⇨ **Choose a diet with plenty of vegetables, fruits, and grain products**. These foods provide the essential vitamins, minerals, fiber, and complex carbohydrates. Since these foods are naturally low in dietary fat, they can help lower your intake of fat.

⇨ **Use sugars only in moderation**. A diet that includes high amounts of sugar has too many calories and may not provide the nutrients your body needs to be healthy. Too much sugar also can contribute to tooth decay.

⇨ **Use salt in moderation**. A diet that is low in sodium can help reduce your risk of high blood pressure.

⇨ **If you drink alcoholic beverages, do so in moderation**. Alcoholic beverages add calories, but provide little nutrition. Alcohol also can contribute to many other health problems and may lead to addiction.

You can see from these dietary guidelines that the key message is moderation. As we progress through the program these guidelines will become more and more familiar to you. Review each of the guidelines again and check to see how many you are now following. At this point in the program I want you to be familiar

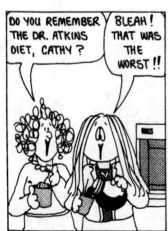
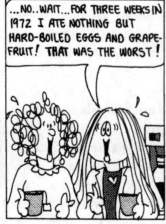
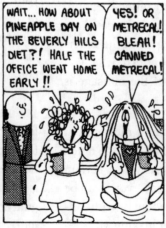
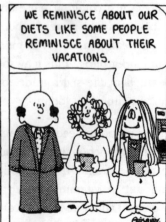

The Food Guide Pyramid

Fats, Oils, & Sweets
Use Sparingly

Key
○ Fat (naturally occurring and added)
▼ Sugars (added)
These symbols show fat and added sugars in foods.

Milk, Yogurt, & Cheese Group
2 - 3 Servings

Meat, Poultry, Fish, Dry Beans, Eggs, & Nuts Group
2 - 3 Servings

Vegetable Group
3 - 5 Servings

Fruit Group
2 - 4 Servings

Bread, Cereal, Rice, & Pasta Group
6 - 11 Servings

with the guidelines so that you can be thinking of how they apply to you and your eating habits.

A Graphic Illustration

The design of the Food Guide Pyramid divides foods into five separate groups as shown on this page. The pyramid also includes a category for fats, oils, and sweets. Each group in the pyramid includes suggested daily servings that are listed beside the groups. Small circles are used throughout the pyramid to identify food groups that contain high-fat foods, and triangles are used to identify foods that have added sugars.

At the top of the pyramid is the section containing foods that should be eaten sparingly. It should not be surprising that this smallest section consists of fats, oils, and sweets. As the food groups progress toward the bottom of the pyramid they become a larger part of your diet. For instance, the bread and cereal group is the largest section. Foods from this group should make up the largest portion of your daily diet.

Many things we eat are a mixture of foods from the five groups. Pizza, for example, has bread (dough), vegetables (tomatoes, peppers, etc.), cheese, and meat in some cases. A chicken pot pie has pastry, vegetables, meat, etc. You will become an expert at identifying the components of combination dishes.

In this lesson, I want you to become familiar with the five food groups in the pyramid. This graphic will become more familiar to you as you continue through the program. In the lessons that follow, I will describe each tier of the pyramid in more detail. At this point in the program do not be concerned with the number of servings you should be eating from the various food groups or how much food it takes to make one serving. I will discuss this and other information about each of the five food groups in later lessons. For now, be aware of the five different

65

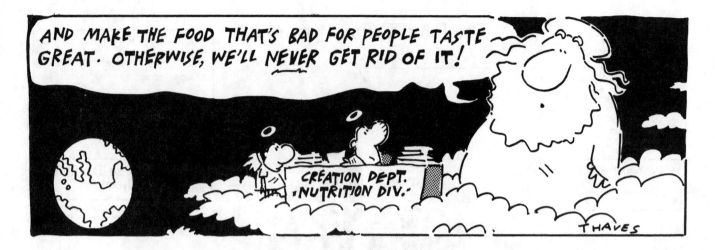

AND MAKE THE FOOD THAT'S BAD FOR PEOPLE TASTE GREAT. OTHERWISE, WE'LL NEVER GET RID OF IT!

CREATION DEPT. ·NUTRITION DIV.·

THAVES

food groups and try to include each group in your diet. In your Food Diary this week, note whether you are eating foods from all five food groups.

The Food Guide Pyramid is a useful way to see that you get balanced nutrition, but it is possible to follow the guide and still take in too many calories to lose weight. Eating the recommended number of servings will generally help the average person maintain his or her weight, but since you want to reduce, the number of servings will have to be reduced. As you find the level of calories you need to lose weight, you will be able to adjust the number of servings from the pyramid.

In thinking about good nutrition while losing weight, both the Food Guide Pyramid and a means of counting calories are important. Within the number of calories you budget for yourself each day, try to choose the right balance of servings across the food groups in the pyramid.

Selecting an Eating Plan: Calorie Counting vs. Exchange Plan

Several food plans are available for eating nutritiously. One prevailing plan is to count calories while eating a specified number of servings in the five food groups in the Food Guide Pyramid. I'll discuss the Food Guide Pyramid in detail in Lesson Five. This approach is one

many individuals are familiar with because counting calories is the way most people learn to judge how they are doing with a weight loss plan. This is the approach used in this program. I introduce it in this lesson and then expand on it in the lessons that follow.

An excellent alternative eating plan is the Exchange Plan developed by the American Dietetic Association (ADA) and the American Diabetes Association. The exchange plan places foods into six categories: starch/bread, meat and meat substitutes, vegetables, fruit, milk, and fat. Within each category, amounts of foods are provided so that in the amount listed, all foods have approximately the same carbohydrate, protein, fat, and calories. A food in a given category, therefore, can be exchanged with any other food in the same category. Copies of the exchange list guide are available for $1.75 each plus $5.00 shipping and handling. If you would like to receive a complete guide for the exchange plan, you can call 1–800–877–1600 or write to:

The American Dietetic Association
P.O. Box 97215
Chicago, IL 60678-7215

Both the calorie counting and exchange plans represent sound nutrition. If you are in a program run by a health professional, he or she may have a preference, so I provide both plans here. Otherwise, choose the plan you feel best meets your need, and then follow it throughout the program. If you choose the exchange plan over the calorie counting approach, you can obtain a copy from the American Dietetic Association as outlined above. You can experiment with the number of servings required for you to lose weight. In the next lesson I will discuss the number of calories you might try to eat each day.

Introducing a New Monitoring Form

This lesson ushers in a new Monitoring Form. An example of a completed form appears at the end of this lesson. The new form has three sections. The section on the top is to record food intake, time, and calories, just as you have done with the Food Diary. There are no longer separate sections for breakfast, lunch, dinner, and snacks. List foods in the order you eat them. This will be a part of the Monitoring Form for the remainder of the program—that's how important it is.

The middle portion of the new form is for recording the behavior changes that have been prescribed for each lesson. For this week, the prescribed activities are:

❶ Increase walking

❷ Note the ABCs of eating

❸ Conquer your food cravings

❹ Set realistic goals

❺ Eat servings from the five food groups

❻ Eat less than _____ calories

You simply mark down whether you follow the recommended behavior most of the time, sometimes, or rarely. Different behaviors will be listed for each lesson.

Some of the techniques you will be trying will be listed under the Most of the Time, Sometimes, or Rarely part of the Monitoring Form, even though the behaviors do not fit neatly in these categories. For example, in Lesson Seven you will be encouraged to shop from a list to avoid impulse buying. However, most people do not shop for food each day, so it is difficult to note each day on the Monitoring Form whether you shopped as you planned. In cases like this, put NA (for not applicable) if Most of the Time, Sometimes, or Rarely do not apply.

The third section, on the bottom, is for you to keep a record of your physical activity and the number of servings you eat from the five food groups of the Food Guide Pyramid. In the lessons that follow, I will discuss the five food groups of the Food Guide Pyramid in more detail. There are also spaces for the type of exercise you do and the number of minutes you do it. This section will also be part of the form from now on. List everything here, like using stairs more than usual, working in the yard, walking, and playing sports.

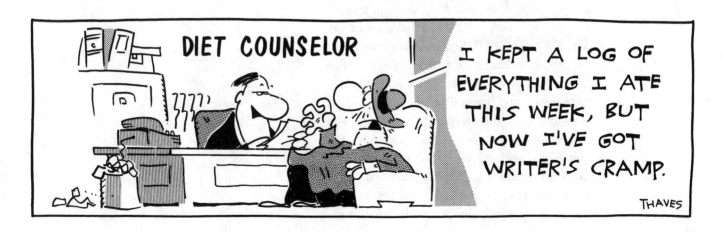

DIET COUNSELOR

I KEPT A LOG OF EVERYTHING I ATE THIS WEEK, BUT NOW I'VE GOT WRITER'S CRAMP.

THAVES

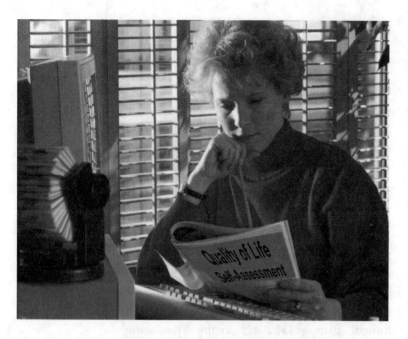

Do not get discouraged with negative (-) numbers in categories that I have not discussed. Simply note these areas for upcoming lessons.

I suspect that your satisfaction has increased in at least one area, if not several. Many people report increased satisfaction the first month with their mood, energy level, general appearance, eating habits, and physical mobility and activity. What is remarkable is that these changes occur relatively quickly and with only a modest weight loss. That is an excellent return on your weight management investment!

Satisfaction may come more slowly in other areas, such as with your social life or leisure and recreational activities. If you have specific desires in these areas, such as wanting to meet new people or taking up tennis or golf, make a plan for how you can start achieving these goals. Do not make the mistake of thinking you have to be at some magical goal weight in order to socialize more or take up a new hobby.

Quality of Life

"One way to assess the changes you are making in your program is to complete and compare your Quality of Life Self-Assessments."

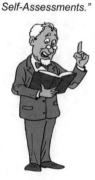

One way of assessing the changes you have made in the first month is to complete the Quality of Life Self-Assessment on page 69. Rate how satisfied you are with each of the 12 areas listed, including your mood, eating habits, and body image. Complete these items based on how you feel today.

Now compare your responses to those before you began the program. Use the form on page 70 to help you make this comparison. In column (b) of the Review of Quality of Life Self-Assessments on page 70, record your ratings from the *Introduction and Orientation* on page 9. In column (c), record your ratings from the Quality of Life Self-Assessment on page 69 in this lesson. Column (d) reflects the positive (+) or negative (-) change in your responses. The positive (+) numbers reflect increased satisfaction with life in the related category. The negative (-) numbers represent decreased satisfaction with life. If you have negative (-) numbers in any of the categories that have been covered in the first four lessons, now is a good time to go back and review this material. Positive (+) numbers in the categories that have been covered in the first four lessons means that you have done well and are ready to move on.

Quality of Life Self-Assessment

Please use the following scale to rate how satisfied you feel now about different aspects of your daily life. Choose any number from this list (1 to 9) and indicate your choice on the questions below.

1 = Extremely Dissatisfied   6 = Somewhat Satisfied

2 = Very Dissatisfied   7 = Moderately Satisfied

3 = Moderately Dissatisfied   8 = Very Satisfied

4 = Somewhat Dissatisfied   9 = Extremely Satisfied

5 = Neutral

1. _____ Mood (feelings of sadness, worry, happiness, etc.)

2. _____ Self-esteem

3. _____ Confidence, self-assurance, and comfort in social situations

4. _____ Energy and feeling healthy

5. _____ Health problems (diabetes, high blood pressure, etc.)

6. _____ General appearance

7. _____ Social life

8. _____ Leisure and recreational activities

9. _____ Physical mobility and physical activity

10. _____ Eating habits

11. _____ Body image

12. _____ Overall quality of life

My Personal Goals for This Week

The main goal for this week is to begin your walking program. Walk as many days as possible by using the guidelines provided in this lesson. Be sure to take it easy if you have not been exercising regularly. Begin using the new monitoring form. It will help you identify patterns and triggers. Remember what you learned the previous week and see if you can develop even more insight into situations which place you at high risk for overeating. Finally, record your weight change on the Weight Change Record in Lesson One on page 25 of this manual.

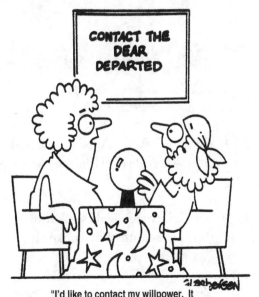

CONTACT THE DEAR DEPARTED

"I'd like to contact my willpower. It died last night at Angelo's Pizza Palace!"

Review of Quality of Life Self-Assessments

	(a)	(b)	(c)	(d)
	Category	Score from Introduction and Orientation Lesson	Score from this Lesson	Change in Scores (column c minus column b)
1.	Mood (feelings of sadness, worry, happiness, etc.)			
2.	Self-esteem			
3.	Confidence, self-assurance, and comfort in social situations			
4.	Energy and feeling healthy			
5.	Health problems (diabetes, high blood pressure, etc.)			
6.	General appearance			
7.	Social life			
8.	Leisure and recreational activities			
9.	Physical mobility and physical activity			
10.	Eating habits			
11.	Body image			
12.	Overall quality of life			

My Self-Assessment

Lesson Four

T F 22. The ABC Approach stands for Alternatives, Behavior, and Consciousness.

T F 23. Everyone should walk with a partner because the company increases pleasure.

T F 24. Shaping refers to encouraging others to help you lose weight.

T F 25. If you eat an equal number of servings from the five food groups of the Food Guide Pyramid, you will have a balanced diet.

T F 26. Eating an extra 10 calories per day will add one pound of weight over a year.

T F 27. Many overweight people are reluctant to exercise because they are embarrassed.

T F 28. A pedometer like the LEARN WalkMaster can be motivational by showing you the small changes in your level of physical activity.

T F 29. Ice cream and several other high-sugar desserts are not allowed in this program.

T F 30. To conquer food cravings, distraction will be helpful for some people and confrontation will be helpful for others.

T F 31. It is helpful to set specific, concrete, and attainable goals at each step of the program.

(Answers in Appendix C, page 271)

Monitoring Form—Lesson Four

Today's Date: _____

TIME	FOOD AND AMOUNT	CALORIES
7:15 am	Apple juice, ½ cup (4 oz)	58
	Special K cereal, 1⅓ cups (1 oz)	111
	Skim milk, 4 oz	43
12:30 pm	Club sandwich	590
	Orange, 1 medium	65
	Coffee, black (4 oz)	0
6:30 pm	Broiled chicken breast, w/o skin (3 oz)	148
	Broccoli, steamed (1 cup)	46
	Butter, 1 t	36
	French bread, 1 slice	81
	Ice tea	0
9:10 pm	Celery, 3 stalks	18
	Skim milk, 8 oz	86
	TOTAL DAILY CALORIES	1,282

PERSONAL GOALS FOR THIS WEEK	MOST OF THE TIME	SOME- TIMES	RARELY
1. INCREASE WALKING		✔	
2. NOTE THE ABCs OF EATING	✔		
3. CONQUER MY FOOD CRAVINGS		✔	
4. SET REALISTIC GOALS		✔	
5. EAT SERVINGS FROM THE FIVE FOOD GROUPS	✔		
6. EAT LESS THAN 1500 CALORIES PER DAY	✔		

FOOD GROUPS FOR TODAY	PHYSICAL ACTIVITY	MINUTES OR STEPS
MILK, YOGURT, AND CHEESE ☑ ☑ ☐	(M) WALKING	2,650 steps
MEAT, POULTRY, ETC. ☑ ☑ ☐	(Tu) WALKING	1,900 steps
FRUITS ☑ ☑ ☐ ☐	(W) LIFECYCLE, WALKING	15 mins 2,435 steps
VEGETABLES ☑ ☑ ☑ ☐ ☐	(TH) WALKING	2,344 steps
BREADS, CEREALS, ETC. ☑ ☑ ☑ ☑ ☐ ☐ ☐ ☐	(F) WALKING	4,120 steps
SERVINGS OF WATER (8 OZ) ☑ ☑ ☑ ☑ ☑ ☑ ☑ ☐	(SA) WALKING, HOUSE WK	5,340 steps
	(SU) YARD WORK	3,500 steps

Monitoring Form—Lesson Four
*Today's Date:*_____

TIME	FOOD AND AMOUNT	CALORIES
TOTAL DAILY CALORIES		

PERSONAL GOALS FOR THIS WEEK	MOST OF THE TIME	SOME-TIMES	RARELY
1. INCREASE WALKING			
2. NOTE THE ABCs OF EATING			
3. CONQUER MY FOOD CRAVINGS			
4. SET REALISTIC GOALS			
5. EAT SERVINGS FROM THE FIVE FOOD GROUPS			
6. EAT LESS THAN _____ CALORIES PER DAY			

FOOD GROUPS FOR TODAY		PHYSICAL ACTIVITY	MINUTES OR STEPS
MILK, YOGURT, AND CHEESE	☐ ☐ ☐	(M)	
MEAT, POULTRY, ETC.	☐ ☐ ☐	(Tu)	
FRUITS	☐ ☐ ☐ ☐	(W)	
VEGETABLES	☐ ☐ ☐ ☐ ☐	(Th)	
BREADS, CEREALS, ETC.	☐ ☐ ☐ ☐ ☐ ☐ ☐ ☐	(F)	
SERVINGS OF WATER (8 OZ)	☐ ☐ ☐ ☐ ☐ ☐ ☐ ☐	(Sa)	
		(Su)	

LESSON FIVE

This lesson begins with a brief discussion on the importance of making small changes in your diet followed by additional information on your quality of life. We then move to a discussion of situations that control eating. After this, I'll talk about how you can perfect your walking program. The notion here is to increase your daily physical activity. I will bring up the idea of working with a partner in your weight management program. Finally, I will discuss what makes up a serving from each of the five food groups of the Food Guide Pyramid.

Small Changes in Your Diet

You may be feeling a bit overwhelmed by all the information you read last week about different methods of following a balanced diet. You learned about the Food Guide Pyramid and the number of servings that you should eat from each of the food groups. Don't be alarmed if your present meal plan would not win an award (or even honorable mention) from the nutrition experts.

Changing your eating habits takes time. For example, if you eat no fruit most days, start by adding just one serving a day, and make it an easy one. You can probably add a small banana to your morning cereal, take an apple with you to work, or have 4 oz of orange juice for an afternoon snack. Each week, try to make one small change you can live with. These small changes will yield big results over the long term.

More on Quality of Life

TAPE 1
SECTION 12

You may have noticed changes in your health in the past month. You may feel more alert and energetic or may be sleeping better. People frequently report such changes with only small weight losses. If you will be seeing your doctor, ask about any changes she or he notices.

Your Health

Your doctor can also assess many changes in your physical health. For example, if your blood pressure, cholesterol, or blood sugar were high before you started this program, they may be slightly lower by now. These reductions are

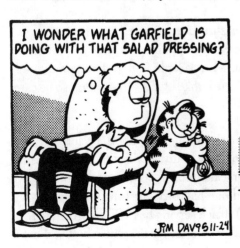

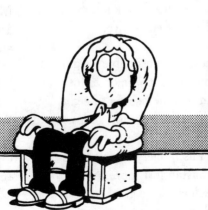

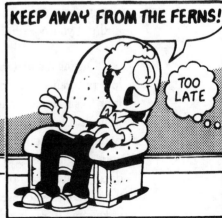

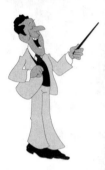
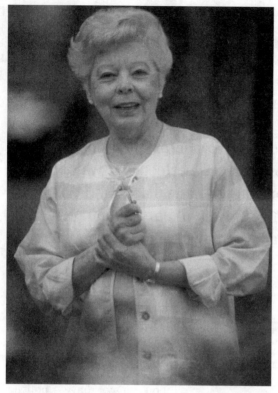

a result of your weight loss and your improved eating and activity habits. Your overall health should continue to improve over the next few months as you progress through the program. What a wonderful accomplishment—to improve your health and well being!

Weight Loss

Improvements in quality of life and physical health are the real measures of success in a program like this, but it's hard not to focus on weight loss. We all like to get things done fast, and people like losing weight fast. If you're losing as you wish, fine. But often people lose slowly and get discouraged. Let's talk numbers and put your weight loss in perspective.

During the first month in reasonable weight loss programs, it is common for women to lose four to six pounds and men to lose six to eight pounds. Don't worry if you've lost more or less; people vary just like cars differ in gas mileage. If your weight loss is in this range, you might be disappointed for not having lost more. Sometimes people who lose slowly have great success at keeping it off. In addition, weight loss of this

magnitude is typical and is cause for celebration, not disappointment. It is important to feel positive about what you have accomplished. This provides motivation and energy to forge ahead.

You may have had the opposite experience the first month and lost far more weight than you had expected. Women who have lost more than 8 pounds and men more than 12 pounds should talk to their doctors. Women should make sure that they eat at least 1200 calories a day and men 1500 calories. Increasing your calorie intake above these levels may be necessary if your weight loss does not slow in the next few weeks. Rapid weight loss can increase the risk of developing gallstones and other health complications.

Calorie Intake

A smaller-than-anticipated weight loss can also result from not decreasing your calorie intake sufficiently. As I discussed in Lesson Two, if you eat 500 fewer calories a day than your body burns, you will lose a pound a week. If, instead, you eat only 250 fewer calories a day, you will lose only about a half-pound a week.

If you lost less than four pounds the first month, plan to pay extra attention to your Food Diary this week. Try to incorporate these tips:

⇨ Record your foods and beverages immediately after consuming them. This will ensure that you remember everything.

⇨ Measure portion sizes to ensure that you are eating the amounts that you think you are. Most people underestimate their daily calorie intake by 20–40 percent, so be careful.

⇨ When reading food labels, be sure to determine how many servings the item contains. For example, a 20-oz soda contains two and one-half servings (one serving equals 8 oz). Each serving has 100 calories or a total of 250 calories for the whole bottle. That is a big difference from thinking that the bottle contains one serving and only 100 calories.

⇨ Keep a running total of your calories throughout the day. That way, you will know if you have enough calories for a second serving at dinner or for a bedtime snack.

Set a calorie goal for the week, not just each day. That way, if you exceed your goal on Thursday, you can eat a bit less on Friday, Saturday, and Sunday—and still make your goal for the week. The closer you come to your calorie goal each week, the better your weight loss will be.

Taking Control of Your Eating

The Food Diaries have helped you discover patterns in your eating, and this section will give you some concrete advice on how to disrupt those patterns. These are classic strategies that have been used successfully by countless people. Let's see if they might work for you.

Many people have situations, times, or activities that stimulate eating. These events become paired with eating so that the event can make you feel hungry. Here are a few examples. You may read the paper every day at breakfast. You may watch television every evening and have a snack. You may always eat when you sit in a certain chair. If eating is paired repeatedly with these events, the events can make you feel like eating. If you sit in your chair, watch TV, or read the morning paper, you will feel like eating, irrespective of physical hunger.

It is important to separate eating from other activities. This will remove the ability of these activities to stimulate eating, freeing you to respond to actual hunger. There are several ways to make this happen. I will present four such techniques below.

Do Nothing Else While Eating

This means reading the paper at another time, eating before or after you watch TV, waiting to read the book, etc. Eating should be a pure experience. Don't contaminate it with extraneous activities. If this seems awkward, it is a sure sign that you are hooked on the association of eating with other activities. The more this technique bothers you, the more you need it.

You may be one of those individuals who does other things while eating. It could be working on a hobby, talking on the phone, writing letters, watching TV, reading a magazine, and so forth. This has two disadvantages. The first is mentioned above; eating can become paired with other activities. Second, the activity distracts you from eating, so you get all the calories but only part of the pleasure.

Calories Should Be Tasted, Not Wasted

Many a food diary shows people who eat half a bag of popcorn, 45 Fritos, 22 pretzels, or

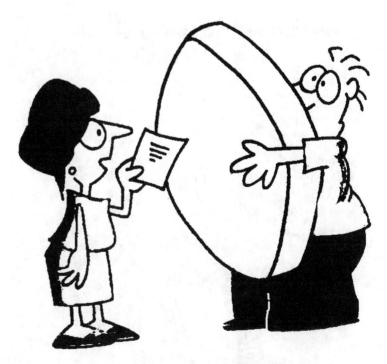

"It says, 'One pill before breakfast controls your appetite all day.'"

three-quarters of a pound of mixed nuts. Many of the calories are wasted, not tasted.

Follow an Eating Schedule

You may have uncovered *time* patterns from your Food Diaries. If you eat many times each day, and if you always feel like eating at those times, a schedule will help. This does not necessarily mean three meals a day at conventional times. It does mean finding a schedule that is convenient for you.

Plan a schedule for your eating. If you eat breakfast at 7:00 a.m., write it down. If you have a mid-evening snack, add it (if necessary). Keep the number of times you eat under control. This may involve eating three conventional meals, but remember to choose a plan you can tolerate.

Following a schedule will help you eat less and think more. You might have a snack planned at 9:00 p.m. If you feel like eating at 8:15, you can wait out the urge, and then see if you are still hungry at 9:00. You may get by with no snack at all! The illustration above is an

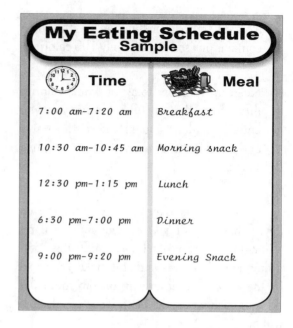

Time	Meal
7:00 am–7:20 am	Breakfast
10:30 am–10:45 am	Morning snack
12:30 pm–1:15 pm	Lunch
6:30 pm–7:00 pm	Dinner
9:00 pm–9:20 pm	Evening Snack

example of an eating schedule made by Judy, one of my clients.

The illustration on page 77 titled "My Eating Schedule" contains blanks for you to plan your eating schedule. List the times and meals you can live with, and do your best to stick with the schedule. There will, of course, be times when you violate your schedule, but do your best. When you feel like eating at times other than your schedule permits, think carefully about whether you are hungry or are responding to associations of eating and other factors.

Eat in One Place

Some people can eat *anywhere*. They eat standing up, sitting down, at the kitchen counter, in an easy chair, lying in bed, or driving the car. They eat in the den, living room, bedroom, basement, and bathroom. One of my former clients even tied Oreo cookies in a bag and hung them with a rope out the window into the shrubs. She could eat with her head hanging out the window! And, this isn't exactly what I have in mind when I say to keep problem foods out of the house.

Here is a hypothetical example I use with my clients. Let's say that for the next 10 years you came to my clinic every day to eat a deli-

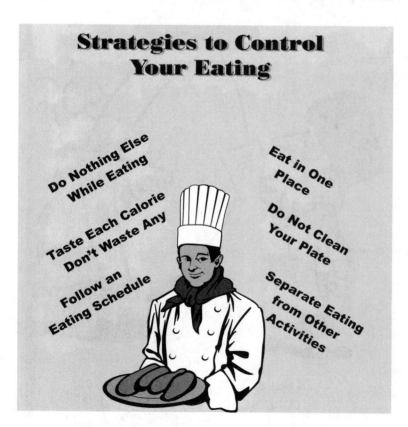

Strategies to Control Your Eating

Do Nothing Else While Eating

Taste Each Calorie Don't Waste Any

Follow an Eating Schedule

Eat in One Place

Do Not Clean Your Plate

Separate Eating from Other Activities

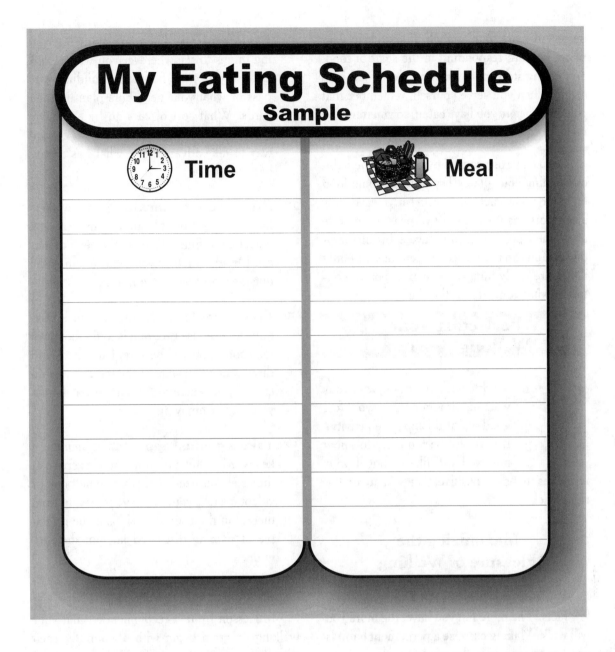

My Eating Schedule
Sample

Time	Meal

cious meal while seated in a yellow chair. At the same time, you would have a chair in your home where no eating would occur. After the 10 years and 3,650 meals, your response to the two chairs would be quite different. You would feel hungry in the yellow chair even after eating. This would not happen in the chair at home.

Select one place in your home where you will eat. Do *all* your eating there, but do *nothing else*. Do not use the place to play chess, pay the bills, plot a way to beat the stock market, or win the lottery.

Do Not Clean Your Plate

It is time to turn the tables on your plate. Until now, you may have been a slave to the rule issued by every mother, "Clean your plate!" It is nice to avoid wasting food, but think for a minute of the folly in cleaning your plate.

When you eat everything on the plate, you are at the mercy of the person doing the serving. Unless the person has mystical powers and knows your body's energy requirements, you will be served too much or too little. Given our cultural tendency to overdo it, you will usually be served more than enough. If you clean your plate, you are responding to the *sight* of food, and eating stops only when no more food is in sight. When you serve yourself, remember that you do so *before* you have eaten, so you might be inclined to serve large amounts.

You can exert control by breaking the habit of cleaning your plate. Try to leave some food on your plate each time you eat. Leave only small portions if you like (two peas or one bite of mashed potatoes), but leave a bit of everything. You can ask for second servings, but only if you are really hungry. This puts *you* in control of what you eat, not the chef.

Perfecting Your Walking Program

TAPE 2
SECTION 10

How are you doing with your walking program? Do you feel good about this positive activity? It may still be too early to know how you will like it, but if your initial reactions are positive, then you are on the right track.

Maximizing the Pleasure of Walking

Walking can be lots of fun if you consider a few facts. The more fun you have, the more you will walk. Making exercise a permanent habit is one key to success in this program.

⇨ **Pay attention**. There are many interesting things to see wherever you walk. Look at the style of the houses or buildings you pass or what your neighbors plant in their yards. What sort of cars go by and what type of people do you see? This is a good way to take advantage of what has always been available.

⇨ **Bring entertainment**. Some walkers like to carry portable radios and cassette players. It is fine to listen to the news or music. Decide whether you want to enjoy the outside world or drown it out.

⇨ **Don't overdo it**. A sure way to undermine an exercise program is to do too much too soon. You will be sore, frustrated, and discouraged. Beware of the tendency to increase your exercise too fast, even though you may be enjoying it.

⇨ **Take a gradual approach**. *Gradual* is a key word in this program. Start exercise at the level you need, not what some book or videotape tells you. Work your way up from there, but do it sensibly. This is the principle of *shaping* discussed later in the program.

Increasing Your Walking

In Lesson Four, I recommended that your walking program begin with 15 minutes each day. If you can do this comfortably, increase the

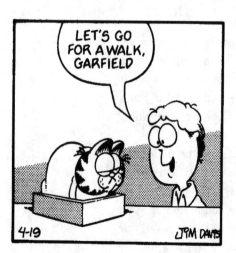

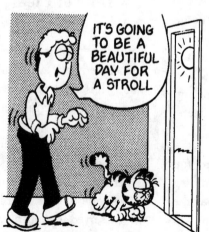

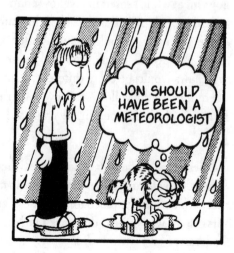

time. Again, your judgment must prevail. Do no more than you can handle, but try to make it a routine part of your day.

I recommend that you add five minutes of walking each day until you reach your goal of one hour of walking per day. As you add time, stop when you feel tired or uncomfortable. For example, you may feel fine when increasing from 15 to 20 minutes, but may feel fatigue or discomfort when going to 25 minutes.

Back up to the 20-minute comfort level and stay there until you are ready to move ahead. Some people will stay at one level for many weeks before moving ahead while others can progress more rapidly. Tailoring these guidelines to your needs is important.

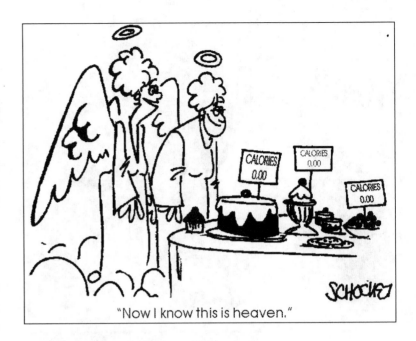

"Now I know this is heaven."

Food and Weight Fantasies

TAPE 3
SECTION 10

Many individuals have fantasies of foods. It is common, for example, to fantasize about having a celebration or "letting go" meal when the program ends. Some people even think about specific foods or the ability to eat large quantities again. Weight fantasies are also common. These usually are visions of a sleek body and huge weight losses.

Food or weight fantasies are a sign of unrealistic expectations. Weight loss is not easy, and pounds do not fly off as we'd like. Food fantasies reveal an expectation that the rigors of going through a program will end some magic day and that old eating habits will return.

You must keep up what you learn. You can eat your favorite foods now, and you will be able to eat them later. You will not, however, be able to return to uncontrolled eating. Identify what you want to eat and eat a small quantity in a controlled manner. Most of all, enjoy it. By not overeating, you will not feel guilty; by eating a small portion, you will not deprive yourself and feel resentful.

Holidays, Parties, and Special Events: A Note

Many people find that their greatest challenge lies in how they handle holidays, parties, and special events. Loads of tempting food are usually available and the hosts want and expect you to eat. Let's face it, celebrating just doesn't seem the same when you have to forego the special foods. Eating out at restaurants can also be challenging.

You can develop ways of being clever that can help you enjoy yourself while keeping control. Because we face so many of these events during a year, being prepared with the necessary skills can be a big help. I deal with these issues in detail in Lesson Fifteen (page 231) in the section called "Holidays, Parties, and Special Events," and in Lesson Twelve (page 183) in the section on "Eating Away from Home." Feel free to read these sections as needed to help with problems you may anticipate.

Solo and Social Changing

Individuals come in many packages with many personalities. Some like to make changes on their own and do not want other people involved. Others like the aid and support they

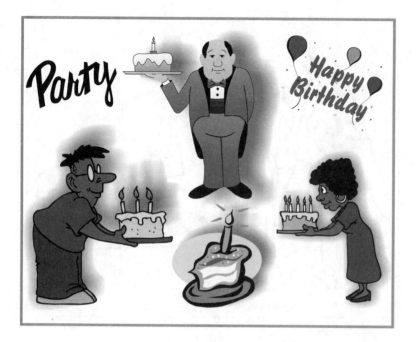

might get from family and friends. I call the first group *solo* changers and the other group *social* changers.

Solo changers like to travel the weight loss path alone. They often do not tell others when they go on a program. They do not enjoy questions about their weight or their eating. No other person knows their weight. Social changers, on the other hand, like company. They talk with others about their program and are pleased when others notice their progress. They might join a program with a friend or enlist someone in the family to exercise with them.

Being a social changer is fine. Being a solo changer is fine. What is important is to determine which type best fits you and to structure your program accordingly. There is much material in this manual about enlisting the aid of family and friends. This is likely to help the social person but not a solo type. Solo changers can be upset when others attempt to assist them, even when the assistance is offered for the right reasons.

Think about whether you are a social or solo person. If you are social, the "Relationships" part of The LEARN Program may be

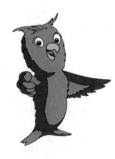

"Some people like to make changes on their own, and others like the aid and support from family and friends."

helpful, starting with the information on partners in the next section.

Think of support from others as a resource to be cultivated. If you are a solo person, decide exactly when and how you would like others to be involved. Support from others is a resource only if you find it helpful. There are many other resources at your disposal.

Would a Partner Help?

Program partnerships can be very powerful. They occur when a person enlists the aid of another. Sometimes the partner is also on a program, but fine partnerships can occur when the partner is thin. How can you tell if a partnership is for you?

First, there are different types of partnerships. The most logical one is with a spouse. A husband or wife can be a real aid, but not in all cases. Many of our clients have formed successful partnerships with coworkers, good friends, neighbors, or relatives.

You may already have a partner in mind. In Lesson Six, you can complete the Support Partner Quiz to determine whether this person would be a good choice.

A program partnership is much like a friendship. It is based on give and take. All the support does not flow from the partner to you. You must reciprocate. There will be good times and bad. Some energy is required to keep the partnership intact, as with any relationship.

Do you think you would profit from a partnership? While you decide, let me explain what scientific studies have shown. There have been about 20 studies on partnership programs, including several that I have conducted with colleagues. In some studies, working with a partner greatly increased weight loss. In others, there was no advantage to the partnership approach. I interpret these inconsistent findings to show that losing weight with a partner is helpful for some, but not for all.

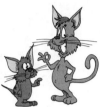

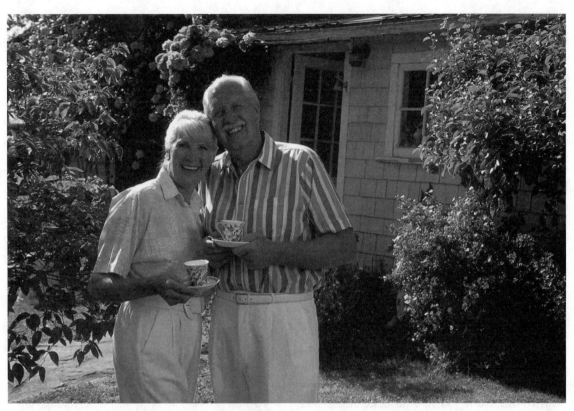

Several examples may illustrate how others can help or hurt. Marjorie enlisted the aid of her husband in her program. He was supportive and showed his concern by walking with her and by not eating treats when she was around. This encouragement helped Marjorie.

Sharon's case was different. Her husband made fun of her and was bitter about her weight problem. He ate in front of her and was nearly always discouraging in his comments. It would have been difficult for Sharon to engage her husband in a partnership. Only you know whether this approach will work for you.

Think about having a weight loss partner. Remember, this person does not have to be overweight. It is important that you feel comfortable with this person and that he or she is able to motivate you. Next, think about your own style and personality. Do you like to do things with others or alone? Can you confide in others or do you keep things to yourself? Could you discuss weight control troubles with another person or would you rather not share them?

Finally, what is your *gut* feeling? Do you think the partnership approach would work for you?

You will have time to ponder these important matters, because guidelines for starting a partnership will appear in the next lesson. Think about your own style and decide if a partnership would help. Sort through your friendships and form a pool of possible partners. The partnership may work for you. Do not feel guilty if you are a solo person. Many people do best this way.

Why Social Support Can Be So Important

TAPE 3
SECTION 4

Many scientists have studied the impact of social networks on health and well-being. In early days, researchers evaluated whether people had friends and interacted frequently with family members. They then studied whether these events were related to health. The problem with this approach is that a person might have a lot of social contacts, but the contacts might not be positive (say in the case of a distressed marriage). More recently, experts have agreed that the quality of a person's relationships is the key. People who have relationships they can count on for emotional support (e.g., love, caring, concern, etc.) and tangible support (e.g., baby-sitting, financial assistance, and other practical issues), live longer, are healthier, and are happier than people who do not have these relationships.

If support can be so helpful, you have to ask yourself two questions:

⇨ Why is it so helpful?

⇨ What can I do to get more support or to take advantage of the support I have?

As for the first issue, support may be helpful for many reasons. Just feeling cared for may help by inspiring you to lead a healthier lifestyle, to do things that make you happier, and perhaps even influence things like your immune system. Whatever the reason, it is clear from many studies that support can be beneficial.

The question then becomes how to get support. Before talking about this, let me first say that support is something that benefits some people more than others. Some people are perfectly content doing things on their own and they do not want or need others involved in their business. This is perfectly fine—in fact, I will speak about different personality types and how some people are more social types and others more solo types. For those who feel they would benefit from support, even if it occurs at a modest level from only one person, there is a lot to discuss.

Servings from the Five Food Groups

The five food groups of the Food Guide Pyramid were introduced in Lesson Four. I can now be more specific about the number of servings to have every day. First, you need to know what constitutes a serving.

It is important to select the correct number of servings from each group to insure the right mix of nutrients. As we continue through the program, the pyramid will become a familiar friend. The average numbers of servings per day recommended for adults are listed in the graphic illustration on page 83. Use this as a guide to structure your diet. Do your best to eat the recommended number of servings every day. I will focus on each of the groups in later lessons and will provide you with lists of servings from each group.

My Personal Goals for This Week

You have several goals this week—some old, some new. Work on maintaining your target calorie level. Make copies of the new Monitoring Form and complete it each day, recording the types and amounts of food you eat. Most women should set a goal of eating approximately 1200 calories a day and men 1500 calories a day. Your Monitoring Form lists the following goals for the upcoming week that include:

❶ Do nothing else while eating

❷ Eat on a planned schedule

❸ Eat in one place

❹ Leave some food on your plate

❺ Eat the correct number of servings from the five food groups of the Food Guide Pyramid

Finally, think about your attitudes toward physical activity, as you prepare to increase your activity this week. Can you see exercise in a more positive light after reading the lesson? Increased activity brings many rewards, one of which is long-term weight management. And, even small increases can help. Remember to record your weight change on your Weight Change Record on page 25 in Lesson One. Good luck on your fifth week.

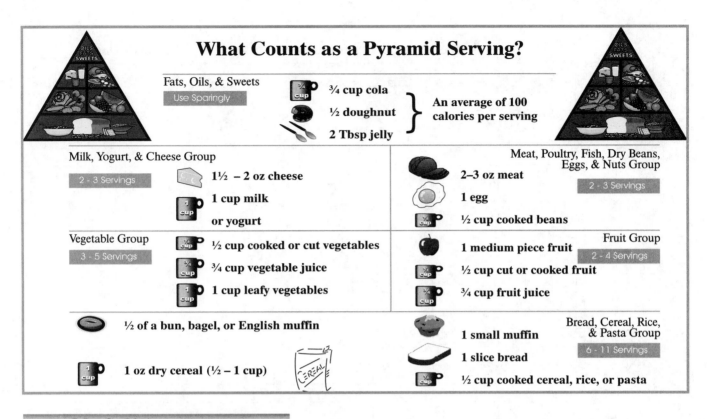

What Counts as a Pyramid Serving?

Fats, Oils, & Sweets
Use Sparingly

¾ cup cola
½ doughnut
2 Tbsp jelly
} An average of 100 calories per serving

Milk, Yogurt, & Cheese Group
2 - 3 Servings

1½ – 2 oz cheese
1 cup milk or yogurt

Meat, Poultry, Fish, Dry Beans, Eggs, & Nuts Group
2 - 3 Servings

2–3 oz meat
1 egg
½ cup cooked beans

Vegetable Group
3 - 5 Servings

½ cup cooked or cut vegetables
¾ cup vegetable juice
1 cup leafy vegetables

Fruit Group
2 - 4 Servings

1 medium piece fruit
½ cup cut or cooked fruit
¾ cup fruit juice

½ of a bun, bagel, or English muffin

1 oz dry cereal (½ – 1 cup)

Bread, Cereal, Rice, & Pasta Group
6 - 11 Servings

1 small muffin
1 slice bread
½ cup cooked cereal, rice, or pasta

My Self-Assessment

Lesson Five

T F 32. Most people get enough exercise to realize the many health benefits of an active lifestyle.

T F 33. Exercise must be done in specific amounts for it to aid you with weight loss.

T F 34. Cleaning your plate is harmful because the server decides how much you will eat.

T F 35. Eating on a schedule is not advisable because it is too regimented.

T F 36. You should find a program partner to be successful at weight management.

T F 37. Weight loss is the best measure of success in The LEARN Program.

(Answers in Appendix C, page 271)

Monitoring Form—Lesson Five

Today's Date: _____

TIME	FOOD AND AMOUNT	CALORIES

TOTAL DAILY CALORIES

PERSONAL GOALS FOR THIS WEEK	MOST OF THE TIME	SOME-TIMES	RARELY
1. DO NOTHING ELSE WHILE EATING			
2. EAT ON A PLANNED SCHEDULE			
3. EAT IN ONE PLACE			
4. LEAVE SOME FOOD ON MY PLATE			
5. EAT SERVINGS FROM THE FIVE FOOD GROUPS			
6. EAT LESS THAN _____ CALORIES PER DAY			

FOOD GROUPS FOR TODAY	PHYSICAL ACTIVITY	MINUTES OR STEPS
MILK, YOGURT, AND CHEESE ☐ ☐ ☐	(M)	
MEAT, POULTRY, ETC. ☐ ☐ ☐	(Tu)	
FRUITS ☐ ☐ ☐ ☐	(W)	
VEGETABLES ☐ ☐ ☐ ☐ ☐	(Th)	
BREADS, CEREALS, ETC. ☐ ☐ ☐ ☐ ☐ ☐ ☐ ☐	(F)	
SERVINGS OF WATER (8 OZ) ☐ ☐ ☐ ☐ ☐ ☐ ☐ ☐	(Sa)	
	(Su)	

You have now had a thorough introduction to the five components of The LEARN Program. We continue our path by dealing with your speed of eating. We'll revisit the Food Guide Pyramid and I'll show you how to estimate portions. You can take the Support Partner Quiz to decide who would be a good weight management program partner. You will learn more about lifestyle activity and I will give you a chart showing the number of calories you burn for various activities. Finally, we'll work on the Attitudes component of LEARN by addressing the topic of negative self-talk. So, if you're ready, let's move on.

Slowing Your Eating Rate

Could you qualify for the Olympic speed-eating trials? Many people, both heavy and thin, eat so fast that their taste buds see only a blur as the food speeds by. This minimizes the enjoyment of food. More importantly, eating rapidly can fool your body's defense against eating too much.

Your body has an internal satiety (fullness) mechanism. When you have eaten enough, the mechanism sends out signals saying "Enough is enough!" Most experts believe this takes about 20 minutes, although it is a very complex process involving the stomach, hormones in the small intestine, brain chemicals, and other factors. If you eat rapidly, you will consume too much food before the mechanism kicks in. You will outpace your body's internal controls.

Slowing down your eating can be like halting a runaway freight train. You have had many meals in your life, so the habit of eating fast has been practiced thousands of times. Be patient and practice the following techniques until the old patterns are replaced by new ones.

Techniques to Slow Your Eating

There are two main ways to slow your eating. Both can help put the brakes on eating and can increase the enjoyment of food.

⇨ ***Put your fork down between bites.*** When you take a bite of food, put your fork down, chew the food completely, swallow, and then pick up the fork for another bite. Do the same with a spoon, and if you are eating finger foods like a sandwich, put the food down between bites.

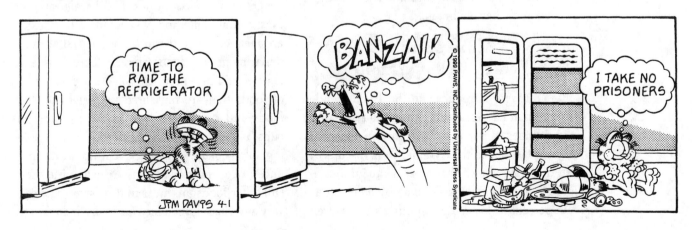

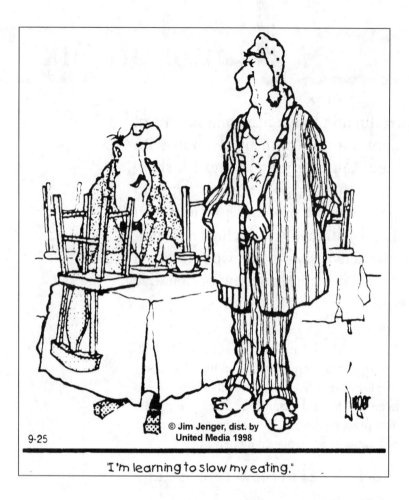

9-25

"I'm learning to slow my eating."

⇨ ***Pause during the meal.*** Take a break during your meal. Start with a brief pause, of perhaps 30 seconds. Gradually increase the time to one, then two, and finally three minutes. This pause gives you time to reflect on what you have eaten, so you can make a conscious decision to proceed with more. This may also help you eat less. One study with animals found that interrupting the meal led to fewer total calories, even though the animals could eat all they wanted after the break.

More on the Food Guide Pyramid

You were introduced to the Food Guide Pyramid in Lesson Four, and in the last lesson the number of servings and portion sizes for each of the tiers in the Pyramid were discussed. Studies have shown that most people underreport their caloric intake—some by as much as 50 percent. This underreporting occurs even when individuals honestly believe they are reporting their portion sizes and calories correctly. These studies highlight the importance of accurately measuring the portion sizes of the foods that you eat. The more accurate you are in recording the calories you eat, the better you will be at determining your body's energy needs. Don't worry, I'm not going to ask you to carry measuring cups and food scales with you everywhere you go. But, I do want to emphasize the importance of accurately measuring portion sizes. Once you master this technique, you can measure portion sizes less and less. It is a good idea, however, to keep these skills polished. So, you may want to measure portion sizes a few days out of every month.

A Food Portion Quiz

On page 87 is a Food Portion Quiz. Take this quiz now to get an idea of how accurately you may be measuring your food portions. This quiz was developed by Dr. Judith Ashley and Frances Poe, both registered dietitians, from the University of Nevada School of Medicine. If you answer "no" to any of the 10 questions, then you may need to improve the accuracy of your measuring abilities. The sections that follow will help you enhance these important skills.

Accurately measuring portion sizes of the foods you eat is important for estimating the total number of calories you eat each day. If you are using the exchange plan, measuring is equally important. Some foods are measured by weight in ounces or grams. Food scales are the most common method of weighing food. Scales are inexpensive and can be purchased at most department or food stores. Cereal, meat, cheese, and dried crunchy snacks are examples of foods that are measured by weight. Other foods and drinks are measured by volume in cups, tablespoons, and teaspoons. Milk, cooking oil, cooked vegetables, cut-up fruit, fruit juices, rice, and dried beans are examples. And still other foods are measured by size. Size can vary anywhere from a measured size in inches to a more subjective food size like a "medium" apple. Measuring portion sizes is most often used with fruits and vegetables. Finally, foods can be measured by item count, such as one slice of bread, one egg, or five crackers.

The Pyramid Guide

As illustrated by the table in Lesson Five on page 83, the Food Guide Pyramid suggests a certain number of daily servings from each of the five food groups, depending upon the number of calories you want to include in your daily diet. On page 88 is the Food Pyramid Servings and Calorie Guide. Following these guidelines will help you eat a balanced diet, achieve optimum nutrition, and help you achieve your target calorie level.

The Importance of the Five Food Groups

The Food Guide Pyramid arranges food groups by the key nutrients that they provide. For example food choices from the Meat, Poultry, Fish, Dry Beans, Eggs, and Nuts Group are high in protein, B vitamins, iron, and zinc. The Milk, Yogurt, and Cheese Group includes foods high in protein and provide other key nutrients like calcium and vitamin D. The Vegetable and Fruit Groups along with the Bread, Cereal, Rice and Pasta Group all provide excellent sources of dietary fiber along with other important vitamins and minerals. Choosing the right number of servings from the different food groups each day helps you achieve a balanced diet.

Visual Guides

As I mentioned earlier, accurately measuring your food portion sizes is a key to controlling the number of calories you eat each day. Of course, it's not always convenient to carry your measuring cups and food scales with you. When was the last time you saw someone in a five-star restaurant taking out the food scales before starting to eat?

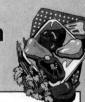

Food Portion Quiz

1. Yes No Do you own a food scale?

2. Yes No Do you have measuring cups and spoons where you serve food?

3. Yes No Do you keep a ruler handy in the kitchen?

4. Yes No Do you know how many ounces the glass you usually use at home holds?

5. Yes No Do you know how much the cup you use at work holds?

6. Yes No Do you know how many ounces are in the hamburgers, chicken, or fish you usually eat?

7. Yes No Do you count the number of strawberries, cherries, nuts, or french fries on your plate?

8. Yes No Do you know how many calories are in an ounce of your favorite cheese?

9. Yes No Do you read food labels to find out how much is in a serving?

10. Yes No Do you compare the calories per serving in possible food alternatives of your favorite foods?

Source: Ashley JM, Poe FE. Too much of a good thing: Keeping an eye on nutrition. *The Weight Control Digest* 1998; 8:742. Reproduced with permission.

The chart on page 88 is a helpful Visual Portion Guide. Study this guide carefully to help you accurately measure the portion sizes of the foods you eat. You may even want to make a copy of this handy guide and carry it with you. Share this information with your family and friends. Many people find it helpful to make estimating portion sizes and calories a part of their meal conversations.

"How much do you really know about the food choices you make each day?"

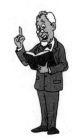

Visual Portion Guide

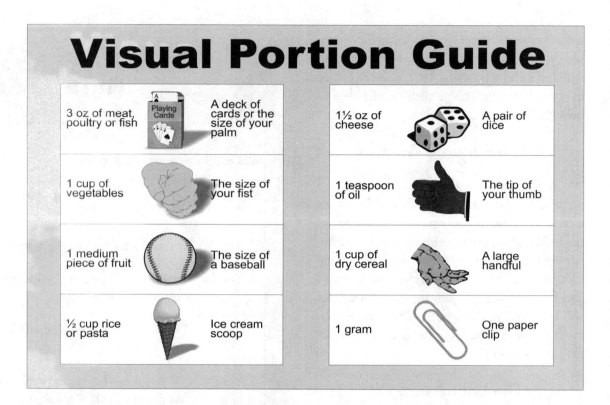

3 oz of meat, poultry or fish	A deck of cards or the size of your palm	1½ oz of cheese	A pair of dice
1 cup of vegetables	The size of your fist	1 teaspoon of oil	The tip of your thumb
1 medium piece of fruit	The size of a baseball	1 cup of dry cereal	A large handful
½ cup rice or pasta	Ice cream scoop	1 gram	One paper clip

Your Target Calorie Level

Back in Lesson Three, you began experimenting with calorie intake to identify the level at which you will lose weight at the recommended rate of one to two pounds per week. Look back now to Lesson Three on page 46 to see what calorie level you selected as your *best guess*.

Now that you are several lessons wiser and have had more experience with your body's response to making changes, it is time to select a more official Target Calorie Level. Enter this number in the space provided on page 89. In the new Monitoring Forms you are using, you will continue to record whether you meet your calorie goal each day. The forms have a space

Food Pyramid Servings and Calorie Guide*					
Food Group	**1200 calories** (number of servings)	**1400 calories** (number of servings)	**1500 calories** (number of servings)	**1800 calories** (number of servings)	**2000 calories** (number of servings)
Bread, Cereal, Rices, & Pasta Group	6	6	7	8	9
Fruit Group	3	3	3	4	4
Vegetable Group	4	4	5	6	6
Milk, Yogurt, & Cheese Group	2 (non-fat)	2 (low-fat)	2 (low-fat)	2 (low-fat)	3 (low-fat)
Meat, Poultry, Fish, Dry Beans, Eggs, & Nut Group	5 oz lean meat (or equivalent)	5 oz medium-fat meat (or equivalent)	5 oz medium-fat meat (or equivalent)	7 oz medium-fat meat (or equivalent)	7 oz medium-fat meat (or equivalent)

* This plan does not leave room for added fat. If you choose lower fat meats and dairy products, you can add some items from the Fats, Oils & Sweets Group.

for you to complete the following item: "Less than _____ calories." The blank spaces are where you fill in your Target Calorie Level. Remember, this is to be the calorie level at which you will lose one to two pounds each week. The number can be modified as you progress through the program. Now, write down your new Target Calorie Level.

My New Target Calorie Level is Less than_____Calories each day.

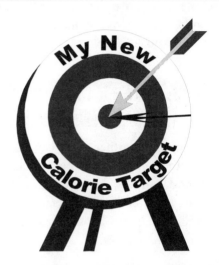

Choosing a Support Person

People who feel they would benefit from the support of another person have a number of choices for doing so. The most extensive involvement is to have a weight management partnership. In this case, you and another person would both be losing weight and would work with each other as support partners. This can work wonderfully in some cases, but again, it is not for everyone.

You can obtain less intensive but equally important support from others, including a spouse, parent, child, friend, coworker, or anyone who encourages you. The person could be involved in a big way, say by asking you each day about your goals and accomplishments, or in a smaller way, by just being there when you ask for help. Who you choose and what you ask them to do is, of course, best decided by you.

I will discuss how to decide whether a given individual would be a good support person. A quiz for this follows. Then I will discuss how to work with such a person and whether it should be in a full-blown partnership or some other type of helping relationship.

A Quiz for Choosing a Support Partner

I promised in the last lesson to give you a quiz for evaluating whether a person would make a good partner to go through the program with you. Your job was to think of possible partners, and then to use the quiz to make a final decision. The Support Partner Quiz is on page 90.

To take this quiz, think of the person you would have as a partner, and answer the questions honestly. First, answer each question either true or false. Beside each of your answers is a number. Write this number in the space provided immediately before each question number. Add the numbers of your responses, then use the scoring guide at the bottom of the quiz.

"For some people, a program partner can be a powerful tool."

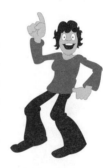

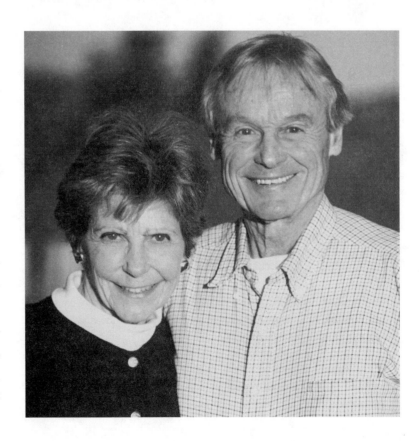

Support Partner Quiz

____1.   It is easy to talk to my partner about weight.

        True—5   False—1

____2.   My partner has always been thin and does not understand my weight problem.

        True—1   False—3

____3.   My partner offers me food when he or she knows I am trying to lose weight.

        True—1   False—5

____4.   My partner never says critical things about my weight.

        True—3   False—1

____5.   My partner is always there when I need a friend.

        True—4   False—1

____6.   When I lose weight and look better, my partner will be jealous.

        True—1   False—3

____7.   My partner will be genuinely interested in helping me with my weight.

        True—6   False—1

____8.   I could talk to my partner even if I was doing poorly.

        True—5   False—1

If you scored between 30 and 34, you may have found the perfect partner. A score in this range indicates that you and this person are comfortable with one another and can work together.

If you scored between 25 and 29, your friend is potentially a good partner, but there are a few areas of concern. Try asking the partner to take the quiz and predict how you answered the questions. This may help you make a decision.

If you scored between 17 and 24, there are potential areas of conflict, and a program partnership with this person could encounter stormy going. Think of another partner.

If you scored between 8 and 16, definitely look to someone else as a partner. A program partnership in this case would be a high-risk undertaking.

These guidelines should help in choosing a partner. Once you have done so, discuss the possibility with the person you have in mind. Below, I will make some specific suggestions on how to proceed.

Let me stress again that you need not have a partner. The decision is left to you. If you do decide on the partner approach, these questions could help in selecting a supportive partner. If you are uncertain about proceeding with a partner, even after taking the quiz, experiment with it. Use what you learn about partnerships to see if you profit from the aid of another person. If not, consider yourself a solo changer and move ahead.

Communicating with Your Partner

The Support Partner Quiz can help you decide whether one or more people might be good support partners. Now you are ready to discuss your program with this person and start the ball rolling. There is a lot you can do to get the most out of this effort.

In later lessons I will discuss methods for dealing with family and friends. This is different from a partnership where someone can be very involved with your program. With the family, there are more ways that support can be provided and sabotage can be prevented. If you feel your family is a problem or can be a useful resource now, it may be helpful to read page 155 in Lesson Ten. In the meantime, let's discuss partnerships.

Here are specific ideas for starting a program partnership. Communicating is the first and most important step. If you and your partner can communicate effectively, you are on the way to a successful partnership. Here are some ideas for making this happen.

It is essential that you and your partner talk together. Sit down and have a friendly talk with the person you have chosen as a partner. Discuss the topics below in an open and honest way.

⇨ **Are you both ready for a partner-ship?** Is your partner ready to listen to requests for help and make the required effort? Is he or she ready to help you during good times and bad? Are you ready to help your partner in return? Some degree of commitment is necessary from both of you.

⇨ **Tell your partner how to help.** A common and crucial mistake is to expect your partner to read your mind. If it is your spouse, you may think he or she should know what you want and need. Most people are not good mind readers, so leave nothing to chance. Tell your partner what he or she can do. Do you want to be praised when you do well or scolded when you do poorly? Should the person avoid eating in your presence? Can your partner help by exercising with you?

⇨ **Make specific requests.** The more specific your requests, the easier it will be for your partner to comply. If your request is vague and general, like "Be nice," your partner is at a disadvantage. A more specific request is better, such as "Please tell me you love me when I lose weight." Instead of saying, "Don't eat in front of me," say "It helps me when you eat your evening bowl of ice cream in the other room." Replace a general statement, like "Exercise with me," with "Please take a half-hour walk with me each morning."

⇨ **State your requests positively.** It is better to ask for something positive than to criticize something negative. Clever changes of words can help. If your partner nags, you can say "It really helps me when you say nice things." If your partner offers you food, you can say "I appreciate the times when you don't offer me food. It is easier to control my eating then." Human nature responds well to the chance to do

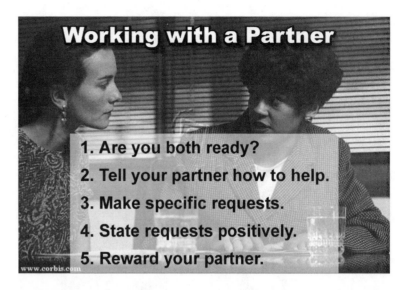

Working with a Partner

1. Are you both ready?
2. Tell your partner how to help.
3. Make specific requests.
4. State requests positively.
5. Reward your partner.

www.corbis.com

something positive, so try this approach with your partner.

⇨ **Reward your partner.** For your partner to help you, you must help your partner. One-way relationships don't last long. If you are going through this program together, you can work out weight-related ways of helping. If your partner is not on a program, be forward, and ask what you can do in return. Remember, being a partner can be challenging, so you need to acknowledge your partner's help.

Use these techniques to start the ball rolling with your partner. Upcoming lessons will give you more ideas for working with your partner. It is important to lay this groundwork first.

"Communicating and feeling comfortable with your program partner is an essential element of a successful partnership."

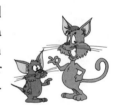

Making Physical Activity Count

TAPE 3
SECTION 9

It is time to distinguish between *lifestyle* and *programmed* activity. Lifestyle activity is simple and can be done in your day-to-day routine. An example would be using stairs rather than an elevator when you go to work. Programmed activity is a traditional exercise regimen of jogging, biking, aerobics, racquetball, and so forth. I will discuss programmed activities beginning with Lesson Eight. For now, let us consider lifestyle activities.

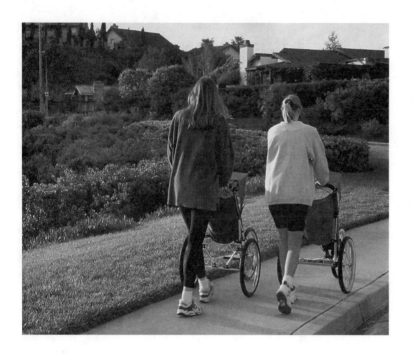

Use the Stairs

Stairs can be a good friend because they are so readily available. Climbing stairs burns more calories per minute than rigorous activities like jogging and cycling. If you work on the fifth floor of a building, take the elevator to the fourth floor and walk the remaining flight. As your condition improves, get off on lower floors. One of my favorite examples is a client who lived in a two-story house with bathrooms on each floor. She decided to use the bathroom on the floor where she wasn't located, which gave her several extra trips per day up and down the stairs.

Park Further Away

When you drive to the mall, don't circle around like a vulture in search of a spot by the door. Park where only the people with new cars pull in—away from the crowd.

Walk More

If you take the bus downtown, get off one or two stops early and walk the extra distance. If someone gives you a ride to the store, have them drop you off a few blocks away. At home, take things up the stairs in several trips instead of letting them accumulate for one trip.

Count All Activity as Exercise

Count everything you do as exercise. When you do housework, turn on a timer and keep moving. Use the vacuum an extra day each

Lifestyle Activity

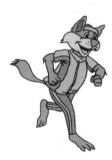

"Count all your activity as exercise—even the fun stuff!"

You can imagine the virtues of lifestyle activity. It is easy, takes little time, does not hurt, does not require special clothes or equipment, and can become habit with little effort. It makes you feel better both psychologically and physically.

The idea here is to sneak in activity whenever possible. The suggestions that follow may help you get started with another part of the assignment for this lesson—*increase your lifestyle activity.*

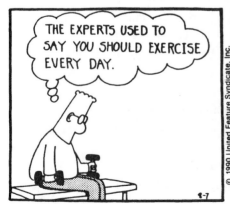

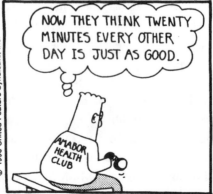

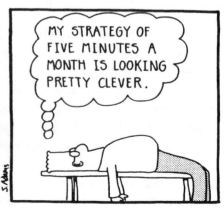

week. Time yourself as you wash the car, rake the leaves, or mow the lawn. You will be surprised how fast the minutes go by, and you will accomplish another task as well.

The beauty of these small bouts of activity is that each one provides an opportunity for you to feel virtuous—to be reinforced for doing something positive. And this is not just a trick—you really are doing something positive. Anything you do to increase your lifestyle activity is beneficial, and makes you feel better. You deserve a pat on the back whenever you make an effort to do something good, and you're the closest one around to do it. My hope is that you will count yourself among the ranks of people who consider themselves exercisers. This can build on itself to the point where you are feeling much better about your body and your physical condition. It doesn't take much to notice improvement.

These are just examples of the general *principle* of increasing lifestyle activity. Think of more methods to fit your own routine. The section that follows, on the calorie values of exercise, may give you more ideas. Be sure to record your lifestyle activities on your Monitoring Form. You deserve credit for doing these activities, so they should show up in your records.

Tracking Your Progress with Activity

When you are making positive changes, it is important to *feel* like you are making progress and to reinforce yourself accordingly. It can help to have a way of assessing how you are doing. The activity section on the monitoring forms at the end of each lesson is an excellent place to begin, but some people like to do more.

Some people like to keep a graph or a log of when they are active. Either could include the number of minutes being active, how fast you do some activity (like walking a certain distance), or how far the activity takes you (distance). Another helpful index of progress can be to use a pedometer. These are available in sporting

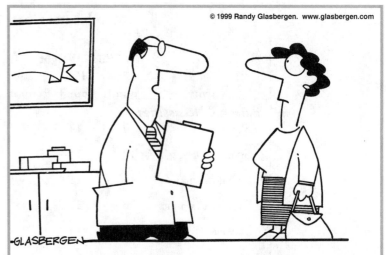

© 1999 Randy Glasbergen. www.glasbergen.com

"If you want to lose weight, you need to change your diet. Eat more greasy food and the fat will slide right off your bones!"

goods stores and have been refined in the last several years to be much more accurate than earlier models. I discussed such a device in earlier lessons when I talked about the LEARN WalkMaster. If you don't have one of these you may want to call 1–888–LEARN–41 to order one or log on to the Internet at www.TheLifeStyleCompany.com. Some devices measure how far you walk and others give the number of steps you take. The ones with the number of steps are nice because you can see evidence of even small increases in activity.

We have worked with individuals who set up reward systems for themselves by making a contract. The contract states that certain rewards (e.g., a movie, a new CD, clothing, etc.) will be given for attaining a certain level of activity. These are fine, but whether or not you have a reward system, it is important to track your activity so you have a sense of how much you are improving. This helps you feel virtuous when you deserve it.

The Calorie Values of Physical Activity

How many calories do you burn when you wash the dishes? Is it more than when you rake leaves? Is it easier to burn calories by swim-

Calorie Values for 10 Minutes of Activity

Activity	Body Weight			Activity	Body Weight		
	125 Pounds	175 Pounds	250 Pounds		125 Pounds	175 Pounds	250 Pounds
Personal Necessities				**Light Work**			
Sleeping	10	14	20	Assembly line	20	28	40
Sitting (watching TV)	10	14	18	Auto repair	35	48	69
Sitting (talking)	15	21	30	Carpentry	32	44	64
Dressing or washing	26	37	53	Bricklaying	28	40	57
Standing	12	16	24	Farming chores	32	44	64
				House painting	29	40	58
Locomotion				**Heavy Work**			
Walking downstairs	56	78	111	Pick & shovel work	56	78	110
Walking upstairs	146	202	288	Chopping wood	60	84	121
Walking at 2 mph	29	40	58	Dragging logs	158	220	315
Walking at 4 mph	52	72	102	Drilling coal	79	111	159
Running at 5.5 mph	90	125	178	**Recreation**			
Running at 7 mph	118	164	232	Badminton	43	65	94
Running at 12 mph	164	228	326	Baseball	39	54	78
Cycling at 5.5 mph	42	58	83	Basketball	58	82	117
Cycling at 13 mph	89	124	178	Bowling (nonstop)	56	78	111
Housework				Canoeing (4 mph)	90	128	182
Making beds	32	46	65	Dancing (moderate)	35	48	69
Washing floors	38	53	75	Dancing (vigorous)	48	66	94
Washing windows	35	48	69	Football	69	96	137
Dusting	22	31	44	Golfing	33	48	68
Preparing a meal	32	46	65	Horseback riding	56	78	112
Shoveling snow	65	89	130	Ping-Pong	32	45	64
Light gardening	30	42	59	Racquetball	75	104	144
Weeding garden	49	68	98	Skiing (alpine)	80	112	160
Mowing grass (power)	34	47	67	Skiing (cross country)	98	138	194
Mowing grass (manual)	38	52	74	Skiing (water)	60	88	130
Sedentary Occupation				Squash	75	104	144
Sitting (writing)	15	21	30	Swimming (backstroke)	32	45	64
Light office work	25	34	50	Swimming (crawl)	40	56	80
Standing, light activity	20	28	40	Tennis	56	80	115
Typing (electric)	19	27	39	Volleyball	43	65	94

ming, jogging, or cycling? Your questions will be answered in the table on page 94.

Several important points are highlighted by the calorie chart. First, any activity uses energy (calories), so any increase in activity can help. Sitting uses approximately 15 calories per 10 minutes, while standing uses 17, and walking briskly uses 60. Even something as simple as standing rather than sitting can use a few extra calories. Second, heavier people burn more calories than other people while doing the same activity, because more energy is required to move the extra weight. Third, several routine activities like using stairs and walking are useful methods of burning calories.

Several facts must be considered when viewing these calorie figures. One is that calorie expenditures vary enormously for many activities, depending on their intensity. Two people shoveling snow may differ greatly in how quickly they shovel, how much snow is lifted with each shovel, and how much they move around while shoveling. Similar differences can occur with skiing, tennis, yard work, and so forth. Therefore, the figures in the table are only averages.

The second fact is that the table shows the calories burned for 10 minutes of continuous activity. If you do an activity for five minutes, divide the value in the table by two. If you are active for 30 minutes, multiply the value by three.

The word *continuous* is important to understanding the table. The table shows that a 125 pound person burns 56 calories for 10 minutes of bowling. This is 10 minutes of nonstop bowling and does not include time to keep score, chat with friends, polish your ball, or visit the snack bar. The 10 minutes for skiing would not include time waiting in the lift line, marveling at the scenery, or falling down! So, to calculate the calories you burn for a given activity, calculate the time you are truly active, and then use the table on page 94 as a guide.

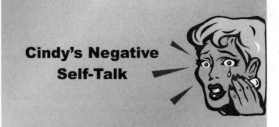

Cindy's Negative Self-Talk

"I knew I wouldn't make it to my goal."

"What good is this 15-pound weight loss when I still have 30 pounds to go?"

"I can only accept myself when I reach my ideal weight."

"The program isn't working anymore."

"I'm just sick that I'm not losing more weight."

The Trap of Negative Self-Talk

TAPE 4
SECTION 3

A person I know, named Cindy, went through a lot of self-doubt at about this stage of the program. She was discouraged because she wasn't losing more weight and was questioning whether she should keep trying. She was on the verge of giving up. When I asked what type of thoughts she was having, she came up with what you see in the chart above.

After some discussion, Cindy came up with more positive ways of looking at things. This helped her get back on track, taking credit for the progress she had made and emphasizing a realistic, attainable set of expectations. Now look at what Cindy was saying to herself in the chart titled, Cindy's More Positive Self-Talk, on page 96.

Think of your weight like a turnstile that moves in only one direction. Losing weight is like the turnstile moving forward. Wouldn't it

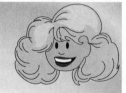
be nice if your weight were like a turnstile in that it never moved in the opposite direction? With the right self-management skills, you can have more confidence that your weight will not bounce back up.

Now, of course, expecting a perfect turnstile is unrealistic, because no person who has lost weight maintains a perfectly stable weight. You can expect some weight fluctuation, created in part by fluctuations in your control over eating and activity. One thing that characterizes successful maintainers is that they set an upper

limit on how much they allow their weight to increase (usually three to five pounds) before they take corrective action. Hence, the turnstile will move mainly in one direction (weight loss) and will accept a little backward movement, but only to a limited degree, before the brakes are applied.

Charting My Progress

Think of the progress you have made. Any weight you have lost is a positive development. Also, remember our discussion on the quality of life. You can measure progress with much more than the scale. Our first order of business is to be sure that these changes are permanent. Therefore, if your weight loss has slowed, pay attention to all you have achieved rather than what you have left to do. Losing more weight is possible for a great many people, so you might find yourself charging ahead, but if not, keep your head high and keep the weight off! Take a few moments to write down the progress you have made since starting the program and all the positive things you have changed. Also, write down all the positive reasons you can think of to maintain changes you have already made and to continue your program. I have provided a table below so that you can take a few minutes now, before continuing with this lesson, to write down your thoughts. So, sharpen your pencil and start writing.

Progress In My Program		
Progress I've Made	Positive Things I've Changed	Reasons I Should Maintain the Changes

My Personal Goals for This Week

One specific goal you can set is to eat more slowly. This helps most people and is worth making a habit. In addition, think of the personal goals you'd like to set at this point, and try your best to reach these goals. Continue walking and find ways to increase your lifestyle activity. If you decide the partnership approach is for you, have a candid and specific talk with your partner. Make it a goal this week to carefully measure your food portion sizes and estimate the calories as accurately as possibly. Finally, keep an eye out for negative self-talk. Set a goal to counter this negative self-talk with positive thoughts and positive self-talk.

My Self-Assessment

Lesson Six

T F 38. Eating rapidly helps you enjoy food more because the taste buds get more stimulation.

T F 39. You should tell your program partner in specific terms how he or she can help.

T F 40. Climbing stairs requires more energy per minute than many traditional exercises, like swimming and jogging.

T F 41. Pausing during a meal increases food intake because the body digests food and sends out signals to eat more.

T F 42. Accurately estimating food portion sizes is not all that important in a weight management program.

T F 43 It is important to reinforce your partner for helping you.

(Answers in Appendix C, page 271)

Monitoring Form—Lesson Six

Today's Date: _____

TIME	FOOD AND AMOUNT	CALORIES

TOTAL DAILY CALORIES

PERSONAL GOALS FOR THIS WEEK	MOST OF THE TIME	SOME-TIMES	RARELY
1. PUT FORK DOWN BETWEEN BITES			
2. PAUSE DURING MEALS			
3. INCREASE LIFESTYLE ACTIVITY			
4. COUNTER NEGATIVE SELF-TALK			
5. MEASURE PORTIONS SIZES OF FOOD SERVINGS			
6. EAT LESS THAN _____ CALORIES PER DAY			

FOOD GROUPS FOR TODAY	PHYSICAL ACTIVITY	MINUTES OR STEPS
MILK, YOGURT, AND CHEESE ☐ ☐ ☐	(M)	
MEAT, POULTRY, ETC. ☐ ☐ ☐	(TU)	
FRUITS ☐ ☐ ☐ ☐	(W)	
VEGETABLES ☐ ☐ ☐ ☐ ☐	(TH)	
BREADS, CEREALS, ETC. ☐ ☐ ☐ ☐ ☐ ☐ ☐ ☐	(F)	
SERVINGS OF WATER (8 OZ) ☐ ☐ ☐ ☐ ☐ ☐ ☐ ☐	(SA)	
	(SU)	

LESSON SEVEN

W e are now far enough into The LEARN Program to reflect on what you have learned, the behaviors you have practiced, and the new outlook on diet and lifestyle changes we have been discussing. Have some of the techniques become habits? Is this a program you can live with? These are the key questions you must consider for the long-term outlook. We have many interesting topics to discuss in this lesson. So, let's begin the lesson with a word about your thoughts.

Thinking Your Way to Success

**TAPE 3
SECTION 1**

I cannot overstate how important your thoughts are. Your thoughts will determine how you feel about yourself, which in turn affects your mood, your interactions with others, and your interpretation of your progress in the program.

People in weight management programs share some common ways of thinking. Examples are expecting too much, being upset with anything less than perfection, and letting small mistakes build to catastrophe. I have seen these take root in hundreds of people. They get in the way, can sour a person's outlook, and can be difficult to change. My job is to help you pull these out by the roots and plant more constructive thoughts in their place. This may sound puzzling to do, but stay with me and I'll explain.

Your Thinking Process

**TAPE 2
SECTION 3**

I discussed goal setting in Lesson Four and concluded that setting unrealistic goals can halt your progress. It is time to explore this matter further. We set goals for everything we do. Although we do not articulate a goal for every activity, hidden within our mind are expectations of how well we should perform. If you mow the lawn, write a letter, buy clothes, or simply talk to a friend, you expect a certain level of performance. If you scalped the lawn, wrote an unintelligible letter, bought gaudy clothes, or said insensitive things to your friend, you would be upset because you expected more—you did not satisfy your internal standard.

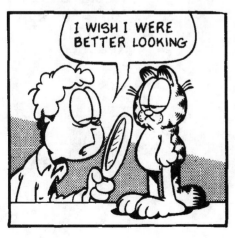

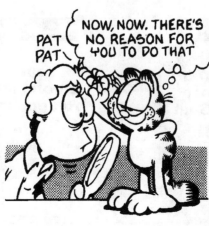

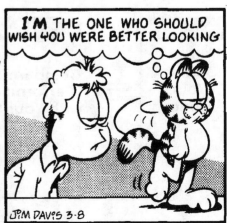

99

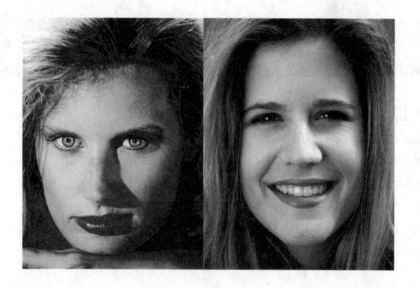

met, the negative emotional response can send your progress into a tailspin.

This occurs in a three-part process. Setting the goals comes first and is often unconscious. You then compare actual performance to that goal. Finally, there is a positive emotional reaction if the goal is achieved and a negative one if it is not. The model below shows this three-step process.

The table on the top of page 101 has a few examples of how this process pertains to weight management goals. These are common examples, so while you are reading, think if these or similar situations occur with you.

This emotional response is what worries me. Many people have enough trouble controlling their eating and exercise without the extra burden of negative feelings and thoughts. You can change the emotional response by altering the two steps that precede it, namely the goal setting and the comparison you make to the goals.

When you have negative feelings, examine them and trace them to the goals you set. If you

"By changing unrealistic goals, you can feel good about your progress."

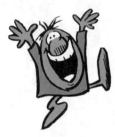

You can see how difficult life would be if your goals were absurdly out of reach. If you expected *Better Homes and Gardens* to lust after your lawn, for the National Archives to enshrine your letter, for a famous designer to covet your clothes, or for your friend to memorialize your words in a book of quotes, you would be crushed by what is otherwise an acceptable performance. Unfortunately, it is just such out-of-reach goals that people losing weight tend to set for themselves about their eating, exercise, and weight loss. When the goals are not

Measuring Up to Your Own Goals

Step 1

Setting Your Goals

⇒

Step 2

Compare Your Performance with Your Goal

⇒

Step 3

Your Emotional Response

Positive if Goal Is Reached +

Negative if Goal Is NOT Reached –

Setting Goal	Comparing Performance	Emotional Response
Will never cheat on a program	Cheating on program does occur	Guilt and resignation
Will be good at sports	Others do better and look better	Embarrassment
Will lose weight each week	Some weeks weight stays stable or goes up	Discouragement and self-blame

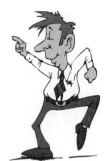

"Goal setting is an ongoing process that is crucial to your weight management program."

feel guilty because you sneak a Snickers, think about your goal, which is probably something like, "I should never cheat on this program." You can examine the comparison to this goal by understanding that you or anyone else could never be satisfied with this as a standard. This will change the emotional response.

Below are the same situations with different goals, comparisons, and emotional responses. Use these examples to analyze your own goals, comparisons, and responses. This can lift the weight of negative feelings from your shoulders.

Shopping for Food

Let's look back on the ABC approach introduced in Lesson Four. The "A" refers to the antecedents that set the stage for eating. One important antecedent is shopping for food. If you buy good foods, you will eat good foods. This may sound obvious, but too few people plan their shopping accordingly.

Having problem foods available in the house, office, car, briefcase, purse, or pocket can be asking for trouble, even if you vow to "eat only a little." If something threatens your restraint, say fatigue or boredom, you can pay a dear price for the decision you made hours or days earlier to buy the food. On the other hand, if your refrigerator resembles a salad bar because of wise shopping, weakened restraint can inflict only minor damage. You can use several clever methods while shopping to make prudent food choices.

⇨ **Shop on a full stomach**. When you are hungry, it is easy to buy impulsively because everything looks appetizing. An innocent trip to the store to buy a few essentials can become an eating excursion. The supermarket to a hungry person is like water to someone stranded in the Sahara. The stores are designed to tempt you. Your restraint is high when you first walk in, but little good it does when you are in the produce section! As you move through the store, your restrain weakens just as you pass the cookie aisle. Desire reaches its peak as you travel down Dessert Lane (the frozen food and ice cream section). Shop only af-

Setting Goal	Comparing Performance	Emotional Response
Will follow the program as much as possible	Meet goal on most occasions	Satisfaction and desire to do better
Will increase level of exercise	Increase is steady and substantial	Pride in doing something positive
Will lose weight most weeks	Lose weight 10 out of 12 weeks	Feel good about hard work

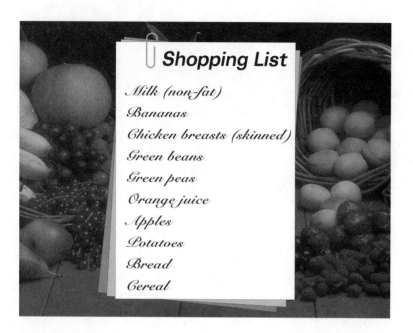

Shopping List

Milk (non-fat)
Bananas
Chicken breasts (skinned)
Green beans
Green peas
Orange juice
Apples
Potatoes
Bread
Cereal

"When you shop for food use a list and buy food that requires preparation."

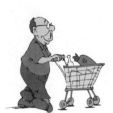

A Shopping Partnership

Partners can often help with your food shopping. There are several ways to do this, as discussed below. If your partner is also on a program, you can swap shopping duties. If not, the partner can help you shop in exchange for favors from you. This was the case with Tom and Sheila. On Saturdays, Tom did yard work while Sheila (the one on a weight loss program) did the food shopping. Sheila had trouble with impulse buying because food beckoned her like the sea nymph sirens beckoned Odysseus. They switched tasks, so Tom did the shopping and Sheila did the yard work. This even added some lifestyle activity to Sheila's routine. Here are a few examples of putting the partnership to work.

⇨ **Shop with a partner**. Shopping can become a social event if your partner journeys with you to the supermarket. You can resist the goodies if you know someone has their eye on your cart. Your partner could help you design your shopping list and could carry it in the store.

⇨ **Switch tasks with your partner.** This is what Tom and Sheila did in the example earlier. Your partner may be willing to do the shopping in exchange for help with another job.

⇨ **Swap shopping duties with your partner**. If your partner is on a program, trade shopping lists. You do your partner's shopping and your partner can do yours. Unless your partner stuffs your bag with treats, you will come away with the foods you need.

The Role of Fat in Your Diet

Fat is what it's all about, right? You want to eat less fat and get rid of body fat. How are dietary fat and body fat different, and what role should fat play in your diet? You might think that fat is just what we see on meats and that it

ter you have eaten. You will be surprised at how much grief this can prevent.

⇨ **Shop from a list**. Prepare a shopping list before you leave the house, and shop only from the list. Decide what to buy *before* you are tempted by the foods in the store. Make the list when you are not hungry.

⇨ **Buy foods that require preparation**. With this age of prepackaged foods, microwave ovens, and fast-food restaurants, you can eat at an instant's notice. Eating requires little thought and can be done impulsively. Buying foods that require preparation can halt this process.

Let's use an example of a common food. If you have a hankering for fried chicken, you could visit the Colonel and procure 1000 calories in an extra crispy three-piece dinner. Little time would separate craving and consumption. If you chose the preparation route, you would buy a whole chicken, cut it, prepare it, then fry it. You could think about how much you wanted the chicken and might eat less (if you eat it at all). In addition, preparing the chicken yourself would give you the option of baking it, which would result in far fewer calories than deep frying.

goes right to our store of body fat. The picture is more complex and very interesting.

The Importance of Fat

Fat plays an important role in everyone's diet and has received a lot of attention lately due to its association with heart disease and cancer. Dietary fat provides *essential* fatty acids that carry fat soluble vitamins (A, D, E, and K) throughout the body and a *semi-essential* fatty acid that helps to prevent growth deficiencies and builds the membranes of cell walls. Fat in your body protects vital organs and prevents excessive heat loss. Fat is also a valuable source of energy, particularly for endurance activities; carbohydrate is used for quick energy. Fat also provides flavoring in many of the foods we eat.

Our bodies can manufacture many of the essential fatty acids we need from carbohydrate or protein, however, there are some that it cannot make—these must be included in the food that we eat. The fat we eat is a combination of fatty acids and glycerol. All fats in foods are mixtures of three types of fatty acids: saturated, monounsaturated, and polyunsaturated. The fatty acids consist of carbon atoms that are attached to oxygen and hydrogen atoms. Each carbon atom has four possible binding sites. When the hydrogen/oxygen atoms are attached to all four binding sites, the fatty acid is *saturated* (i.e., the carbon atom is saturated with the maximum number of hydrogen/oxygen atoms). When the hydrogen/oxygen atoms are attached to less than all four binding sites, the fatty acid is said to be *unsaturated*. You can visually identify saturated fats because they are usually solid at room temperature and come primarily from meat and dairy products, although they are also found in some vegetable fats, such as coconut, palm, and palm kernel oils.

When two nearby carbon atoms are each missing one molecule from one of their four binding sites, a double bond can be formed between the two atoms. When this happens the fat is considered to be *monounsaturated*. Monounsaturated fats are found mainly in olive, pea-

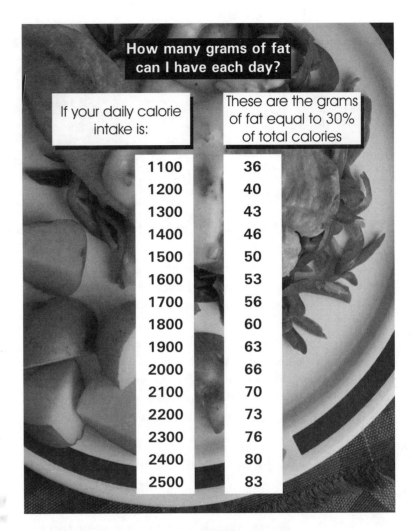

How many grams of fat can I have each day?

If your daily calorie intake is:	These are the grams of fat equal to 30% of total calories
1100	36
1200	40
1300	43
1400	46
1500	50
1600	53
1700	56
1800	60
1900	63
2000	66
2100	70
2200	73
2300	76
2400	80
2500	83

nut, and canola oils. If more than one double bond is formed, the fat is said to be *polyunsaturated*. Polyunsaturated fats are generally liquid or soft at room temperature and are found mainly in safflower, sunflower, corn, soybean, and cottonseed oils and some fish.

This distinction between saturated and unsaturated fats is important for health reasons. Again, the saturated fats are easy to distinguish because they are usually solid at room temperature and come primarily from animal sources (butter, lard, meat). High consumption of these fats has been associated with heart disease and is likely related to increased risk for colon and breast cancers.

On the other hand, monounsaturated and polyunsaturated fats are usually liquid or soft at room temperature and are from vegetable

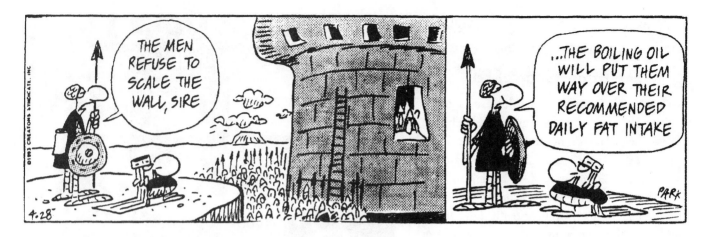

sources (vegetable oils, margarine). These are generally healthier than the saturated fats. This is why so many people have switched from butter to margarine, reduced their intake of high-fat meats like beef and pork, and cook more with vegetable oils. The best unsaturated oils are corn, soy, sunflower, and safflower (the most highly unsaturated oil). A noteworthy point is that all fats contain the same number of calories.

How Much Fat Should I Eat?

There are three basic facts to remember for your diet. The first is that fat provides a lot of energy, which is bad news for a person trying to lose weight. Fat contains twice the calories (nine per gram) of either protein or carbohydrate. You will get more calories from the fat on a single steak than from an equal amount of pure sugar.

Second, the amount of fat you eat is associated with risk for several serious diseases. The average American gets close to 40 percent of total calories from fat. This is 10 percent above the recommended limits of no more than 30 percent of total calories from fat. The chart on page 103 provides the grams of fat for different calorie levels that equal 30 percent of the calorie levels. Saturated fat should be limited to less that 10 percent of calories, or about one-third of total fat intake. Reducing your fat intake should help with weight and with general health.

Third, I mentioned earlier that fat calories are more easily converted to body fat than are calories from other sources. Therefore, keeping

Calculating My Daily Fat Intake		
(Example)		
Total Daily Calorie Intake (calories)		1500
Target Percentage of Total Calories	x	30%
Daily Calories from Fat		450
Number of Calories in One Gram of Fat	÷	9
Daily Grams of Fat		50

Calculating My Daily Fat Intake		
Total Daily Calorie Intake (calories)		_____
Target Percentage of Total Calories	x	_____
Daily Calories from Fat		
Number of Calories in One Gram of Fat	÷	_____
Daily Grams of Fat		_____

Fat from the Different Food Group Choices

Foods	Servings	Grams of Fat
Fats, Oils, and Sweets		
Butter, margarine, 1t	–	4
Chocolate bar, 1 oz	–	9
Cola, 12 fl. oz	–	0
Cream cheese, 1 oz	–	10
Fruit drink, 12 fl oz	–	0
Fruit sorbet, ½ cup	–	0
Gelatin dessert, ½ cup	–	0
Mayonnaise, 1T	–	11
Salad dressing, 1T	–	7
Salad dressing, reduced calorie 1T	–	A
Sherbet, ½ cup	–	2
Sour cream, 2T	–	6
Sugar, jam, jelly, 1t	–	0
Milk, Yogurt, and Cheese Group		
Cheese, cottage 4 percent fat, ½ cup	¼	5
Cheese, process, 2 oz	1	18
Cheese, Mozzarella, part skim, 1 ½ oz	1	10
Cheese, natural, cheddar, 1 ½ oz	1	14
Ice cream, ½ cup	⅓	7
Ice milk, ½ cup	⅓	3
Milk, chocolate 2 percent, 1 cup	1	4
Milk, low-fat, 2 percent, 1 cup	1	5
Milk, skim, 1 cup	1	Trace
Milk, whole, 1 cup	1	8
Yogurt, frozen, ½ cup	½	2
Yogurt, non-fat plain, 8 oz	1	Trace
Yogurt, low-fat fruit, 8 oz	1	3
Yogurt, low-fat plain, 8 oz	1	4
Meat, Poultry, Fish, Dry Beans, Eggs, and Nuts Group		
Beef, ground, lean, cooked	3 oz[B]	16
Bologna, 2 slices	1 oz[B]	16
Chicken, with skin, fried	3 oz[B]	13
Dry beans and peas, cooked, ½ cup	1 oz[B]	Trace
Egg, 1	1 oz[B]	5

Foods	Servings	Grams of Fat
Lean meat, poultry, fish, cooked,	3 oz	6
Peanut butter, 2T	1 oz[B]	16
Nuts, ⅓ cup	1 oz[B]	22
Vegetable Group		
French fries, 10	1	8
Potatoes, scalloped, ½ cup	1	4
Potato salad, ½ cup	1	8
Vegetables, cooked, ½ cup	1	Trace
Vegetables, leafy, raw, 1 cup	1	Trace
Vegetables, non leafy, raw, chopped, ½ cup	1	Trace
Fruit Group		
Avocado, ¼ whole	1	9
Fruit juice, unsweetened, ¾ cup	1	Trace
Fruit, raw or canned, ½ cup	1	Trace
Whole fruit: medium apple, orange, banana	1	Trace
Bread, Cereal, Rice, and Pasta Group		
Bread, 1 slice	1	1
Breakfast cereal, 1 oz	1	A
Cake, frosted, 1/16 average	1	13
Cookies, 2 medium	2	19
Crackers, plain, small, 3–4	1	3
Croissant, 1 large (2 oz)	2	12
Danish, 1 medium (2 oz)	2	13
Doughnut, 1 medium (2 oz)		11
Hamburger roll, bagel, English muffin, 1	2	2
Pancakes, 4" diameter, 2	2	3
Pie, fruit, 2-crust, 1/6 8" pie	2	19
Rice, pasta, cooked, ½ cup	1	Trace
Tortilla, 1	1	3

A Check product label.

B Serving sizes vary with the type of food and the meal.

Source: Adapted from Home and Garden Bulletin Number 252, U.S. Department of Agriculture, 1992.

The Food Guide Pyramid

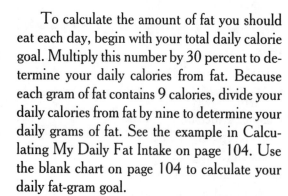

Fats, Oils, & Sweets
Use Sparingly

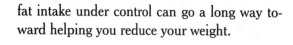

Key
○ Fat (naturally occurring and added)
▼ Sugars (added)
These symbols show fat and added sugars in foods.

Fats, Oils, & Sweets
Use Sparingly

Milk, Yogurt, & Cheese Group
2 - 3 Servings

Meat, Poultry, Fish, Dry Beans, Eggs, & Nuts Group
2 - 3 Servings

Vegetable Group
3 - 5 Servings

Fruit Group
2 - 4 Servings

Bread, Cereal, Rice, & Pasta Group
6 - 11 Servings

"Dietary fat should be eaten sparingly. Keep an eye out for the hidden fat in foods."

fat intake under control can go a long way toward helping you reduce your weight.

To calculate the amount of fat you should eat each day, begin with your total daily calorie goal. Multiply this number by 30 percent to determine your daily calories from fat. Because each gram of fat contains 9 calories, divide your daily calories from fat by nine to determine your daily grams of fat. See the example in Calculating My Daily Fat Intake on page 104. Use the blank chart on page 104 to calculate your daily fat-gram goal.

Sources of Fat

We generally don't realize how much fat we eat. About 60 percent of the fat we eat cannot be seen (hidden fat) because it is contained in other food products, such as meat, cheese, nuts, breads, etc. In determining the amount of fat in your diet, it is important to account for both visible and hidden fat.

The chart on page 105 provides you with a sampling of foods from the five food groups of the Food Guide Pyramid. This chart includes the number of servings of each food and the

amount of fat for each. Use this chart along with a calorie guide to help you reduce your dietary fat.

Dietary Fat Adds Up

The fat in some foods adds up quickly. As mentioned earlier, fat contains more than twice the calories of protein or carbohydrate. One gram of fat has 9 calories, whereas 1 gram of carbohydrate or protein has only 4 calories. One teaspoon (one pat) of butter or margarine has 4 grams of fat; that's 36 calories of fat for every teaspoon. It is important to watch out for those extras that contain high amounts of fat. For example, a bologna-and-cheese sandwich made with two slices (2 oz) of bologna, two slices (2 oz) of cheese, and 2 teaspoons of mayonnaise, counts up to about 36 grams of fat, approximately 324 calories. A similar sandwich, however, made with lean beef, lettuce, tomato, and low-fat mayonnaise, and served with a cup of nonfat milk instead of cheese, has only about 6 grams of fat, or 54 calories.

Reducing the Fat in Your Diet

There are many tips available for lowering the amount of dietary fat we eat every day. The first step is to determine a target intake of fat as we did in the calculation on page 104. Next, you should become aware of the fat content of the foods that you eat. In addition to reading food labels, there are many good books available that can help you. Here are some additional tips that will help you decrease the level of fat in your diet.

From the Milk, Yogurt, and Cheese Group

Use skim or low-fat milk (2 grams of fat per serving) instead of whole milk (16 grams of fat per serving) for drinking as well as cooking. Also, use nonfat or low-fat fruit yogurt (2 grams of fat per serving) over whole-milk yogurt (7 grams of fat per serving). Frozen yogurt or ice milk (2 to 3 grams of fat per ½ cup) is a nice substitute for ice cream (7 grams).

From the Meat, Poultry, Fish, Dry Beans, Eggs, and Nuts Group

Eat modest portions of meat, poultry, and fish. Three cooked ounces is the recommended portion size. Choose lean cuts of meat, such as sirloin tip and round steak, and choose lean and extra lean ground beef, center cut ham, loin chops, and tenderloin. Limit your use of processed meats that tend to be high in fat. When in doubt, read the food label. If the fat content is not listed on the food product, be extra cautious. If cholesterol is a problem, limit your use of organ meats (liver, kidneys, brains, etc.) and limit the number of egg yolks to three or less per week. Legumes (dried beans and peas) are good alternative sources of protein and have little or no fat. Use them in mixed dishes instead of meat, or combine them with a small portion of meat or poultry.

From the Vegetable and Fruit Groups

Fruits and vegetables provide a good supply of fiber, vitamins, and minerals—all with low fat and no cholesterol. Use them generously at mealtime and for snacks. For both cooked and fresh vegetables (including salads) try seasonings and substitute flavorings, such as herbs, spices, or a splash of lemon instead of butter or salad dressings. Remember, there are 4 grams of fat in each teaspoon of butter, margarine, or mayonnaise. Cutting out the salad dressing can save up to 9 grams of fat for each tablespoon.

From the Bread, Cereal, Rice, and Pasta Group

Use rice, pasta, and other grain products as the mainstay of a low-fat eating plan. Small portions of meat, fish, and poultry go a long way when combined with grain products. Eating whole-grain products will help you maximize your intake of fiber and other nutrients. Choose a dinner roll (2 grams of fat) rather than a croissant (12 grams of fat).

Cooking Tips to Reduce Fat

Trim away all visible fat from meat before cooking. Remove skin and fat from chicken and turkey before cooking. Use nonstick pans and sprays for cooking. In sauces, salads, and soups, substitute low-fat or nonfat plain yogurt for sour cream or mayonnaise. Broil or bake meats instead of frying.

Fat in Snacks and Desserts

Eat plenty of fresh fruit and vegetables every day. Pop popcorn in a microwave or air popper. To add flavor, spray the popcorn lightly with hot vegetable oil or vegetable spray and add seasoning salts. Sorbet, flavored ice, and frozen fruit bars are a nice snack. Danish, doughnuts, cookies, and frosted cakes are high in fat and should be eaten sparingly. Also, potato chips and other crunchy snacks are often high in dietary fat. Be sure to read the food label for the fat content of these foods.

Planning Healthy Meals

Many excellent resources are available for planning healthy meals. These include cookbooks and guides for buying, preparing, and serving healthy foods. These are handy aids because losing weight conjures up impressions of deprivation and boring food. A trip to the bookstore can help prevent this boredom. The fol-

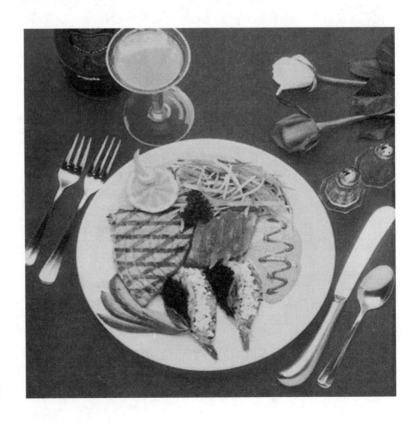

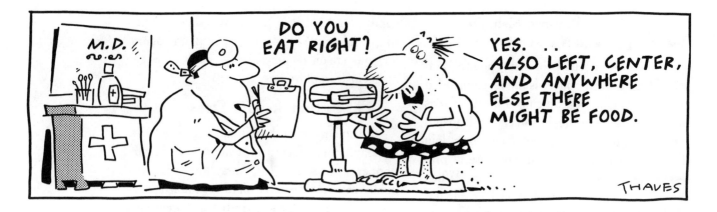

lowing books are filled with ideas and recipes that can help you eat delicious foods while reducing calories, fat, sodium, cholesterol, and increasing fiber. Get those taste buds ready!

American Heart Association Quick and Easy Cookbook. New York: McKay, 1998.

Better Homes and Gardens Low Fat, Bold Flavors. Des Moines, Iowa: Meredith, 1999.

Betty Crocker's New Choices: A Fresh Approach to Eating Well. Foster City, Calif.: IDG Books Worldwide, 1999.

Cooking Light Annual Recipes 1999. Oxmoor House, 1999. 1–800–633–4910 to order.

Cooking Light 2000: Annual Recipes. Oxmoor House, 1999. 1–800–633–4910 to order.

Fat Free Living Cookbook From Around the World. Scottsdale Ariz.: Fat Free Living, 1999.

Light Basics Cookbook. New York: William Morrow & Co., 1999.

Quick & Easy Menus: More Than 130 Low-Fat Recipes. Oxmoor House, 2000. 1–800–633–4910 to order.

5 Ingredient 15 Minute Cookbook: Cooking Light. Oxmoor House, 1999. 1–800–633–4910 to order.

Impressive Reasons to Be Active

TAPE 2
SECTION 6

Previously, I mentioned that people who are regularly active tend to lose weight better over the long term. Scientists have used nearly every known psychological and medical test to predict who will lose weight and keep it off. The most consistent finding is that exercise is associated with weight maintenance. In addition, some impressive new studies suggest that regular physical activity may even increase our learning ability.

Weight Maintenance

An impressive example of the research on this topic is a study by Kayman, Bruvold, and Stern published in the *American Journal of Clinical Nutrition.* They studied people in a large Health Maintenance Organization who had taken part in a weight loss program. Many months after the program, the individuals were contacted to see what distinguished those who had maintained their weight loss from those who regained.

As the graph on page 109 shows, exercise was a key factor. Of those who maintained their weight loss, 92 percent were getting regular physical activity. Only 34 percent of the regainers were exercising.

The effect of physical activity on weight maintenance could occur in many ways. There may be physical effects on metabolism or other factors, but almost certainly the psychological

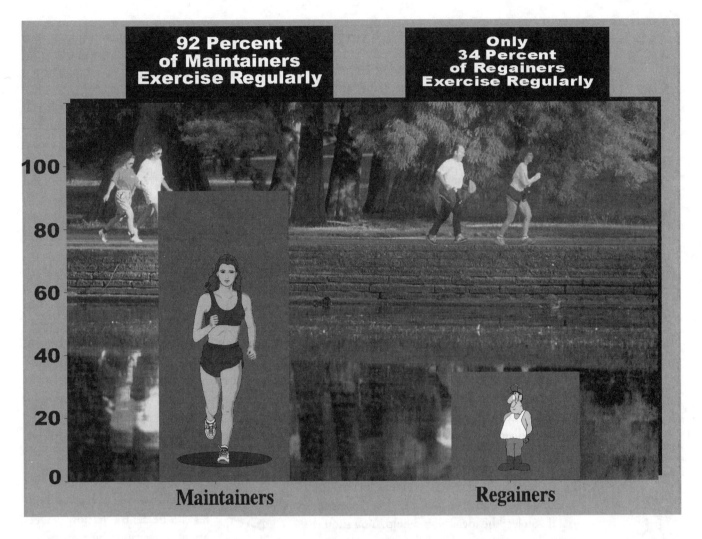

advantages of activity are operating. When you are active, even in a modest way, you are doing something positive—you are making a statement to yourself that you are committed to lifestyle change. This goes a long way in making you feel good and in boosting your confidence for weight management. So, if you are in this for the long run, regular physical activity is one of the best companions you can have.

Learning Ability

Some new and very exciting studies now suggest that regular physical activity can have a positive impact on the brain. Although more research needs to be done, this is very exciting news. In studies with both humans and animals, researchers have found that exercise increases learning ability, improves mood, and keeps brains cells alive longer. Exercise increases blood flow to the brain as well as the levels of a brain-cell growth hormone. This stimulates the growth of new brain neurons while prolonging the survival of existing brain cells. The researchers found that the new brain neurons develop in the part of the brain responsible for new memory.

I cannot emphasize enough the importance of regular physical activity. I hope that you have increased your activity level since beginning this program and that you are now feeling the positive effects of a more active lifestyle. The evidence is now overwhelming that physical activity is both a powerful weight management tool and an important instrument of overall well-being and good health.

Continuing Walking and Lifestyle Activity

Let's review your progress with walking and lifestyle activity. This is a good time to look back at the section on the "Benefits of Exercise" from Lesson Two. As you may recall, being active brings many physical and emotional benefits. Two of the most important benefits, at this stage of your program, are that exercise may help control appetite and may bolster self-confidence.

Remember that exercise is one predictor of who will keep weight off over the long run. On average, people who exercise are more likely to maintain their weight loss long after a program ends. There are exceptions, however. Some people exercise and do not lose weight, and others lose weight without exercising. Where you fit in this scheme may not be evident for many months, but increasing your activity now may pay nice dividends later.

"Continuing your walking program and other lifestyle activity is a key ingredient of your weight management program."

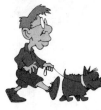

How much are you walking, and do you enjoy it? Lesson Five contained ideas for making walking pleasurable, so please review that material if you feel the ideas would help. You should be walking between 15 and 60 minutes each day. It is best to walk as much as possible without feeling discomfort. If you tire from walking, take several short walks rather than one long

one. Having two brisk 30-minute walks or four 15-minute walks can help you as much as an hour walk in a single bout.

What types of lifestyle activities have you been doing? Have you found opportunities to use stairs, to park some distance from your destination, or to do some extra walking? These lifestyle activities are nice because they remind you that you are doing something positive.

One reason I use the term *lifestyle* activity is the hope of developing permanent habits. Each trip up the stairs may not make you lose a pound, but summed over many days, months, or years, the effect can be powerful. New habits can be difficult to acquire, so it is important to practice and then practice some more. Some of my clients say they now search out stairs wherever they go and feel that an opportunity is missed when they must use an elevator or escalator.

Your Body and Your Self-Esteem

**TAPE 4
SECTION 1**

How we feel about our bodies can be central to how we feel about ourselves. Our view of our own body is called body image, and unfortunately, body image is negative for most people, especially for women and people who are overweight. This is not surprising considering the enormous pressure in our society to be thin and for women to be valued for how they look rather than for who they are as people. Many, many people internalize these social norms, find a major difference between the way they look and the way they think they should look, and then hurt themselves emotionally as a result. It really isn't fair, because the social norms present an ideal that is unrealistic and even unhealthy.

Let's look at how this might work for a young woman; I'll call her Ann. As Ann approaches puberty, she is full of energy, is athletic, enjoys being active, has fun, and takes pleasure in what her body can do for her. Yet,

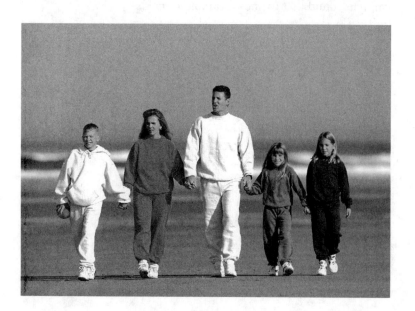

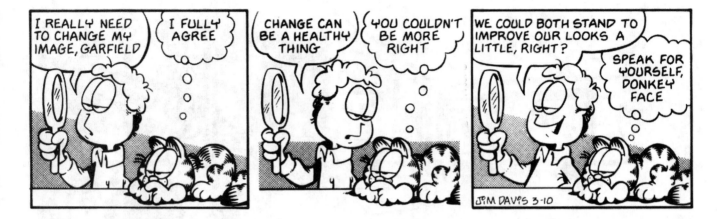

she is increasingly aware of the need to be thin. She is not prepared for this pressure to be so intense at the very time puberty causes her body to deposit more fat. Instead of accepting and enjoying the changes in her body, she feels her body is betraying her. Natural processes like eating and exercise become a battleground. She must restrict what she eats and must now exercise, not for fun, but for the purpose of losing weight. Ann may enter into a fight with her own body that will never end.

As Ann enters her 20s and then passes the 30-, 40-, and 50-year benchmarks, two things are likely to happen. One is that she will be dissatisfied with her body. She will overlook its virtues—that it allows her to be active, to move places, and to feel sensual. Instead, she will focus on the disparity between ideal and actual and will feel it is her fault that she does not look perfect.

The second event is that Ann will let her body image have too much impact on her self-esteem. Our self-esteem is made up of how we evaluate ourselves on many dimensions (as a parent, child, brother or sister, employer or employee, friend, etc.). Our looks influence us all, but for some people, appearance creeps into the heart of self-esteem. It can crowd out other positive influences, so that no matter how good we are at other things, there is always this looming matter of how we look.

Having a Positive Body Image

Having a positive view of your body, no matter how imperfect, is really important. If you dislike how you look and accept society's unrealistic beauty standards, you will be unhappy with what you accomplish in this program or any others. The risk is that you will make very positive changes in eating, activity, and weight, but feel you are still far from your goal and, therefore, will despair over your lack of success. This is a setup for disappointment, frustration, and giving up.

The Body Image Workbook, written by Dr. Thomas F. Cash for the general public, is an excellent book on this topic. The book is published by New Harbinger Publications and can be purchased by calling 1–800–736–7323. The book contains many good ideas for evaluating how we feel about our bodies, how this affects the way we feel about ourselves in general, and how we can respond.

In his book, Cash discusses fundamental assumptions people make about their appearance and their lives. Some of these are shown in the table on page 113, "Faulty Assumptions about Appearance."

These assumptions lead to an overestimation of how appearance governs one's life and to an overemphasis on changing appearance to improve well-being. With these common assumptions, a person can be continually dissatis-

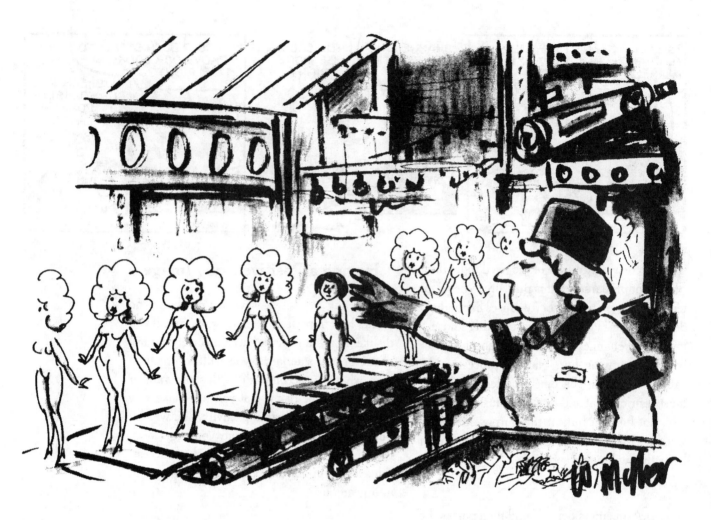

fied with his or her appearance, and no weight loss is enough.

So, what can you do to be happier about the way you look? The book by Cash includes exercises and ways to evaluate whether your body image is changing. Here are some ideas that may be helpful.

⇨ **Get accustomed to seeing your body**. Most people who do not like their bodies do everything they can to avoid looking at them. Mirrors, especially full-length mirrors, store windows, and other places are avoided. Stop avoiding and find a way to believe that your body can be your friend.

⇨ **Challenge the faulty assumptions about appearance and life**. To equate appearance with happiness is to give the body much more power than it deserves. You can be a smashing success at many

things in life (most notably being a good person), irrespective of appearance. Appearance is only one aspect of our lives.

⇨ **Confront what is realistic for you as an individual**. Given what you have looked like during your adult life, given how your parents looked, and given how difficult it might be for you to lose to an "ideal" weight, be candid, and consider how you might "realistically" look. Perhaps you can do more, perhaps not.

⇨ **Uncouple body image from self-esteem**. The assumption that how you look is who you are can be very damaging.

⇨ **Focus on how your body is a gift**. Your body can do many fine things for you. It allows you to live, to move, to accomplish what you'd like, not to mention how good it feels when you relax, work out, and engage

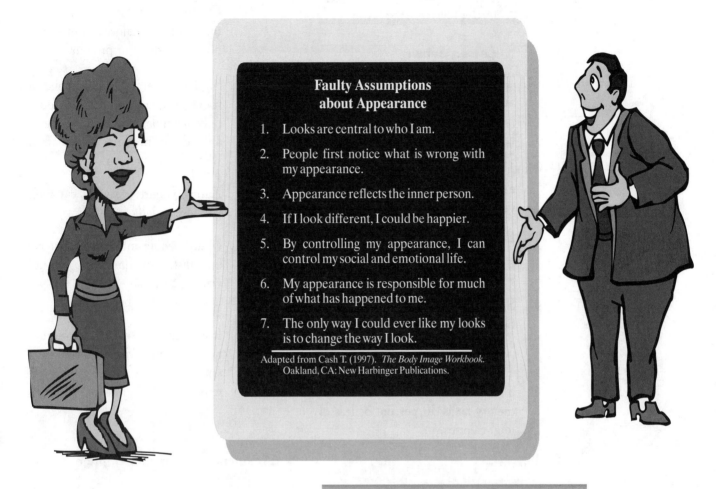

**Faulty Assumptions
about Appearance**

1. Looks are central to who I am.

2. People first notice what is wrong with my appearance.

3. Appearance reflects the inner person.

4. If I look different, I could be happier.

5. By controlling my appearance, I can control my social and emotional life.

6. My appearance is responsible for much of what has happened to me.

7. The only way I could ever like my looks is to change the way I look.

Adapted from Cash T. (1997). *The Body Image Workbook.* Oakland, CA: New Harbinger Publications.

in sensual activities with another person. The body gives you many gifts of living and is, therefore, a gift itself. If you focus on the virtues of your body, it becomes less of an adversary. Being friends with your body is central to your long-term happiness.

None of these will be easy, because how you feel about yourself is the product of years and years of experiences, thoughts, attitudes, and feelings. Just vowing to be happier with the way you look is not enough. You must challenge the faulty assumptions constantly. You must make a concerted effort to reward yourself for looking good, and then practice this new way of thinking for days, weeks, and months. It takes a lot to undo the powerful messages you have been exposed to, so please keep at it. You deserve to feel good about yourself, no matter what you weigh.

My Personal Goals for This Week

Your monitoring form contains entries from the new behaviors discussed above. The first three relate to changes with shopping: shop on a full stomach, shop from a list, and buy foods that require preparation. This is also the time to examine your goals and emotions. Your nutrition goal for the week will be to keep your fat intake to 30 percent or less of total daily calories. Challenge the faulty assumptions you have about your body. And, of course, set goals in other areas that you feel are important (an activity goal, a nutrition goal, etc.). Don't forget to record your weight change on the Weight Change Record in Lesson One on page 25. Good luck this week!

My Self-Assessment

Lesson Seven

T F 44. Thoughts and attitudes often occur automatically when we are confronted by certain situations and cannot be changed.

T F 45. It is wise to shop for food when you are hungry to test the new restraint you have learned.

T F 46. Buying foods that require preparation can increase your awareness of eating and help you eat less.

T F 47. Since too much dietary fat has been linked to heart disease and other health-related risks, it's best to eliminate all fat from your diet.

T F 48. The recommended daily intake of dietary fat is 30 percent or less of total calories.

T F 49. One gram of fat contains more than twice the calories of one gram of carbohydrate or protein.

T F 50. Saturated fat is usually solid at room temperature and is found only in animal foods, such as meats and dairy products made from whole milk or cream.

T F 51. Eating yogurt everyday can help you lose weight.

T F 52. Many people internalize society's unrealistic standards for beauty, weight, and shape and are likely to have a negative body image.

T F 53. It is possible to weight more than the ideal, and even be fairly heavy, and still have good self-esteem and reasonable body image.

(Answers in Appendix C, page 271)

Monitoring Form—Lesson Seven *Today's Date:* _____

TIME	FOOD AND AMOUNT	CALORIES
TOTAL DAILY CALORIES		

PERSONAL GOALS FOR THIS WEEK	MOST OF THE TIME	SOME-TIMES	RARELY
1. SHOP ON A FULL STOMACH			
2. SHOP FROM A LIST			
3. BUY FOODS THAT REQUIRE PREPARATION			
4. CHALLENGE FAULTY APPEARANCE ASSUMPTIONS			
5. EAT LESS THAN _____ CALORIES PER DAY			
6. EAT LESS THAN _____ GRAMS OF FAT EACH DAY			

FOOD GROUPS FOR TODAY	PHYSICAL ACTIVITY	MINUTES OR STEPS
MILK, YOGURT, AND CHEESE ☐ ☐ ☐	(M)	
MEAT, POULTRY, ETC. ☐ ☐ ☐	(Tu)	
FRUITS ☐ ☐ ☐ ☐	(W)	
VEGETABLES ☐ ☐ ☐ ☐ ☐	(Th)	
BREADS, CEREALS, ETC. ☐ ☐ ☐ ☐ ☐ ☐ ☐ ☐	(F)	
SERVINGS OF WATER (8 OZ) ☐ ☐ ☐ ☐ ☐ ☐ ☐ ☐	(Sa)	
	(Su)	

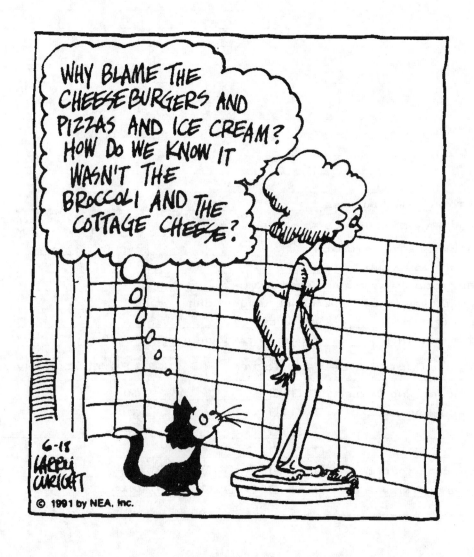

I have spoken mainly of walking thus far, but there are many other activities you might like to try. Having several activities available increases the chance that being active will be fun, and having fun is one key to making physical activity a permanent part of your life. I'll introduce you to a new activity formula for all Americans. In this lesson, we begin our discussion of the different type of nutrients in the foods we eat and look at the Milk, Yogurt, and Cheese Group of the Food Guide Pyramid. Also in this lesson, I will speak about storing food to help you keep temptation under control. The topic of Attitudes comes up as I talk about a specific area of attitude change, something I call internal attitude traps. Here I begin to show you how to challenge thoughts that hold you back and replace them with positive ways of thinking. We have a lot to cover in this lesson, but it is all very interesting.

A New Activity Formula for Americans

TAPE 3
SECTION 3

The work of experts in the exercise field has provided a growing body of evidence that regular, moderate-intensity physical activity can result in substantial health benefits. One of the primary benefits is protection against coronary heart disease. Other health benefits may include protection against several other chronic diseases, such as adult-onset diabetes, hypertension, certain cancers, osteoporosis, and depression.

While most of us would readily agree that regular physical activity is beneficial, most of us

are not physically active on a regular basis. Only about 22 percent of adults in this country engage in leisure time physical activity. About 24 percent of adults are completely sedentary, and the remaining 54 percent are inadequately active. They too would benefit from more regular physical activity. With all of this scientific evidence, why are we a nation of inactivity? Two reasons come to mind.

We live in a high-tech society. The more technologically advanced we become, the more inactive we become. Cars, garage-door openers, portable telephones, television, remote controls for most electrical devices, and many other labor-saving gadgets have changed the way we

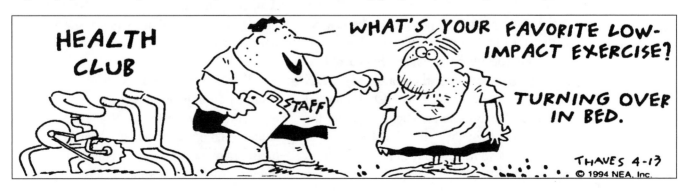

"Most people do not get enough exercise."

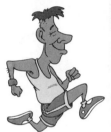

Fitness in America

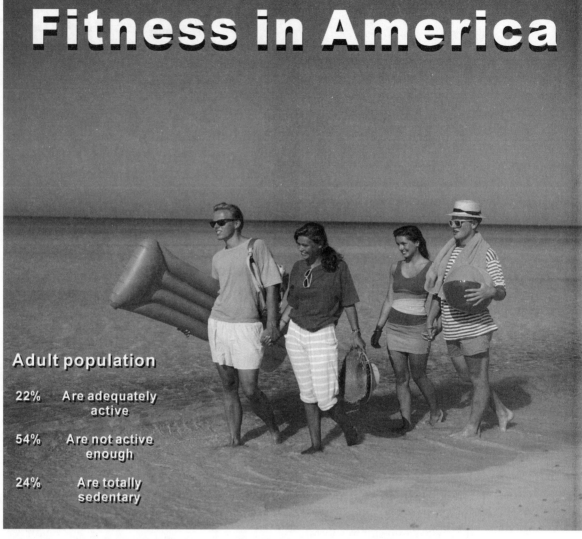

Adult population

22% Are adequately active

54% Are not active enough

24% Are totally sedentary

work, take care of our homes, and use our leisure time. Technology entices us to be inactive. Further, our environment presents many obstacles and barriers to physical activity. Walking to the corner store is difficult if there are not adequate sidewalks, and riding a bicycle or walking to work is difficult because people living in the suburbs are further from their work.

The second reason people may be inactive is that they have a misconception about exercise. Many people have thought that the old exercise prescription for working out hard is **THE** prescription for exercise. It is NOT! This led to the belief that if a person could not follow the prescription, then they should not exercise at all. The following new guidelines may help to dispel this old myth.

New Guidelines for Exercise

In July of 1993, the American College of Sports Medicine and the U.S. Centers for Disease Control and Prevention, in cooperation with the President's Council on Physical Fitness and Sports, released new exercise guidelines and recommendations for Americans. The new guidelines recommend 30 minutes or more of moderate-intensity physical activity on most days of the week (at least five days).

This is great news! Six, 5-minute walks count as 30 minutes of activity. Activities that also can contribute to the 30-minute total include walking up stairs, gardening, cleaning house, raking leaves, and walking part or all of the way to and from work. The recommended

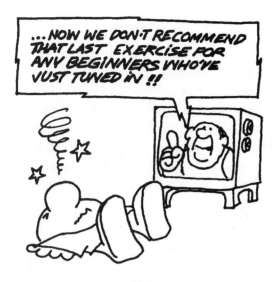

30 minutes of physical activity may also come from planned exercise or recreation, such as jogging, riding a bicycle, playing golf or tennis, or swimming. A brisk two-mile walk is another way to achieve 30 minutes of physical activity.

As you can see, there are many reasons to increase your physical activity. The best advice is to build physical activity into your daily routine—make it part of your lifestyle, just like eating, working, and sleeping. The physical and psychological aspects of a more active lifestyle can be quite rewarding.

The Importance of Food

TAPE 3

SECTION 10

In simple terms, food is energy; it is the fuel our body uses to enable us to carry on our daily activities. Like most energy sources, quality is as important as quantity, and having the right mixture of nutrients at the right time is also important. Some nutrients have energy (calories) and others do not, but both are critical to our bodies. The nutrient needs of our bodies are comparable to the different needs of our automobiles. Gasoline and diesel fuel provide fuel or energy. Oil, water, transmission fluid, and other lubricants are also critical to a car's operation, but they do not provide energy.

Our bodies need over 45 different nutrients every day. These nutrients are essential for our health and must be provided in the food we eat. There are six classes of these nutrients listed in the table on page 120, and they can be divided into two categories:

❶ Nutrients with energy (calories)

❷ Nutrients without energy

Nutrients with energy include carbohydrates, proteins, and fats. In Lesson Seven, I discussed the role of fat in your diet; proteins and carbohydrates will be covered in later lessons. The nutrients without energy include minerals, vitamins, and water.

Nutrients Without Energy

Three classes of nutrients that are essential to our bodies are contained in the food that we eat and provide no energy (calories). These nutrients include minerals, vitamins, and water.

Minerals

Our bodies contain over 60 different minerals, 22 of which are essential. The amount needed of the different minerals varies greatly. The 22 essential minerals are classified by their presence in the body as either *Macronutrients* (those needed in larger amounts) and *Micronutrients* (those needed in smaller amounts). It is important to remember that this classification

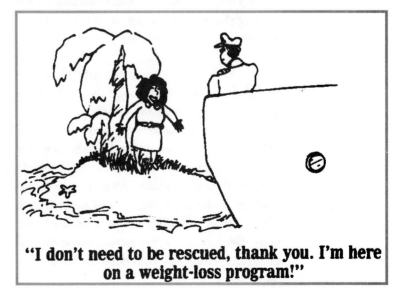

"I don't need to be rescued, thank you. I'm here on a weight-loss program!"

The Six Classes of Nutrients

Nutrients with Energy (Calories)

1. **Carbohydrates**—starches, sugar, and fiber
2. **Protein**—includes 22 amino acids
3. **Fats**—saturated, monounsaturated, and polyunsaturated fatty acids

Nutrients Without Energy

4. **Minerals**—22 in total

7 Macronutrients	*15 Micronutrients*	
calcium	arsenic	manganese
chlorine	boron	molybdenum
magnesium	cobalt	nickel
phosphorus	copper	selenium
potassium	chromium	silicon
sodium	fluorine	vanadium
sulfur	iodine	zinc
	iron	

5. **Vitamins**

Fat Soluble	*Water Soluble*
vitamin A-RDA 5000 IU	vitamin C-RDA 60 mg
vitamin D-RDA 100 IU	vitamin B_1 (thiamine)-RDA 1.5 mg
vitamin E-RDA 30 IU	vitamin B_2 (riboflavin)-RDA 1.7 mg
vitamin K	vitamin B_3 (niacin)-RDA 19 mg
	vitamin B_6 (pyridoxine)-RDA 2.0 mg
	vitamin B_{12} (cobalamin)-RDA 6 μg
	folacin-RDA 400 μg

6. **Water**

is based upon the amount in the body and not on importance. For example, a deficiency in cobalt, which comprises only two parts per trillion of body weight, can have more damaging effects than a deficiency in calcium, which accounts for two percent of body weight.

Minerals serve many functions. They help to aid in the growth of body tissue, transmit nerve impulses, regulate muscle contraction, maintain water balance in the body, form parts of essential body compounds, maintain the acid-base balance in the cells, and facilitate many biological reactions. Minerals are found together in the foods we eat and interact with each other as well as with other nutrients in the body. Because of this interaction and combination, certain foods are considered better sources than others.

Vitamins

Vitamins are also essential nutrients that are needed to sustain life. They are required for the regulation of the body's metabolism and for the transformation of energy (protein, carbohydrates, and fat) in the body. Some vitamins help to form important enzymes, and others act as catalysts to speed certain chemical reactions. There are two types of vitamins:

❶ **Fat soluble**

❷ **Water soluble**

Fat Soluble Vitamins

The four fat soluble vitamins are A, D, E, and K. These vitamins are found in dietary fat and are stored in the body's fat tissue if consumed in excess amounts. Because these vitamins are stored, high doses can be toxic. You should be cautious of people who promote large quantities of these vitamins. No more than the Recommended Daily Allowance (RDA) is suggested.

Vitamin A is essential for the growth of skin, bones, and teeth. It is also important in vision. Vitamin D is essential for bone and tooth development. In addition, it helps the body utilize calcium and phosphorus. Vitamin E is essential for the functioning of red blood cells and helps the body utilize the essential fatty acids. Vitamin K is used by the liver to produce prothrombin, a factor in blood plasma that combines with calcium to help in blood clotting.

Water Soluble Vitamins

Water soluble vitamins consist of seven primary vitamins: vitamin C and the B complex vitamins that include vitamin B_1 (thiamine), vitamin B_2 (riboflavin), vitamin B_3 (niacin), vitamin B_6 (pyridoxine), folacin, and vitamin B_{12} (cobalamin). Unlike the fat soluble vitamins, these are absorbed in the body's water, and excess amounts are usually excreted.

Vitamin C is used by the body for teeth, bones, cells, and blood vessels; it is essential for good health. Vitamin B_1 is essential for the heart and nervous system and plays an important role in carbohydrate metabolism. A deficiency of this vitamin can result in beriberi and certain nervous disorders. Vitamin B_2 is also important in carbohydrate metabolism and body tissue repair. It is necessary for the skin and helps prevent light sensitivity in the eyes. A deficiency of this vitamin in the diet can lead to stunted growth and loss of hair. Vitamin B_3 (more commonly known as niacin) is important for metabolism and absorption of carbohydrates in the body and plays an important role in converting food to usable energy. Vitamin B_6 aids in the metabolism of protein, carbohydrate, and fat. Vitamin B_{12} is essential for normal growth and neurological function. This vitamin also helps prevent anemia. Folacin is also important because it helps the body metabolize food and is useful in preventing certain anemias.

As a general rule, nutrition experts believe that people in the U.S. receive an adequate supply of minerals and vitamins if they eat a balanced diet. Following the dietary guidelines of the Food Guide Pyramid will help insure a balanced diet. Therefore, most people do not need or benefit from mineral or vitamin supplements, much less the mega doses promoted by some people, including seemingly credible nutrition stores. *The LEARN Healthy Eating and Calorie Guide* (see page 303) has specific dietary recommendations for the essential vitamins and minerals.

Water

Many people overlook the importance of water in their diets, not realizing that water is an essential nutrient. Considering that water makes up about 60 percent of your body and that water is needed by every cell in your body, water is indeed an important nutrient and should be consumed generously. Most people in the U.S. do not consume enough water. As a rule of thumb, about 4 cups of water should be consumed for every 1000 calories eaten. For most adults, this is equivalent to about 10 cups (2½ quarts) of water each day.

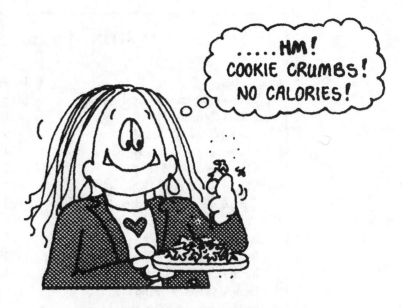

Milk, Yogurt, and Cheese in Your Diet

The second tier of the Food Guide Pyramid represents foods that come essentially from animal sources—milk, yogurt, and cheese; and meat, poultry, fish, dry beans, eggs, and nuts. The focus in this lesson will be on the Milk, Yogurt, and Cheese Group.

Food items in this group include milk, yogurt, and cheese. These foods are good sources of protein and carbohydrate, but can provide large amounts of unwanted dietary fat (see the food list on page 122). In addition, foods from the Milk Group are good sources of vitamin A, vitamin D, and calcium. Vitamins A and D are essential for the growth and development of skin, bones, and teeth. Calcium is an essential mineral for good health. Approximately 2 percent of the body is calcium, most of which is teeth and bones. Food items from the Milk Group are the best source of calcium and generally supply the greatest amount of calcium in our diet. One cup of milk (8 fl oz), for example, provides 500 International Units (IUs) of vitamin A (i.e., 10 percent of the 5000 RDA) and 100 IUs of vitamin D (i.e., 25 percent of the 400 RDA). The same cup of milk also provides about 313 mg of calcium (i.e., 30 percent of the 1000 mg RDA).

Milk, Yogurt, and Cheese

Description	Calories	Protein (g)	Carbohydrate (g)	Fat (g)
Cheese, American processed—2 oz	212	12.6	1.0	17.8
Cheese, cheddar—1½ oz	171	10.6	.6	14.1
Cheese, Colby—1½ oz	168	10.0	1.0	13.7
Cheese, cottage, creamed—2 cups (16 oz)	434	52.4	11.2	19.0
Cheese, cream—1½ oz	149	3.2	1.2	14.9
Cheese, mozzarella—1½ oz	120	8.3	.9	7.2
Cheese, mozzarella part skim—1½ oz	108	10.4	1.2	6.8
Cheese, ricotta whole milk—½ cup (4 oz)	216	14.0	3.8	16.1
Cheese, ricotta part skim— ½ cup (4 oz)	171	14.1	6.4	9.8
Ice cream, 10% fat—1½ cup (12 oz)	404	7.2	48.0	21.5
Ice cream, 16% fat—1½ cup (12 oz)	524	6.2	48.0	35.6
Ice milk, vanilla—1½ cup (12 oz)	276	7.8	43.5	8.4
Ice milk, soft serve—1½ cup (12 oz)	335	12.0	57.6	6.9
Milk, skim—1 cup (8 oz)	86	8.4	11.9	Trace
Milk, 1%—1 cup (8 oz)	104	8.5	12.2	2.4
Milk, 2%—1 cup (8 oz)	125	8.5	12.2	4.7
Milk, whole—1 cup (8 oz)	150	8.0	11.0	8.0
Yogurt, nonfat—1 cup (8 oz)	90	10.0	13.0	Trace
Yogurt, light—1 cup (8 oz)	100	9.0	17.0	Trace
Yogurt, low-fat—1 cup (8 oz)	144	11.9	16.0	3.5
Yogurt, skim—1 cup (8 oz)	127	13.0	17.4	Trace
Yogurt, whole—1 cup (8 oz)	139	7.9	10.6	7.4
Yogurt, frozen 1 cup (8 oz)	210	6.2	33.2	6.2

Note: This table should be used as a guide for the foods listed. Since food values vary by brand name it is important to read the food labels for these foods.

Cheese items have proportionally more calories from protein than carbohydrate. Milk and yogurt, on the other hand, provide more carbohydrates per serving than protein.

How Many Servings?

The Food Guide Pyramid suggests two to three servings per day from the Milk Group. For most people, two servings from this group is sufficient; however, for teenagers, young adults, and women who are pregnant or breast feeding, three servings per day is recommended. It is important to know what makes up a serving size. Many people may know that servings from this group are important, yet most do not know how many servings are optimal.

How Much Is a Serving?

The guide here lists single serving portions for many common food items from this group. The following items count as a single serving:

1½ oz processed cheese

1 cup (8 oz) milk

1 cup (8 oz) yogurt

1½ oz natural cheese

½ cup (4 oz) ice cream

½ cup (4 oz) cottage cheese

Eating food items from the Milk Group should be balanced during the day. In other words, it is best not to eat all of the required servings at the same time. An example of balance would be to have a cup of milk at breakfast (with cereal or in a glass), cheese or yogurt for lunch, and a serving of milk, yogurt, cheese, or ice cream for dinner.

Watch out for Fat

Most products from the Milk Group come from animal sources. As such, these food items also contain cholesterol and fat. The fat content as well as the number of calories in each serving can vary greatly. For instance, one serving of skim milk (8 fl oz) has 86 total calories, compared to one serving of ice cream (12 oz) which can have as many as 524 calories. Moreover, the one serving of skim milk has only a trace (less than 1 percent) of fat. Compare this to the ice cream with 35.6 grams of fat—that is 61 percent of total calories from fat!

Storing Foods (Out of Sight, Out of Mouth)

The less you see and think about food, the easier it will be to control eating. Where and how you store food can influence what and how much you eat.

Let's examine two approaches to the same problem to illustrate this point. Suppose salted nuts are your passion and you bring home a one-pound bag from Tiny's Nut House. You could make the nuts a constant temptation by keeping them in an open dish, using the classic dodge that, "I need them in case someone drops by."

Another approach would be to keep the nuts out of sight. This would put some effort between the nuts and you. You could lock them in a safe that is stored in your attic behind 24 boxes of old papers and books. In which case would you eat more nuts?

The attic example is far-fetched, but it does show how the accessibility of food can influence whether you eat. Storing food wisely and keeping it out of sight can be helpful. Here are some ways to follow through.

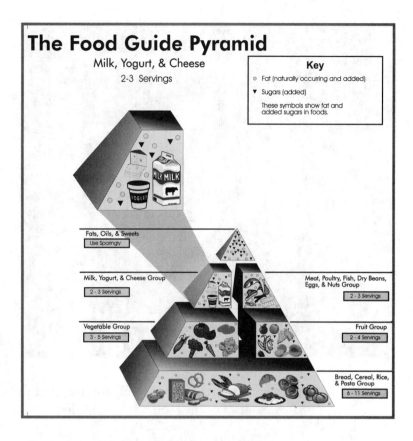

Hide the High-Calorie Foods

High-calorie impulse foods should be stored out of sight. Put the ice cream under the frozen peas and behind the chicken breasts so you won't see it each time you open the door. Store the cookies on a high shelf behind the sel-

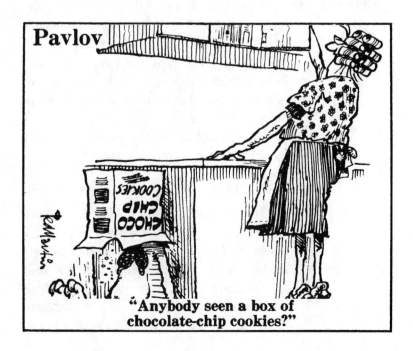

"Anybody seen a box of chocolate-chip cookies?"

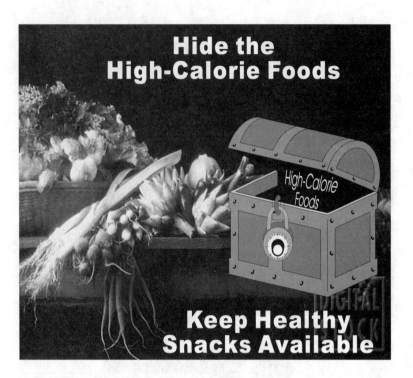

Hide the High-Calorie Foods

Keep Healthy Snacks Available

reach for the celery, carrot sticks, raisins, apples, cauliflower, vegetable soup, or oranges.

Compulsive Eating and Binge Eating

TAPE 2
SECTION 7

Doctors increasingly recognize that a small but significant minority of overweight individuals struggle with episodes of compulsive eating or binge eating. Overeaters Anonymous popularized the most widely used term for this problem—compulsive overeating. Researchers have called this binge eating.

The official definition of binge eating has two features. The first is eating what others would consider a large amount of food and the second is feeling out of control. When this happens with sufficient frequency (two times a week or more) and over a sufficient period of time (six months) a person can qualify for a diagnosis called Binge Eating Disorder. I hasten to add that some people have binges many more times than this, and some people have fewer or less frequent binges but still have a troubling problem. If you think you may have a problem with Binge Eating, you can log onto the www.TheLifeStyleCompany.com website and complete the Binge Eating Questionnaire. This an be found under the tab "Self-Assessments You Can Do" on the home page. Completing this questionnaire can help you decide if you need additional help with binge eating problems.

In the early stages of research on binge eating, some experts felt that individuals who ate compulsively needed treatment for this type of eating disorder in addition to whatever help they needed for weight. More recently, research has shown that individuals who participate in a program like The LEARN Program stop binge eating as well as people who get a program focused specifically on the binge eating, but in addition, lose more weight. Therefore, if you have a problem with binge eating, you may

"The less you see and think about food, the easier it will be to control eating."

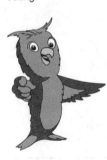

dom-used guest dishes, and put the potato chips on a low shelf behind the colander.

This leads back to Antecedents (discussed in Lesson Four). Bringing problem foods in the house and having them available are steps that precede eating. It would, of course, be preferable to intervene at the earliest step and not buy the foods at all. If you do buy the foods, keeping them out of the way is the next logical step.

Keeping food out of sight serves two purposes. If you don't see it, you may not be stimulated to eat. Also, putting some effort between you and the food stops automatic eating and gives you time to change your mind. You can help the cause even more by storing foods in opaque containers. Keeping the brownies in a plastic bowl will make them less tempting than having them in a clear cookie jar.

Keep Healthful Snacks Available

Because Sherlock Holmes would now have trouble finding the high-calorie foods in your house, you can use the space vacated by goodies to store healthful foods. When you buy fresh fruits and vegetables at the store, cut them up immediately after you get home so they are readily available to eat. If you get an urge to eat,

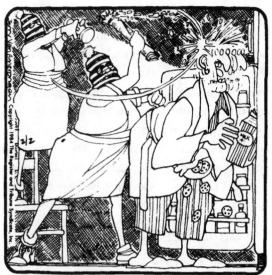

Since joining Diet Watchers Anonymous, Noel Cramer continues to be surprised at just how comprehensive the group's services are.

Support Organizations for Eating Disorders
(Potential Help for Compulsive Eating/Binge Eating)

United States

National Eating Disorders Organization
6655 S. Yale Avenue
Tulsa, OK 74136
918-481-4044

American Anorexia/Bulimia Association
293 Central Park West, Suite 1R
New York, NY 10024
212-575-6200

**National Association of Anorexia Nervosa
and Associated Disorders**
P.O. Box 7
Highland Park, IL 60034
708-831-3438

Anorexia Nervosa and Related Eating Disorders
P.O. Box 5102
Eugene, OR 97405
503-344-1144

Canada

National Eating Disorder Information Centre
200 Elizabeth Street
College Way
Toronto, Ontario M5G 2C4
416-340-4156

Bulimia, Anorexia Association
3640 Wells Street
Windsor, Ontario N9C 1T9
519-969-2112

United Kingdom

Eating Disorders Association
Sackville Place
44 Magdalen Street
Norwich
Norfolk NR3 1JU
01603-621414

find that this program helps control overeating and promotes weight loss.

There will be some people who need additional help. If by this time in the program you are having problems with eating compulsively, you might examine whether additional resources would be helpful. I suggest three approaches.

The first approach is to use a book entitled *Overcoming Binge Eating* written by Dr. Christopher Fairburn, a leading authority from Oxford University in England. The book is an excellent guide that has been tested thoroughly and brings the best of science to the reader in a useable and friendly format. The book is published by Guilford Press in New York and can be ordered by calling 1–888–LEARN–41. This is the best such guide of its type available today.

The second, but more expensive, alternative is to seek counseling. If you choose this option, try to see someone with special experience in treating eating disorders. Several organizations can provide the names of professionals in your area who have experience with eating disorders, although there is no guar-

antee that such professionals are truly skilled. These organizations are listed in the table above. The two approaches that have been proven effective for binge eating are cognitive behavior therapy and interpersonal psychotherapy, so you might ask the professional you contact if he or she offers one of these.

A final approach is to consider help from Overeaters Anonymous (OA). While OA has not been evaluated, it does offer strong support and a focus on compulsive eating. For some people, the support, the around-the-clock help

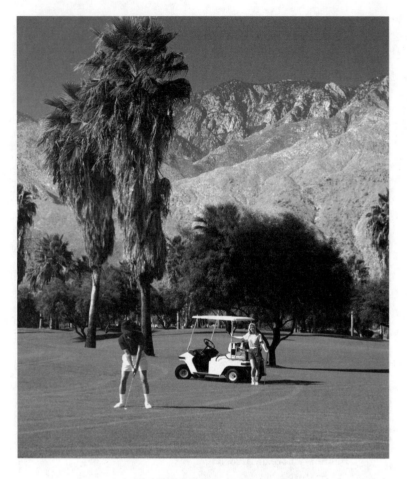

available from a sponsor, and the group meetings can be quite helpful.

Selecting and Starting a Programmed Activity

TAPE 3
SECTION 9

I cannot emphasize enough the importance of regular physical activity. In recent years, researchers have found many important reasons to be active, and the many benefits of exercise are very impressive. Regular physical activity in moderate amounts is one of the most powerful means at your disposal to reduce risk for heart disease and other serious illnesses. Being active can put more life into every step you take, give you more energy, make you feel better about your body, and improve your mood. Best of all, it can really help you lose weight and maintain the weight loss. I suggest you reread the section on Impressive Reasons to Be Active from Lesson Seven on page 108 to get the full rationale.

If you know that activity is good for you and would like to do more, then you need to look at what gets in the way and what might be done. What often gets in the way is embarrassment, being timid about exercise, thinking that you couldn't possibly do as much as necessary, and practical issues such as time. I have given you enough ammunition throughout this program to challenge and defeat each of these obstacles. It's a great time to rise above the barriers and start the activity. Here's how to do it.

Choosing the Best Activity

There are many activities to choose from. Several possibilities will be discussed below. There are four factors to consider in making your decision.

⇨ *Select something you can do*. Consider your current physical condition when choosing an activity. Basketball is strenuous and is not advisable if you are not in tip-top condition. Pick something where you can move at your own pace. Walking, cycling, and swimming are good examples.

⇨ *Select something you would like to do*. Hiking may be something that always caught your fancy, so go ahead and try. If you are turned off by swimming, don't do it just because you think you should. It helps to like the activities you choose.

⇨ *Select a solo or social activity*. We covered this earlier in our discussion of walking. In your choice of an activity, consider whether you would like to exercise alone (jogging, swimming, cycling) or with other people (tennis, golf, aerobics class). If you are a social person, having others around can be an incentive to participate.

⇨ *Do not be embarrassed*. This is easier said than done. Many heavy people avoid exercise completely or avoid it when they can be seen by others. They are embarrassed about their bodies, their clothes, and their poor physical condition. Try to put

Programmed Activities

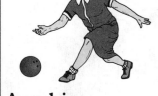

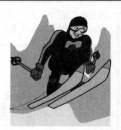

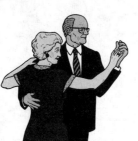

Aerobics

Badminton

Bowling

Cycling

Dancing

Golf

Hiking

Jogging

Join a Spa

Racquetball

Rollerblading

Rowing

Running

Skating

Skiing

Softball

Squash

Stair climbing

Swimming

Tennis

Treadmill

Walking

Weights

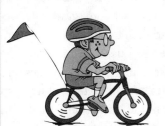

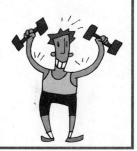

this aside. Take a deep breath, and ask yourself which is more important, avoiding embarrassment or losing weight.

A Helpful Tip

Let me pass along a tip drawn from my own experience. I exercise regularly and try to have a number of activities to choose from. I run, ride a bike, play tennis, and do strength training. Mixing up these activities provides me with choice and variety, both of which help minimize boredom. I can watch TV, listen to music, or both while doing some of these things, so I sometimes save the exercise when I know there is something I might like to see on the television.

Most people can probably find more than one activity as possibilities. If an outside activity is not possible, then an inside alternative might fit the bill. The key is whether you will still be active months or years from now. Whether this occurs depends in large part on whether you enjoy it, and whether you enjoy it may depend on variety and the presence of other interesting things.

Warming Up and Cooling Down

Warming up before exercise and cooling down afterwards is important. This will help stretch your muscles to avoid strains and pulls. It will also help your heart and circulatory system make the transition from rest to exercise and then back to rest. You should warm up and cool down at least five minutes for a 30-minute bout of exercise.

In general, a good warmup for most activities is the same activity performed at lower intensity. Walking slowly is a good warm up for brisk walking, and brisk walking can serve as a warmup for running. Here are several additional warm-up exercises. Please note that some exercises may be problematic if you have certain conditions. Trunk twists may create difficulty if you have back problems. Check with your phy-

"Programmed activities should be something you enjoy and will do over and over again."

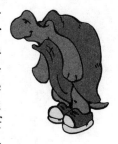

127

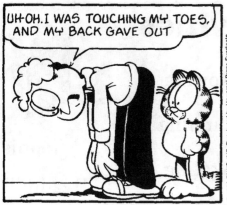
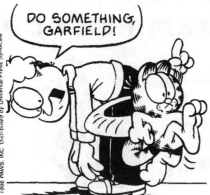
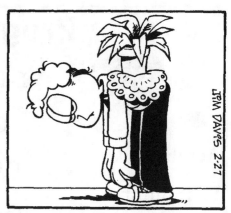

UH-OH. I WAS TOUCHING MY TOES, AND MY BACK GAVE OUT

DO SOMETHING, GARFIELD!

sician or a sports medicine specialist if you have such problems.

⇨ **Trunk Twists**. Stand with your feet shoulder-width apart. Extend your arms to the side so they are horizontal. Twist your trunk to the right as if you are trying to look over your right shoulder. Then reverse directions and move your trunk so your left arm extends to your right. This exercise should be done slowly or as a held stretch to avoid jerking the muscles.

⇨ **Toe Touches**. Stand with your feet a little more than shoulder-width apart. Bend at the waist and slowly attempt to touch your toes with your fingertips. Keep your knees bent and do not bounce the upper body. Hold the stretch for a few seconds. Return to the standing position and then repeat. If you have back problems, the sit-and-reach exercise may present fewer difficulties.

⇨ **Sit-and-Reach**. Sit on the floor with your legs straight out in front of you. Slowly reach to touch your toes, and hold the reach for a few seconds. As with the toe touches, keeping the legs bent is important to avoid strain on the knees and back.

⇨ **Arm Circles**. In the standing position, hold your arms out to the side of your body in a horizontal position. Roll your arms up, back, and then down to produce backward circles.

When you begin your programmed activity, be it cycling, swimming, walking, or anything, begin slowly and gradually increase your pace. To end your exercise session, gradually decrease the pace, and then finish with some combination of the exercises described above. The warming up and cooling down activities are worth the little extra time they take. They can prevent nagging injuries that could keep you away from exercise for a long time.

Cardiovascular Training

Exercise physiologists have done extensive research to show how much exercise is necessary to improve cardiovascular condition. This refers to the efficiency of your heart, blood vessels, and general circulatory and respiratory systems. From this research was born a formula known to millions of people. This three-part formula deals with *how much*, *how often*, and *how long* you must exercise to get this training effect. Keep in mind that this formula for cardiovascular training is much different than the activity needed to reach a moderate level of fitness as I discuss later in Lesson Eleven on page 171.

This is what aerobics is all about. An activity is *aerobic* if the body uses large amounts of oxygen (i.e., if the heart, lungs, and blood vessels are working hard). As a result of this hard work, these parts of the body become conditioned. This conditioning is associated with greater life expectancy, lowered risk of heart disease, and other positive effects.

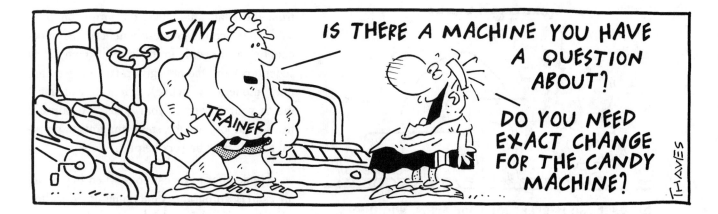

What about the F.I.T. Approach?

The question then is "How much and what type of activity should I do?" The answer to this question comes from the American College of Sports Medicine (ACSM), an authoritative organization of professionals in exercise physiology and sports medicine.

The ACSM has published a position paper entitled, "The Recommended Quantity and Quality of Exercise for Developing and Maintaining Cardiorespiratory and Muscular Fitness in Adults." *Cardiorespiratory* fitness refers to the condition of your heart (cardio) and lungs (respiratory).

The ACSM document focuses on the F.I.T. principle (Frequency, Intensity, and Time). These are important for cardiovascular conditioning, while frequency and the number of repetitions is important for increasing muscular strength. The five main components to the ACSM guidelines:

① *Frequency of Training*. Exercising three to five days per week is recommended.

② *Intensity of Training*. During a bout of exercise, your heart rate should be 60–90 percent of maximum. You can estimate your maximum heart rate by subtracting your age from 220. For instance, for a person who is 40 years old, maximum heart rate would be 180 beats per minute (220–40). During a workout, this person would want the heart to beat 108–162 times per minute (this is 60–90 percent of the maximum of 180 beats per minute).

③ *Duration of Training*. The recommended duration of activity is 20–60 minutes of continuous aerobic activity. High-intensity activities require less duration. The ACSM notes that total fitness can be attained with programs of longer duration and that lower intensity exercise is easier to sustain over a longer time.

④ *Type of Activity*. Recommended activities are those that use large muscle groups, are rhythmic and aerobic, and can be maintained continuously. Examples are walking, hiking, running, jogging, cycling, cross-country skiing, dancing, skipping rope, rowing, swimming, stair climbing, skating, and endurance-game activities.

⑤ *Resistance Training*. To improve muscle strength, 8–12 repetitions of 8–10 exercises that focus on the major muscle groups are recommended for a minimum of two days per week.

If you are sufficiently fit to focus on these issues, these guidelines should be helpful. If not, it is important to emphasize small and gradual changes in physical activity, remembering that any activity is helpful.

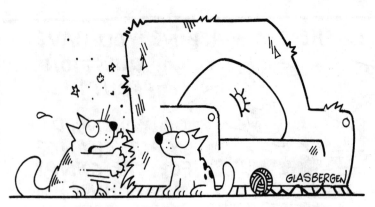

"This exercise is great for your arms, shoulders, chest and back. Do four sets of 15 repetitions, then move on to the yarn ball for your aerobics."

Do You Need This?

Vigorous activity is required to get your heart rate to this target zone of 60–90 percent of maximum. Keeping it there for 20 minutes can be difficult for some people. Take your pulse the next time you go for a walk. Use the procedure described in Lesson Thirteen on page 207 to take your pulse, except take your pulse immediately after you stop walking. Count the beats in 10 seconds, then multiply by six for the number of beats per minute. The level is probably below the 60–90 percent demanded by the formula.

The important question is, "Do you need to do this much?" The answer is "yes," if you want to get the training effect. The answer is an emphatic "no," if you are exercising to boost your weight loss or to reach the moderate level of fitness (I discuss this later in Lesson Eleven). Any exercise is better than no exercise. Low levels of activity can help, so you may be better off ignoring the formula. I presented it here to clarify the numbers that are widely cited. Exercise in any amount carries many benefits, so do not be discouraged if you do not meet the standards set by the formula.

It is also essential to remember that the high level of exercise needed to improve cardiorespiratory fitness is not necessary to lower risk. You will see this in Lesson Eleven

from the Blair study (see the graph on page 172) in which the greatest benefit to health occurs between people in the least fit (completely sedentary) and the next group (people who are only moderately active). Hence, you must match your activity to your goals. To improve health and lose weight, small amounts of physical activity may be very helpful.

Remember to be cautious when beginning an exercise program. Guidelines for deciding whether you need medical screening are listed in Lesson Three (page 50). Review the guidelines and consult a physician if these or any other factors suggest any problems. Most people without a specific health problem can safely begin a program of at least brisk walking.

You should always warm up and cool down before and after exercise. The body does not like abrupt changes, so you must warm up to prepare it for vigorous activity and cool down in the transition from exercise to rest. You may want to review the section about warming up and cooling down that I presented earlier in this lesson.

Danger! An Exercise Threshold Attitude

Many people on weight loss programs labor under the insidious influence of a dangerous attitude—the exercise threshold. They feel they must do a magic amount of exercise for it to have any value. One client asked me, "Is it enough that I walked around the block after dinner last night?" Implicit in the word "enough" is that exercising below this threshold has no value. You must banish this concept from your mind!

The threshold concept was born from the cardiovascular training idea discussed above. If you will forgive me for stating it again—***any exercise is better than no exercise***. Walking around the block is not as impressive as running a marathon, but it's better than watching reruns of *Gilligan's Island* and munching on corn chips. If you walk two blocks, it is better than one block, but not as good as three blocks. Do anything to be active. Remember, small amounts of exercise add up, so do not feel you must strain to accomplish some arbitrary level.

Internal Attitude Traps

We all talk to ourselves, albeit silently. I discussed this earlier when I talked about goal setting and emotions. How you view your lifestyle changes can help or hinder you greatly. There are several common traps you may encounter. If you are prepared with counter thoughts and attitudes, your job will be easier.

Countering the Traps

You might visualize the part of yourself that pressures you to eat. You can be more than a match for this part, but only if you are conscientious and face the problem directly. What follows are some common traps, called *fat thoughts*. I will give you material for possible counter measures.

Internal Trap Number 1: "The diet is the key."

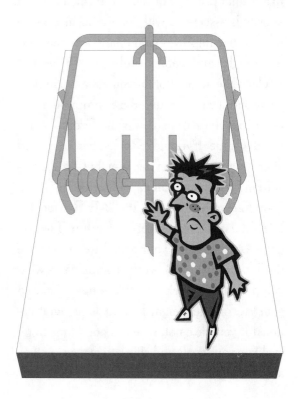

Fat Thought: The diet and this program are the only reasons I lose weight. When the program is over, I will have real trouble keeping the weight off.

Counter: I am losing weight because of my own efforts. Just because the program ends does not mean my new habits will vanish. The program helps me along, but I get the credit.

Internal Trap Number 2: "Is this worth the effort?"

Fat Thought: I have been on my program for weeks, and I still have lots of weight to lose. I can't wait till this program ends so I can get back to normal.

Counter: Stop this right now! Who said this would be easy? It took a long time to gain the weight, and it will take a long time to lose it. I would like to lose fast and easy, but facts are facts. I don't want to let down now and waste my effort. I can stick with it.

Internal Trap Number 3: "I have done this before."

Fat Thought: I have heard this nutrition stuff before, and we covered behavior modification in the last program I was in. It didn't help me then and will not help me now.

Counter: I have never been taught these things in such a concentrated way, and my motivation to learn may be different now. I know deep down this is the only way to get permanent results, so putting down the approach just means I have trouble doing the work. Only I can do it, so I must forge ahead.

Try to recognize these and other internal traps. The fat thoughts you have lived with for years will do their best to control your attitudes and eating. Now you can blast them with a counterattack.

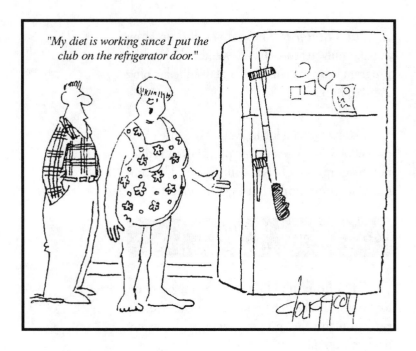

"My diet is working since I put the club on the refrigerator door."

Rating Your Diet

In Lesson Two, you took a short quiz to rate your diet. It is now time to take the same quiz again and see if your diet has improved. On page 287 in Appendix E, is the Rate Your Diet Quiz for Lesson Eight. Take a few moments now to take the quiz. How does your total score now (on page 290) compare with your total score a few weeks ago (on page 286)? Hopefully your score has improved and you're on your way to being a nutrition whiz.

My Personal Goals for This Week

As you set your personal goals for this lesson, focus on your attitudes. The internal attitude traps trip up lots of people, so see if the material in these sections applies to you. Are there traps your mind sets for you that you know in advance will cause problems in certain situations? This is also a good time to think about physical activity and to have goals that can lead to a regular program of activity. Remember that activity is associated with long-term success, so being active improves your chances of conquering weight and eating problems. Focus this week on the amount of fat you eat and check to make sure you are eating the appropriate number of servings from the Milk Group of the Food Guide Pyramid. Remember to record your weight change on the Weight Change Record in Lesson One on page 25. Also, now is a good time to look back at the "My Reasonable Weight Loss" worksheet in Lesson Two on page 42 to see how your actual weight change during the first eight weeks compares to what you planned in week two. If you have achieved your reasonable weight loss goals, congratulations! If you have not, now is a good time to re-evaluate your goals and check to make sure they are reasonable.

"Countering those destructive attitude traps is important for success."

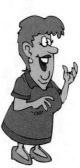

Quality of Life Self-Assessment

It is time again to complete the Quality of Life Self-Assessment. I ask you to do this about once a month to track changes in important areas of your life. Following a healthier diet, being more physically active, and losing weight can have multiple benefits. The problem is that we are so focused on the scale that we overlook some of the most important benefits of all. Having more energy and more self-confidence are just examples. One reason we do this self-assessment periodically is to keep you going even when the scale seems stuck. If the assessment shows change, things are going well and you have cause to feel good. Compare your score today with the scores from the Quality of Life Self-Assessments you filled out in the Introduction and Orientation (page 9). Remember, the scale is only one index of your success. In Lesson Nine, we'll revisit these scores and I'll have you complete a score comparison worksheet.

My Self-Assessment

Lesson Eight

T F 54. Thirty minutes of incremental moderate-intensity physical activity per day is now recommended for Americans.

T F 55. All nutrients that we eat contain calories.

T F 56. Keeping high-calorie foods stored out of sight can decrease impulsive eating.

T F 57. One cup (8 oz) is equal to one serving from the Milk Group of the Food Guide Pyramid.

T F 58. The recommended number of daily servings from the Milk, Yogurt, and Cheese Group is two to three.

T F 59. Fat thoughts can hinder a person's efforts to lose weight.

T F 60. Warming up and stretching before exercise is to strengthen your muscles.

T F 61. To get a cardiovascular training effect, there must be the right combination of frequency, intensity, and time.

T F 62. By Lesson Eight in this program, nearly everyone has developed a plan of regular, vigorous physical activity.

T F 63. Binge eating is characterized by eating large amounts of food with an accompanying sense of loss of control.

(Answers in Appendix C, page 271)

Quality of Life Self-Assessment

Please use the following scale to rate how satisfied you feel now about different aspects of your daily life. Choose any number from this list (1 to 9) and indicate your choice on the questions below.

1 = Extremely Dissatisfied   **6 = Somewhat Satisfied**

2 = Very Dissatisfied   **7 = Moderately Satisfied**

3 = Moderately Dissatisfied   **8 = Very Satisfied**

4 = Somewhat Dissatisfied   **9 = Extremely Satisfied**

5 = Neutral

1. _____ Mood (feelings of sadness, worry, happiness, etc.)
2. _____ Self-esteem
3. _____ Confidence, self-assurance, and comfort in social situations
4. _____ Energy and feeling healthy
5. _____ Health problems (diabetes, high blood pressure, etc.)
6. _____ General appearance
7. _____ Social life
8. _____ Leisure and recreational activities
9. _____ Physical mobility and physical activity
10. _____ Eating habits
11. _____ Body image
12. _____ Overall quality of life

Monitoring Form—Lesson Eight

*Today's Date:*_____

TIME	FOOD AND AMOUNT	CALORIES
TOTAL DAILY CALORIES		

PERSONAL GOALS FOR THIS WEEK	MOST OF THE TIME	SOME-TIMES	RARELY
1. HIDE HIGH-CALORIE FOODS			
2. WATCH OUT FOR FAT			
3. EXPERIMENT WITH PROGRAMMED ACTIVITIES			
4. DAILY SERVINGS FROM THE MILK GROUP			
5. EAT LESS THAN _____ CALORIES PER DAY			
6. EAT LESS THAN _____ GRAMS OF FAT EACH DAY			

FOOD GROUPS FOR TODAY	PHYSICAL ACTIVITY	MINUTES OR STEPS
MILK, YOGURT, AND CHEESE ☐ ☐ ☐	(M)	
MEAT, POULTRY, ETC. ☐ ☐ ☐	(TU)	
FRUITS ☐ ☐ ☐ ☐	(W)	
VEGETABLES ☐ ☐ ☐ ☐ ☐	(TH)	
BREADS, CEREALS, ETC. ☐ ☐ ☐ ☐ ☐ ☐ ☐ ☐	(F)	
SERVINGS OF WATER (8 OZ) ☐ ☐ ☐ ☐ ☐ ☐ ☐ ☐	(SA)	
	(SU)	

Welcome to Lesson Nine of The LEARN Program. I hope the first eight weeks of your program have gone well and that you are well on your way to managing your weight. In this lesson, you will be learning more about positive attitudes, additional techniques for controlling your eating, and more about nutrition. We have covered a lot of material the past two months, and I hope you are pleased with how much you have learned. We still have much more to cover. The topics we will be covering over the next eight weeks are very interesting. So, if you're ready, let's move on.

A Two-Month Review

TAPE 3
SECTION 7

This lesson marks another milestone in your weight management program. For two months now, you have been using The LEARN Program. I hope you have made meaningful changes in your diet, fitness level, and overall health. Congratulations on your progress! You deserve much credit for all your hard work. Let's briefly review your efforts in these important areas.

Reviewing Your Quality of Life

How is your quality of life today compared with two months ago? Has your attitude about weight management and health in general improved? At this point in the program, many people have begun to change the way they view weight management. Many of the people I have

worked with over the years start focusing more on healthy lifestyle habits and less on the scale. As they continue to make better dietary and activity choices they feel better about themselves and their ability to control what they eat and how much exercise they do. This feeling is a powerful motivational tool.

The key is to make your changes continue to work for you—weaving them into the very fabric of your lifestyle. This way of thinking will help you lose weight, maintain the weight loss you have achieved, and feel better about yourself. On page 136 is a Review of Quality of Life Self-Assessments for you to complete. This is a similar form you completed in Lesson Four, on page 70. This worksheet will help you see the important progress you have made over the past two months and may highlight some areas that need additional work. Take time now

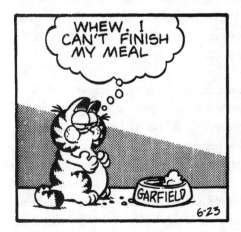

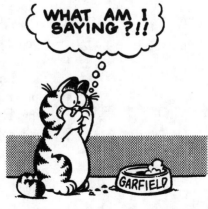

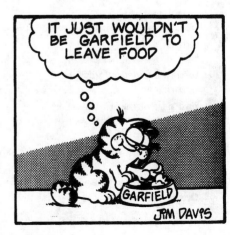

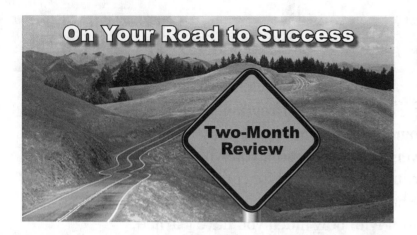

On Your Road to Success

Two-Month Review

to compete this worksheet before continuing with the lesson. This is an important part of the program.

Eating and Activity Habits

We have not reviewed your eating and activity habits is detail in the last few lessons, but I hope you are still focused on them. Keeping your Monitoring Forms and increasing your physical activity can be two keys to long-term success. Your Monitoring Forms will tell you if you are eating the appropriate number of calories and exercising enough. In addition, continue to use your records to identify patterns in your eating.

Are you measuring and weighing your food portions? This is something you don't have to do everyday, but is a helpful strategy to do every now and them. People often feel frustrated when they *believe* they are eating 1500 calories per day and not losing weight, when in reality, they may be eating over 2000 calories per day. Remember, it is easy to "underestimate" your calorie intake by as much as 60 percent. If you have not been measuring or weighing your food portion sizes, now may be a good time to dust off the food scale and measuring cups. During a meal at home, fill your plate as you normally would and write down the serving sizes of your meal. Then, before you start to eat, measure each portion size carefully. How close were you to estimating the correct portion sizes?

Some people dislike keeping the Monitoring Forms. They say that it takes too much time, is too bulky to carry through the day, or prevents them from enjoying their meals. If this is true for you, then stop using my forms and develop one of your own. You may want to use a 3" x 5" spiral pad or index cards. Similarly, you may want to develop your own records on weekends or at times when you usually eat more. There are dozens of ways that you can track the foods you eat. Find one that works for you if you don't like mine.

I hope that you are enjoying your walking program or whatever other activity you are doing. Remember, the object is to make sure that you enjoy the activities you are doing by choosing activities you enjoy, setting modest goals, and focusing on additional ways of making activity pleasurable. Take a few minutes to review your activity during the past two weeks. Are

Review of Quality of Life Self-Assessments

	(a) Category	(b) Score from Introduction and Orientation Lesson	(c) Score from Lesson Eight	(d) Change in Scores (column c minus column b)
1.	Mood (feelings of sadness, worry, happiness, etc.)			
2.	Self-esteem			
3.	Confidence, self-assurance, and comfort in social situations			
4.	Energy and feeling healthy			
5.	Health problems (diabetes, high blood pressure, etc.)			
6.	General appearance			
7.	Social life			
8.	Leisure and recreational activities			
9.	Physical mobility and physical activity			
10.	Eating habits			
11.	Body image			
12.	Overall quality of life			

you as active as you would like to be or could have been? If not, try to determine the barriers that keep you from being active. Review the "Barriers to Physical Activity" section in Lesson Four on page 55.

Weight Loss

After eight weeks on The LEARN Program, most people have lost about 4 to 6 percent of their starting weight. Look back to your Weight Change Record on page 25 and see where you are. Also, look back at the "My Reasonable Weight Loss" worksheet you completed in Lesson Two on page 42. Is your weight change at the end of week eight close to your goal weight projected on the worksheet? If not, now is a good time to make adjustments in your reasonable weight loss goal for the next eight weeks.

If you weighed 200 pounds before the program, I suspect you have lost about 8 to 12 pounds. If you have lost substantially less than this (less than 3 percent of your starting weight) or much more (more than 10 percent of your starting weight), you may want to talk with your doctor. While rapid weight loss is exciting, it can increase the risk of gallstones and other complications.

More likely, your health has continued to improve with weight loss. If you have high blood pressure or blood sugar, these conditions have probably improved even more since the first month of the program.

It is important to honestly assess your progress at this point in the program. If you have done well and feel successful, congratulate yourself and tell yourself how proud you are of your accomplishments. Too often, people make key lifestyle changes and overlook them or fail to take credit for all their hard work. You deserve the credit and recognition. If you feel there are areas you still need to work on for topics already covered, take time to go back and work on them. Much more interesting information in ahead.

Serving and Dispensing Food

Here are five questions I like to ask to determine whether a person reacts to the site, smell, or thought of food.

❶ **Do you feel like eating dessert when it looks appetizing, even after eating a large meal?**

❷ **Is there always room for something you like?**

❸ **Do you get excited about a buffet?**

❹ **If you drive by a bakery or fast-food place and smell the food, do you want to eat regardless of whether you are hungry?**

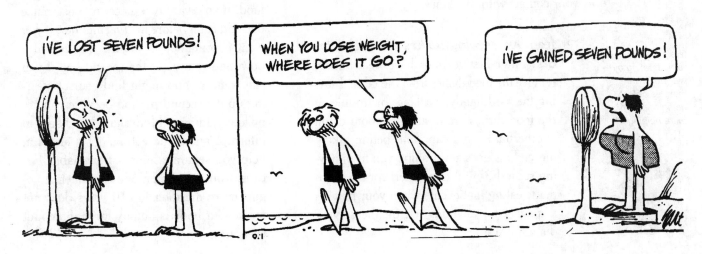

5 Do you feel like eating when you see a picture of a delicious dessert in a magazine?

If you answer "yes" to these questions, you may be high in externality. This means you are sensitive to external cues or signals, namely the sight, smell, or suggestion of food. If this describes you, join the crowd. There are millions like you, both heavy and thin. It may be very helpful for you to reduce your exposure to food. If this description does not fit you, read on anyway. These techniques may help you corral your desire to overeat.

The methods you learned earlier for buying and storing food were designed to reduce exposure to food. We have been moving forward in the sequence of antecedents. We began with the first step (shopping). We then moved a step closer to eating (storing food). We will now move even closer by discussing serving and dispensing food.

I will describe several techniques for serving food. All follow a general principle, which is to interrupt the sequence of events associated with eating. Some techniques will apply to you more than others. You can use the principle to develop techniques of your own.

The following techniques are designed to help you control eating when your exposure to food cues is at its peak. The aim is to minimize your contact with these cues.

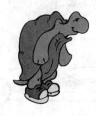

"Help slow your rate of eating by waiting five minutes before going back for extra helpings."

⇨ **Remove serving dishes from the table**. After first servings have been made, remove the food dishes from the table. Having the food handy is asking for trouble. If the food dishes are in another room or on another table, you can *think* before taking more. This does not prohibit you from having seconds, but it does interrupt the automatic eating that occurs when your plate is a magnet for anything left on the serving dishes.

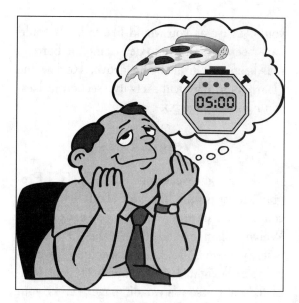

⇨ **Leave the table after eating**. This may sound antisocial, but some people are helped by leaving the table after dinner. This reduces the time you are exposed to food and to the circumstances of eating. If you finish long before the others, you may be eating too fast, and slowing down would help. If not, perhaps the others can retire to another room with you for the post-meal chat. This technique can work in concert with the previous suggestion to remove serving dishes from the table. If *all* the dishes are gone, it is not necessary to leave the table because exposure to food signals will be low. If food remains, bid the table farewell and depart for safer surroundings.

⇨ **Serve and eat one portion at a time**. Make and serve yourself only one portion of food. If you want two pieces of toast, make one and eat it before making another. If you want a container of yogurt, put half in a bowl and return for the second half if you still want it. You might find yourself passing up the second portion because you are no longer hungry. Here again is a chance to interrupt automatic eating. This also can help you separate hunger from habit. Because you have eaten one container of yogurt every morning for 10 years does not mean your body is hungry for that amount every day.

⇨ *Follow the five-minute rule*. Wait five minutes before going back for extra helpings. This will help you slow the rate of eating and will give you time to decide how much food you really need.

⇨ *Avoid being a food dispenser*. Are you the gatekeeper of food in your house? Do the kids get their snacks from you? Do you prepare all the food? This is a disadvantage because your routine brings you in contact with food many times each day.

Drop the job of being a food dispenser. Have the children pack their own lunches, if possible. Your spouse can manage snacks without you and may be willing to help even more by taking on some of the responsibility you have for distributing food.

More on Activity

We are now in Lesson Nine and have covered much of the introductory information on both lifestyle and routine activity. Much has been said about the importance and benefits of regular activity.

Are You Being More Active?

By this time in the program, my hope is that you are exercising daily. If this is possible for you, make it your goal, and do your best to make some time for exercise each day. Of course, missing a day here and there does not mean you have failed in your program. Daily activity is, however, a nice goal to strive for.

Look back over your Monitoring Forms, and see if your level of exercise has changed. Have you found something you like? Do you use this exercise regularly? Does the exercise help you stick to your eating plan and lose weight?

If you are having trouble with the exercise, read over the exercise sections in the earlier lessons. Let me remind you that people who are still exercising a year or two after they enter a

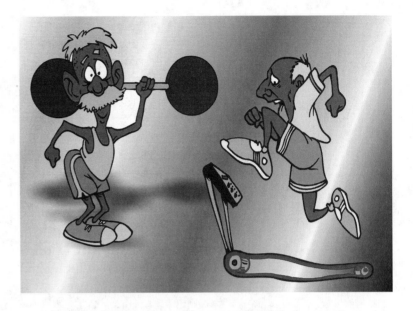

program tend to be the ones who have lost weight and kept it off.

People resist exercise for several good reasons. For some people, exercise is physically difficult to manage, and for others, strong negative feelings about sports and exercise present a psychological barrier. Another common problem is a busy lifestyle and the difficulty of budgeting time each day to be physically active.

These are all understandable reasons not to exercise. I hope you find the reasons in favor of exercise to be more compelling. It could mean a great deal to you, both now and in the future.

Consider this a pep talk. I really do feel that exercise is important, and I would like to do whatever is possible to encourage you to be active.

Matching Your Activity to Your Goals

In the previous lessons, I discussed various reasons to be active. Some people aim to improve their cardiovascular fitness and choose aerobic activities. Some want to increase strength and improve their physique, so they work out with machines or use free weights. Others want to use exercise to speed weight loss, so they do whatever they can to keep mov-

"Match your activity goals to the right exercise. If you want to increase strength, choose an exercise like free weights or if you want to speed weight loss, choose jogging or walking."

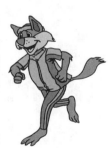

The Benefits of Various Exercises

	Developing Cardiovascular Fitness	Developing Strength	Muscular Endurance	Developing Flexibility	Controlling Body Fat
Archery [1]	1	2	1	1	1
Badminton [1]	2	1	2	2	2
Baseball [1]	1	1	1	1	1
Basketball— half court [1,2]	2	1	2	1	2
vigorous	4	1	3	1	4
Bowling [1]	1	1	1	1	1
Canoeing [1]	2	1	2	1	2
Fencing [2]	2	2	3	2	2
Football [2]	2	3	2	1	2
Golf (walking) [1]	2	1	1	2	2
Gymnastics [2]	2	4	4	4	2
Handball [1,2]	3–4	1	3	1	3–4
Horseback Riding [1]	1	1	1	1	1
Judo/Karate [1,2]	1	2	2	2	1
Mountain Climbing [1,2]	3	3	3	1	3
Pool/Billiards [1]	1	1	1	1	1
Racquetball [1,2]	3–4	1	3	1	3–4
Rowing, Crew	4	2	4	1	4
Sailing [1]	1	1	1	1	1
Skating—ice [1,2]	2–3	1	3	1	2–3
roller [1,2]	2–3	1	2	1	2–3
Skiing—cross-country [1,2]	4	2	3	1	4
alpine (downhill)	1	2	2	1	1
Soccer [2]	4	2	3	2	4
Softball [1,2]	1	1	1	1	1
Surfing [1,2]	2	1	3	2	2
Table Tennis [1]	1	1	1	1	1
Tennis [1,2]	2–3	1	2	1	2–3
Volleyball [1,2]	2	2	1	1	2
Waterskiing [1,2]	2	2	2	1	2

[1] Indicates lifetime sport.

[2] Indicates fitness needed to prevent injury.

4=Excellent   3=Good   2=Fair   1=Poor

Adapted from Corbin CB, Lindsey, R, editors. *Fitness for Life, 3rd Ed.* New York: Scott Foresman & Co.; 1993.

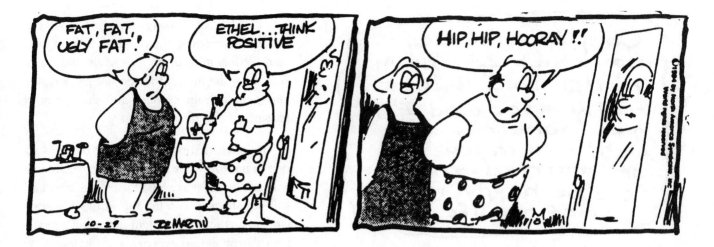

ing, usually with walking or jogging. Each type of activity is valuable, but for different purposes.

By now you have a good idea about what you hope to accomplish with exercise. The table presented on page 140 entitled, "The Benefits of Various Exercises," shows the strong and weak points of different activities. This may be helpful as you match your exercise to your goals.

From the table, it is apparent that the activities useful for controlling body weight also earn high marks for cardiovascular fitness. This is because the movement activities like jogging and cycling require effort (calories) for a sustained time and also give the heart a workout.

Remember, however, that cardiovascular fitness improves only when the right combination of frequency, intensity, and duration are present (see Lesson Eight). To utter once again the most oft-repeated sentence in this book: Any exercise is better than no exercise!

The Myth of Spot Reducing

Many people would need a computer to count the number of sit-ups they have done to tighten the tummy, leg exercises to trim the thighs, and contortions of the neck to wipe out a double chin. The trouble is, these things don't work, yet millions still fall for slick advertisements or books that promise ways of reducing specific parts of the body.

Where your body stores fat depends on genetic and hormonal factors. Women tend to store fat below the waist, on their hips, thighs, and buttocks. When they become heavy, they also store it above the waist. Men tend to store fat above the waist, in the abdomen. When you lose weight, your body burns fat, but you have little control over where it happens.

Exercises will help you with muscle tone. This can improve appearance somewhat. Doing sit-ups will tighten the muscles in your abdomen and will help you look a little less flabby, but they cannot force your body to take fat from there.

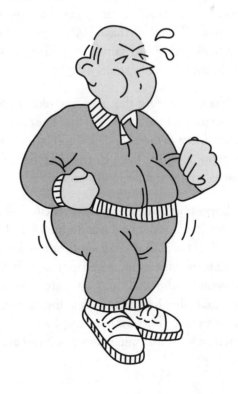

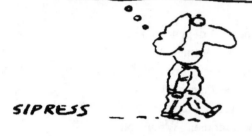

Oh please, scale, say that I'm down to 110, so I'll look really good and I'll meet someone, and we'll fall in love and get married and I'll be happy for the rest of my life...

SIPRESS

Impossible Dream Thinking

Along with Negative Self-Talk and Internal Attitude Traps, Impossible Dream Thinking ranks high as an attitude barrier to losing weight. In a later lesson, I'll discuss another attitude trap—Dichotomous Thinking. Impossible Dream Thinking occurs when you fantasize or dream about impossible accomplishments. You might have 100 pounds to lose on Thanksgiving and fantasize wearing a size nine to the office Christmas party.

Before you turn the page and skip to the next section, let me assure you that most people are not aware of these thoughts. Yet, after some reflection, most see them clearly. Maybe a few more examples will bring this home.

Impossible Dream thinking occurs when you daydream about how wonderful life will be after weight loss. It is common for those losing weight to imagine an improved marriage, better job, wonderful social life, intimate relationships, and other happy endings to their struggle to lose weight. These things may be possible, but it is unlikely that weight loss alone will make them happen.

This type of thinking also occurs when you imagine succeeding at a program without hard work. When most begin a program and fantasize about the future, they do not picture pain and puffing from exercise and the agony of passing up chocolate mousse.

It does no harm to hope for the best and aspire to improve your life. However, weight loss will usually not make a bad marriage good and will not shoot you to the top of the corporate ladder. Getting your weight down can actually be a disappointing experience if the fantasy is not fulfilled. This is what happened with one of my clients, Audrey.

Audrey was one of my first overweight clients. She was 28 years old and was working on an advanced degree in chemistry. She had been heavy since childhood and had been in no serious relationships. She was lonely and yearned to settle down with a stable and loving partner.

Audrey lost weight rapidly and seemed happy about her progress. She spoke often, but in a joking way, about how she would meet the person of her dreams when she got thin. I would easily spot it now, but at the time, I did not realize how serious she was about this fantasy. When she reached her goal, she steadily became more depressed because no spectacular romance evolved. Clearly, there were problems other than weight that prevented the relationships from developing, but Audrey saw weight loss as her salvation. Fortunately, I worked with Audrey on these problems, and she eventually did find the romance she was seeking.

This is a dramatic example of Impossible Dream Thinking. This specific case may not parallel your situation, but think honestly about whether you are harboring impossible dreams.

For many people losing weight, life does change in dramatic and positive ways. I hope this happens for you and that what you hope will happen actually occurs. Please remember, however, that weight loss may not automatically change your life.

Here are four ways to deal with Impossible Dream thinking. They can help keep your spirits high.

❶ *Counter the impossible dreams*. Pinpoint your Impossible Dreams and counter them with more rational expectations. Methods for developing counter statements were discussed in Lesson Eight on page 131 in the section on Internal Attitude Traps.

❷ *Set short-term goals*. Concern yourself with what you will do today and tomorrow, not what life will be like when you lose weight. This gives you many chances to experience success because you will be making small accomplishments in route to a larger goal. It will also prevent unrealistic fantasies from dominating your thoughts.

❸ *Focus on behavior, not weight*. Remember that your behavior must change before weight can change, so give yourself credit for following the program. You will have something to feel good about every day and will not be so discouraged by weight setbacks.

❹ *Set flexible goals*. If your goals don't work, set new ones. If you vowed to walk three miles each day but cannot, walk one or two miles every other day and work your way up. This puts the focus on short-term changes in behavior, so Impossible Dream Thinking will fade to the background.

Something for Your Partner to Read

TAPE 3
SECTION 4

In earlier lessons, I discussed ways to select a partner and to ask for help. One way to help your partner help you is to make specific suggestions. I often encounter partners who ask for guidance on what they can do. Most are genuinely interested in helping and need only suggestions.

This section is written for *you and your partner*. Have your partner read it and then discuss the material together. Decide on concrete

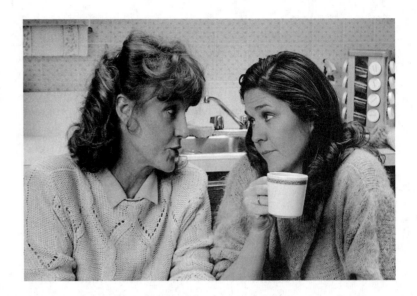

ways your partner can help and implement these right away.

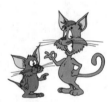

"Communication with your partner is essential to a positive relationship."

Partners can model good eating habits. A partner may help you immensely by doing what you are trying to accomplish. Eating slowly is a good example. A partner can exercise with you, can help keep food out of sight, and can display a positive attitude. This will remind you to do the same and will be a visible sign that your partner is trying to help.

Partners can praise your efforts. A pat on the back and a few kind words can go a long way. Your partner should not wait for you to lose weight to be kind to you, and he or she should not focus just on your weight change. When you make positive changes in eating or exercise, your partner can acknowledge it with supportive comments. By waiting only for changes in your weight, your partner misses many opportunities to help.

Partners can help with the weigh-in. Not everyone on a program will want a partner to know his or her weight, but if the relationship can tolerate this knowledge, having your partner present at a regular weigh-in can help. This gives your partner an idea of how you are doing. You may like this additional motivation. The partner must be forewarned, however, that weight loss will not occur every week. If the weigh-ins are more frequent than once per week, fluid shifts will give false indications about your progress in the program.

Partners can be rewarded in return. I explained earlier that the person in the program must be kind to the partner in exchange for the partner's support. This is a basic rule of relationships. In fact, many people feel better knowing that they are doing something nice for their partner. I also explained how you should be frank with your partner in asking for support and should be specific in these requests. These same rules apply to the partner. Your partner should tell you in specific terms what he or she can do to be nice. An example of a specific request might be, "I would like you to go to the movies with me once each week."

More Facts about Vitamins

Do you take vitamins? Chances are, the answer is yes. Do you need the vitamins you take? Chances are, the answer is no. Pretty bold statement, right?

The amount of money made on vitamins is unbelievable. The amount of fraud and exploitation is intolerable. An example from my own experience shows this. I once stopped in a health food store hoping to find some fruit. Upon entering, the owner was prescribing an assortment of vitamins to a woman who had arthritis and heart disease. She seemed to have little money but was willing to risk it on the hope the fellow might be right. What he told her was not only false, but could have harmed her, because he was prescribing high doses of fat soluble vitamins.

When asked why he thought this would help the woman, his response was "prove that it doesn't." He felt no burden to show that his advice was safe and effective. He then asked if I had cancer, diabetes, poor vision, or impotence (!) and pointed to shelves of vitamins that looked like alphabet soup.

This fellow was in his own small business, but similar hoaxes occur nationwide in chain stores. Many malls, shopping centers, and downtown shopping districts have such stores that seem official because of their fancy displays, nice signs, and wholesome appearance. Yet, they sell vitamins and other products some people don't need.

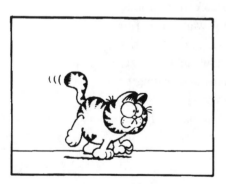
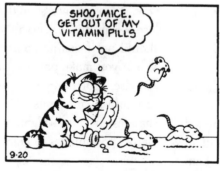
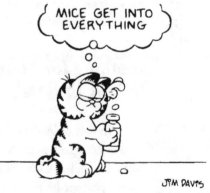
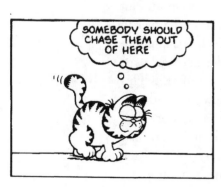
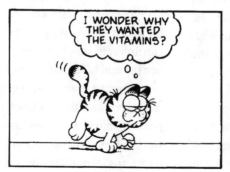
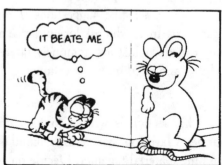

Perhaps some straightforward talk about vitamins will help clarify this confusing situation. Before I tell you what vitamins are and what they do, let me state my beliefs about vitamins and weight loss, a belief shared by every nutrition expert I have consulted:

THERE IS NO EVIDENCE THAT ANY VITAMIN OR COMBINATION OF VITAMINS HELPS PEOPLE LOSE WEIGHT

To review from Lesson Eight on page 120, vitamins are required for the transformation of energy in the body and for the regulation of metabolism. They do not produce energy themselves, but are crucial to the body's energy process. Some vitamins are needed to form important enzymes and others act as catalysts (they speed chemical reactions).

There are two main types of vitamins: fat soluble and water soluble. The fat soluble vitamins are vitamins A, D, E, and K. They are absorbed in fat tissue and are not excreted by the body if you take too much. They can be toxic.

The water soluble vitamins are vitamin C and the B-complex vitamins, which include thiamin, riboflavin, and niacin. These are absorbed in the body's water. Excess amounts can usually be excreted through the urine, so taking more than your body needs is wasting money because the vitamins simply pass through your body.

More information on specific vitamins can be found in *The LEARN Healthy Eating and Calorie Guide* mentioned throughout this manual (see page 303). This guide includes the functions of each vitamin, their sources in foods, and facts about vitamins and health.

Nutrition experts feel, as a general rule, that most people in developed countries, particularly the U.S., receive adequate vitamins if they eat a balanced diet. Most people need no vitamin supplement at all, much less the mega

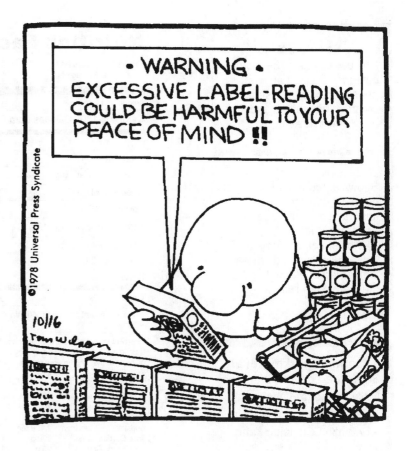

doses prescribed by someone with unproven ideas.

Because you are exercising and eating less, taking a multiple vitamin each day probably will not hurt and may help remedy any deficiency created by the change in food intake. But again, if you are careful with the foods you choose, this may not be necessary.

Reading Food Labels

By now it should be apparent that one of the keys to eating right is portion control (i.e., calories). Learning how to use and apply a calorie guide is one way you can control the number of calories you eat each day. Another helpful tool is the food label. The U.S. government has passed legislation requiring almost all food products to include a standardized labeling system. Food labels can be very helpful, and you should know what they mean to you. The following discussion will help you understand how to read and use food labels.

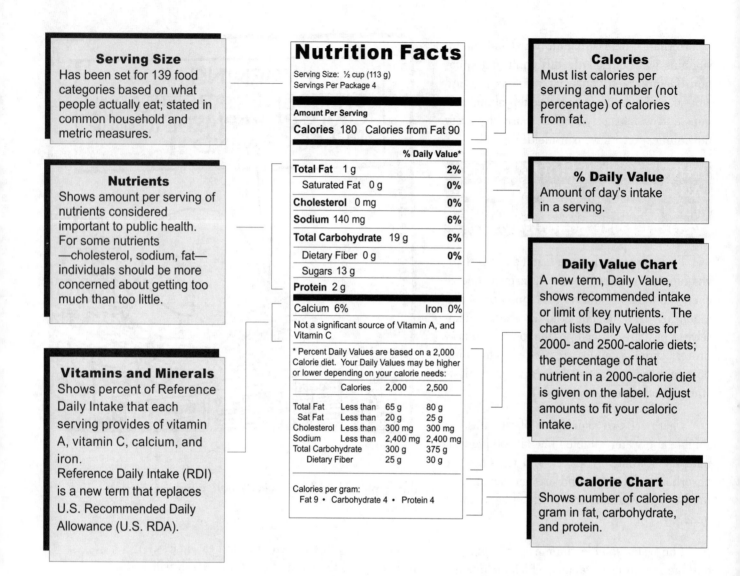

Serving Size
Has been set for 139 food categories based on what people actually eat; stated in common household and metric measures.

Nutrients
Shows amount per serving of nutrients considered important to public health. For some nutrients —cholesterol, sodium, fat— individuals should be more concerned about getting too much than too little.

Vitamins and Minerals
Shows percent of Reference Daily Intake that each serving provides of vitamin A, vitamin C, calcium, and iron.
Reference Daily Intake (RDI) is a new term that replaces U.S. Recommended Daily Allowance (U.S. RDA).

Calories
Must list calories per serving and number (not percentage) of calories from fat.

% Daily Value
Amount of day's intake in a serving.

Daily Value Chart
A new term, Daily Value, shows recommended intake or limit of key nutrients. The chart lists Daily Values for 2000- and 2500-calorie diets; the percentage of that nutrient in a 2000-calorie diet is given on the label. Adjust amounts to fit your caloric intake.

Calorie Chart
Shows number of calories per gram in fat, carbohydrate, and protein.

Nutrition Facts

Serving Size: ½ cup (113 g)
Servings Per Package 4

Amount Per Serving

Calories 180 Calories from Fat 90

	% Daily Value*
Total Fat 1 g	2%
Saturated Fat 0 g	0%
Cholesterol 0 mg	0%
Sodium 140 mg	6%
Total Carbohydrate 19 g	6%
Dietary Fiber 0 g	0%
Sugars 13 g	
Protein 2 g	

Calcium 6%	Iron 0%

Not a significant source of Vitamin A, and Vitamin C

* Percent Daily Values are based on a 2,000 Calorie diet. Your Daily Values may be higher or lower depending on your calorie needs:

		Calories	2,000	2,500
Total Fat	Less than		65 g	80 g
Sat Fat	Less than		20 g	25 g
Cholesterol	Less than		300 mg	300 mg
Sodium	Less than		2,400 mg	2,400 mg
Total Carbohydrate			300 g	375 g
Dietary Fiber			25 g	30 g

Calories per gram:
Fat 9 • Carbohydrate 4 • Protein 4

Food label reform was enacted in 1990 to serve three primary purposes. The first is to help Americans choose a more healthful diet. The second is to decrease the confusion about advertising descriptions and other misleading information that has prevailed for years. Finally, the labeling requirements offer an incentive for food companies to improve the nutritional quality of their products.

Under the label reform regulations, most foods now require nutrition labeling. Nutrition information is voluntary for many raw foods, including the 20 most frequently eaten fresh fruits and vegetables and raw fish. Although currently voluntary, the Nutrition Labeling and Education Act of 1990 (NLEA) states that if voluntary compliance is insufficient, nutrition information for such raw foods may become mandatory.

The Nutrition Facts Panel

The food label includes a nutrition facts panel as shown in the diagram above. The heading of the panel includes the title "Nutrition Facts." This title alerts consumers that the label meets the requirements of the label regulations. The panel includes certain items that are mandatory and other items that are voluntary. The panel includes terms that may be unfamiliar to may people. References are made to Daily Values (DV) and comprise two sets of dietary guidelines: Reference Daily Intakes (RDIs) and Daily Reference Values (DRVs). To help make the label less confusing, however, only the term Daily Value is used.

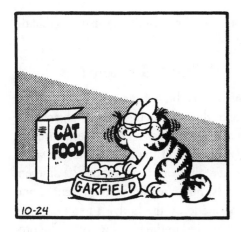
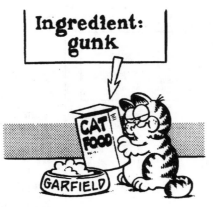
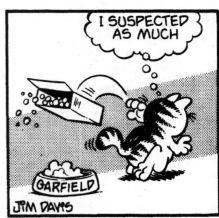

Reference Daily Intakes

The term Reference Daily Intakes (RDI) replaces the more familiar term U.S. Recommended Daily Allowance (U.S. RDA). The values for the RDIs remain the same as the old U.S. RDAs, at least for now. A major revision is currently underway to replace the RDI with revised recommendations called Dietary Reference Intakes (DRI). Until DRI can be established for all nutrients, the more familiar RDI values will continue to appear on food labels and will be used by health professionals.

Daily Reference Value

Under the label reform regulations, DRVs are established for those nutrients that contain energy (calories). These include fat, carbohydrate (including fiber), and protein. It is important to understand these percentages so that they are not mistaken as percentages of total calories. The DRVs are based on the number of calories consumed per day. As a common reference, 2000 calories is established as a daily intake. The DRVs for the energy nutrients and calculated in the following manner:

⇨ *Fat is based on 30 percent of calories.*

⇨ *Saturated fat is based on 10 percent of calories.*

⇨ *Carbohydrate is based on 60 percent of calories.*

⇨ *Protein is based on 10 percent of calories.* The DRV for protein applies only to adults and children over four years of age. RDIs for protein have been established for special groups.

⇨ *Fiber is based on 11.5 grams of fiber per 1000 calories.*

The DRVs also include sources for some non-energy nutrients, including cholesterol, sodium, and potassium. In addition, the DRVs for fats, cholesterol, and sodium represent the highest limits that are recommended. These values are as follows:

⇨ **Total fat: less the 65 g**

⇨ **Saturated fat: less than 20 g**

⇨ **Cholesterol: less than 300 mg**

⇨ **Sodium: less than 2400 mg**

Ingredients List

The ingredients list of the food is required on the food label. Food components are listed in order by weight from the most to the least.

Take a few minutes to carefully read through the illustration of the food label on page 146. Knowing how to read a food label can save you time in the grocery store isles and give you a leg up on good nutrition.

The Food Guide Pyramid

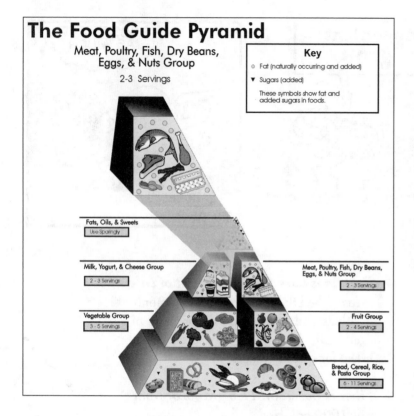

Meat, Poultry, Fish, Dry Beans, Eggs, & Nuts Group
2-3 Servings

Key
- Fat (naturally occurring and added)
- ▼ Sugars (added)

These symbols show fat and added sugars in foods.

Fats, Oils, & Sweets
Use Sparingly

Milk, Yogurt, & Cheese Group
2 - 3 Servings

Meat, Poultry, Fish, Dry Beans, Eggs, & Nuts Group
2 - 3 Servings

Vegetable Group
3 - 5 Servings

Fruit Group
2 - 4 Servings

Bread, Cereal, Rice, & Pasta Group
6 - 11 Servings

The Importance of Protein

Protein is a popular topic of conversation. I hear about high-protein diets and low-protein diets. I also hear about liquid protein, protein bread, and protein supplements. What is this fuss about?

Protein is the most abundant material in the body aside from water. It has many functions and is found in all cells. It plays many roles:

⇨ Protein is contained in hemoglobin, which carries oxygen in the blood.

⇨ Protein is related to DNA (deoxyribonucleic acid), which provides the genes with the code to transmit heredity.

⇨ Protein is used to build muscle and all other body tissue.

⇨ Protein is an important part of insulin, which regulates blood sugar.

⇨ Protein is used to build the enzymes that digest our food.

What Is Protein?

Proteins are built from approximately 20 amino acids that are put together in long chains. Protein can be synthesized or manufactured by the body, but only if the *essential* amino acids are present at the same time. Of the 20 different amino acids, nine are considered *essential* and cannot be made by the body. Therefore, they must be provided in the foods we eat. The protein our body uses best contains these amino acids. The 11 *nonessential* amino acids can be synthesized by the body, but only if the building blocks are present. These building blocks include the nine essential amino acids, nitrogen, and calories.

You may have heard about *high-quality* and *low-quality* proteins. High-quality proteins are those the body can use to function properly, because they contain all of the essential amino acids. Low-quality proteins have one or more essential amino acids missing.

Sources of Protein

Meat and dairy products contain high-quality proteins and do not have to be supplemented with other proteins because they contain all nine of the essential amino acids. Plant proteins usually lack one or more of the essential amino acids, but can provide adequate amounts of the essential and nonessential amino acids. Vegetarian diets can provide adequate protein if the sources are reasonably varied and the caloric intake is enough to meet the individual's energy needs.

Eating a variety of legumes and grains will provide high-quality protein. Legumes include dried peas and beans, such as black-eyed peas, chick peas (garbanzo beans), kidney beans, lentils, lima beans, navy beans, and soybeans. Soy protein has been shown to be nutritionally equivalent in protein value to proteins of animal origin. Nuts are also in this category, but they contain high amounts of fat. Grains include

Meat, Poultry, Fish, Dry Beans, Eggs, and Nuts

Description	Calories	Protein (g)	Carbohydrate (g)	Fat (g)
Beef:				
Chuck arm, lean braised (3 oz)	191	28.0	0	7.9
Ground, lean broiled (3 oz)	231	21.0	0	15.7
Round, lean broiled (3 oz)	204	23.0	0	11.6
Sirloin, lean broiled (3 oz)	229	23.5	0	14.3
Chicken:				
Dark, w skin roasted (3 oz)	215	22.0	0	13.4
Dark, w/o skin roasted (3 oz)	174	23.3	0	8.3
Light, w skin roasted (3 oz)	189	24.7	0	9.2
Light, w/o skin roasted (3 oz)	147	26.3	0	3.8
Fish:				
Flounder/sole, baked (3 oz)	173	25.7	0	7.0
Haddock, baked (3 oz)	95	20.6	0	.8
Lobster, steamed (3 oz)	83	17.4	1.1	.5
Shrimp, breaded & fried (3 oz)	206	18.2	9.8	10.4
Shrimp, boiled (3 oz)	84	17.8	.0	.9
Trout, baked (3 oz)	129	22.4	.0	3.7
Tuna, canned in water (3 oz)	111	25.1	.0	.4
Pork:				
Chop, lean center broiled (3 oz)	190	16.0	0	13.0
Ham, cured roasted (3 oz)	239	17.4	0	18.2
Loin, lean braised (3 oz)	266	25.3	0	17.5
Almonds, dry roasted (1 oz)	167	4.0	6.0	14.7
Black-eye peas, boiled (½ cup)	99	6.6	17.8	4.5
Chick-peas, boiled (½ cup)	135	5.9	27.2	1.4
Great northern beans, boiled (½ cup)	105	7.4	18.6	.4
Kidney beans, boiled (½ cup)	113	7.7	20.2	.4
Lima beans, boiled (½ cup)	121	7.3	19.6	.6
Navy beans, boiled (½ cup)	130	7.9	23.9	.5
Pink beans, boiled (½ cup)	125	7.0	23.0	.4
Pinto beans, boiled (½ cup)	93	5.5	17.5	.4
Pigeon peas, boiled (½ cup)	102	5.0	19.0	.3
Split peas, boiled (½ cup)	116	8.0	20.0	.4
Egg, raw whole (1 large)	79	6.1	.6	5.6
Peanut butter (1 T)	94	3.9	3.5	8.0
Peanuts, dry roasted (1 oz)	164	6.6	6.0	13.9
Pecans, dry roasted (1 oz)	187	2.0	6.0	18.5
Rice, long grain brown (1 cup)	232	4.9	49.7	1.2
Rice, long grain white (1 cup)	223	4.1	49.6	.2

Note: Each of the food items listed above counts as one serving. This table should be used as a guide for the foods listed. Since food values vary by brand name it is important to read the food labels for these foods.

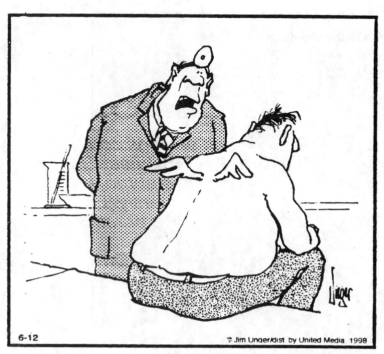

"Chicken for breakfast, chicken for lunch, chicken for dinner. What d'you expect?"

barley, corn, oats, rice, sesame seeds, sunflower seeds, and wheat.

Protein rarely exists by itself (egg whites or albumin is the exception) and is most often accompanied with mixtures of fat in foods like meat, fish, poultry, and milk products. Protein contains 4 calories per gram; this is the same caloric content by weight as carbohydrates. One ounce (28 grams) of lean meat, fish, or poultry contains approximately 7 grams of protein and 3 grams of fat (a total of 55 calories), whereas protein foods with higher fat content provide as much as 70–120 calories per ounce and 5–10 grams of fat per ounce.

How Much Protein Should You Eat?

Some health experts believe that Americans eat too much protein and that they should cut back. A major benefit would be a reduction in total fat, because the most popular protein foods (meat, fish, and poultry) also provide significant amounts of fat. We must remember, however, that protein in the diet is essential. Recommended amounts of protein range from 10–15 percent of total calories or approximately 50–75 grams of protein per day for adults. To see how your daily protein intake fits the guidelines for a healthy diet, multiply your target calorie level by 15 percent, the maximum recommended protein calories per day. For example, if your target caloric intake is 1200, $1200 \times .15 = 180$. Because there are 4 calories in every gram of protein, divide 180 by 4; $180 \div 4 = 45$. You know that you need to eat about 45 grams of protein daily to meet the government's recommended guidelines. For most people, the main source of dietary protein will come from the Meat, Poultry, Fish, Dry Beans Eggs, and Nuts Group of the Food Guide Pyramid.

The Meat, Poultry, Fish, Dry Beans, Eggs, and Nuts Group

The food items in this group include meat, poultry, fish, dry beans, eggs, and nuts. Meat, poultry, and fish provide good sources of protein, B vitamins, iron, and zinc. Dry beans, eggs, and nuts are similar to meats in providing protein and most vitamins and minerals.

How Much Is a Serving?

As a general rule, 2 to 3 oz of cooked lean meat, poultry, or fish count as one serving from the Meat and Protein Group. A 3-oz piece of meat is about the size of an average hamburger, a deck of cards, or the amount of meat on half a medium chicken breast. For other foods in this group, count ½ cup of cooked dry beans, one tablespoon of peanut butter, or one egg as 1 oz of meat (i.e., ⅓ of a serving). As an example, 6 oz for the day (two servings) may come from:

1 egg (counts as 1 oz of lean meat) for breakfast;

2 oz of sliced turkey in a sandwich at lunch; and

3 oz cooked lean hamburger for dinner.

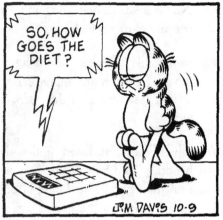 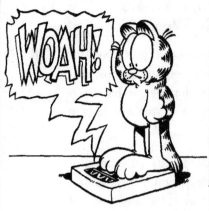 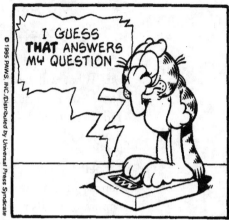

How Many Servings?

The Food Guide Pyramid suggests two to three servings per day from the Meat and Protein Group. The total from all servings should be the equivalent of between 5 and 7 oz of cooked lean meat, poultry, or fish per day. The table on page 149 shows items from this food group.

Watch out for Fat

As mentioned earlier, the best sources of protein come from animal products, such as dairy, meat, poultry, fish, and eggs. However, these food sources can be high in saturated fat and cholesterol. These tips will help reduce fat in your diet:

⇨ Choose lean meat, fish, poultry without skin, dry beans, and peas. These foods are the choices that are lowest in dietary fat.

⇨ Prepare meats in low-fat ways; trim away all the visible fat and boil, roast, or broil these foods instead of frying them.

⇨ Eat egg yolks sparingly—they are high in cholesterol. Use only one yolk per person in egg dishes and make larger portions by adding extra egg whites.

⇨ Remember, nuts and seeds are high in fat, so they should be eaten in moderation.

⇨ For beef, roasts and steaks of round, loin, sirloin, and chuck arm are lean choices.

⇨ For pork, roasts and chops of tenderloin, center loin, and ham are the leaner choices.

⇨ For veal, all cuts are generally lean, except for ground veal.

⇨ Lamb roasts and chops of leg, loin, and fore shanks provide the lean cuts.

⇨ Fish and shellfish are generally low in fat; however, those canned or marinated in oil are higher.

⇨ For chicken and turkey, both light and dark meat are lean choices provided the skin has been removed.

A New Weight Change Record

Each week you have been recording your weight change on the My Weight Change Record worksheet in Lesson One on page 25. This worksheet should now be completed. On page 154 is a new Weight Change Record for you to continue to record your weight change for Lessons Nine through Sixteen.

My Personal Goals for This Week

Set goals that are personally relevant for you. What will be most helpful in your program? Are there some techniques we have covered in earlier lessons that you are having trouble with?

Setting specific goals for a regular form of exercise such as walking, jogging, cycling, and swimming is also helpful. The goal you set might be to increase the number of days you engage in this activity or the number of minutes you do the activity. And, as we say in each lesson, keep up the goal setting for the changes you feel are most important. Focus this week on your eating and activity habits. Practice the techniques I discussed in the serving and dispensing food section of this lesson. Avoid falling into the impossible dream thinking trap. Also this week, become an avid reader of food labels. Try to include the correct number of servings from the Meat, Poultry, Fish, Dry Beans, Eggs, and Nuts Group of the Food Guide Pyramid. Continue to watch your diet for fat, and don't forget to record your weight change on the My Weight Change Record in on page 154.

My Self-Assessment

Lesson Nine

T F 64. It is best to take all of what you will eat in one serving so you will not need additional helpings.

T F 65. No exercise can help you lose fat in specific parts of the body.

T F 66. Impossible Dream Thinking is having fantasies and images about weight loss, life as a thin person, etc.

T F 67. The Total Fat listed under the heading "% Daily Value" on the Nutrition Facts Panel of the Food Label indicates the percentage of calories from fat for one serving of the food.

T F 68. It is fine to eat as much protein as you can to manage your weight because protein is good for you.

T F 69. The only way to get high-quality protein in your diet is to eat foods from the Meat, Poultry, Fish, Dry Beans, Eggs, & Nuts Group of the Food Guide Pyramid.

T F 70. If a partner is working with you to lose weight, it is important to reward him or her for the help he or she provides.

(Answers in Appendix C, page 271)

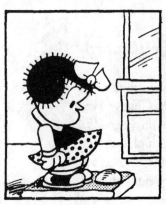
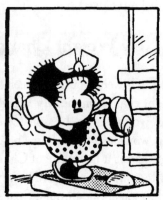
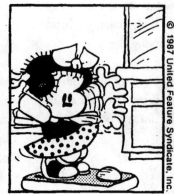
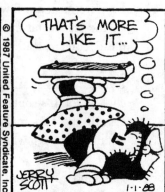

Monitoring Form—Lesson Nine *Today's Date:_____*

TIME	FOOD AND AMOUNT	CALORIES

TOTAL DAILY CALORIES

PERSONAL GOALS FOR THIS WEEK	MOST OF THE TIME	SOME-TIMES	RARELY
1. LEAVE THE TABLE AFTER EATING			
2. SERVE AND EAT ONE PORTION AT A TIME			
3. FOLLOW THE FIVE-MINUTE RULE			
4. AVOID BEING A FOOD DISPENSER			
5. DAILY SERVINGS FROM THE MEAT GROUP			
6. EAT LESS THAN _____ CALORIES PER DAY			
7. EAT LESS THAN _____ GRAMS OF FAT EACH DAY			

FOOD GROUPS FOR TODAY	PHYSICAL ACTIVITY	MINUTES OR STEPS
MILK, YOGURT, AND CHEESE ☐ ☐ ☐	(M)	
MEAT, POULTRY, ETC. ☐ ☐ ☐	(Tu)	
FRUITS ☐ ☐ ☐ ☐	(W)	
VEGETABLES ☐ ☐ ☐ ☐ ☐	(Th)	
BREADS, CEREALS, ETC. ☐ ☐ ☐ ☐ ☐ ☐ ☐ ☐	(F)	
SERVINGS OF WATER (8 OZ) ☐ ☐ ☐ ☐ ☐ ☐ ☐ ☐	(Sa)	
	(Su)	

My Weight Change Record
(Weeks 9–16)

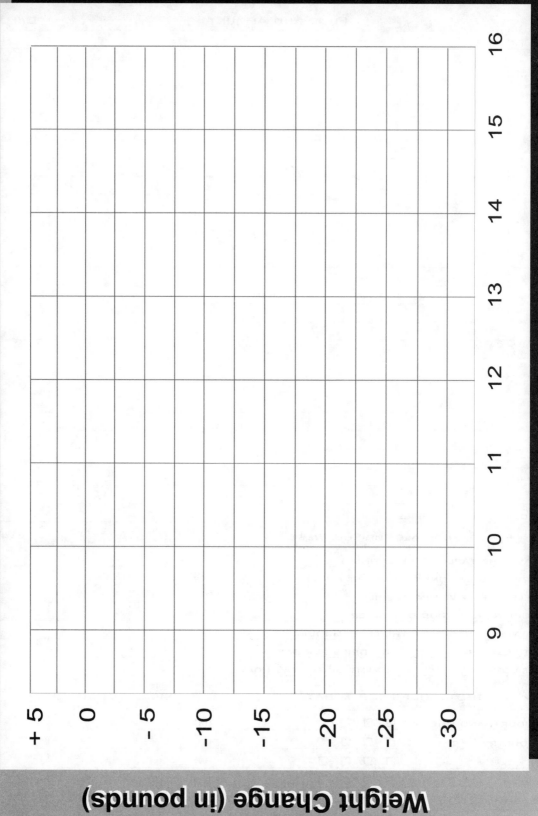

Weight Change (in pounds)

| | +5 | 0 | −5 | −10 | −15 | −20 | −25 | −30 |

Week

9 10 11 12 13 14 15 16

LESSON TEN

I would now like to raise the potentially touchy but important issue of family relationships. We'll also cover the testy issue of pressures to eat from other people. This can be helpful because offers and even demands to eat from others can be hard to resist. We then move to a new category of attitude traps—the imperatives. Stress and eating are often coupled, so we'll spend some time discussing this important issue. On the exercise front, I discuss the benefits of jogging and cycling as possible physical activities. Under nutrition, you will be learning more about water soluble vitamins and the important role of carbohydrates in your diet. We have a full agenda for this lesson, so if you're ready, let's begin.

For You and Your Family to Read

Some time ago, I traveled to Argentina and was invited to speak before a large meeting of a group called FAMALCO in Buenos Aires. Loosely translated, FAMALCO stands for "Families Anonymous of Relatives Fighting Against Obesity." This group was an outgrowth of ALCO, a large, nationwide, self-help group for obesity patterned after Alcoholics Anonymous (AA), in the same way Overeaters Anonymous in North America is patterned after AA. FAMALCO is similar in nature to AL-ANON, which is for families of alcoholics. The innovative nature of FAMALCO was inspiring. It is unfortunate

that no such group exists in our country. I would like to share what can be learned from this experience with you and your family, *so please ask your family to read this*.

The FAMALCO meeting began with moving testimonials from husbands, wives, children, and parents of people struggling with their weight. Some of the family members expressed sorrow about the weight problem, while others related dismay, sympathy, anger, and hostility. One thing common to all was the pain, suffering, and frustration experienced by both the overweight person and the family. FAMALCO allowed the family members to discuss these issues with others in the same situation and provided many opportunities for the

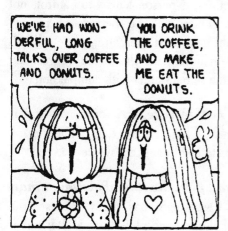

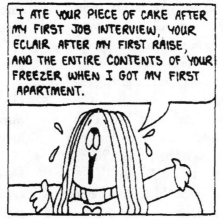

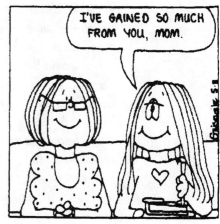

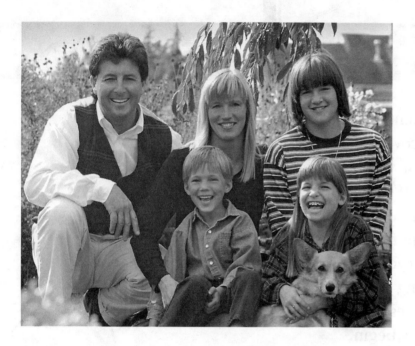

families to learn new ways to help the family member and to help themselves.

This meeting reinforced my belief that families can be a great resource for a person losing weight, but that harmony between the individual and the family requires a special effort from both parties. Communication is the first step. The burden falls to the person losing weight to express how he or she feels and how the family can help. This is sometimes difficult when the person resents the family's response to his or her weight. However, you must communicate by talking to your family and expressing your feelings.

The same responsibility applies to the family. The overweight person may have only a superficial knowledge of how the family feels. When the family finally expresses their feelings, the individual is likely to be relieved because the cards are on the table. This permits open discussion, positive communication, and suggestions from the person losing weight and his or her family about how they might help each other. I now recommend that the family and you read the section in Lesson Six, page 90 on "Communicating with Your Partner." The guidelines presented there can be used to begin and sustain the communication.

When I completed my lecture before FAMALCO, the audience responded with a warm, loud ovation. I assured the audience that I had learned at least as much from them as they had learned from me. I was even more certain of this when I listened to the speaker following me, Dr. Alberto Cormillot.

Dr. Alberto Cormillot is a prominent physician and public official in Buenos Aires, known all over Argentina for his work on weight loss. He developed a comprehensive approach to overweight that would rival any in the world. In his talk, Dr. Cormillot listed a number of things the family should or should not do. They are as relevant in our country as they are in his.

Things the Family Should Avoid

⇨ *Do not hide food from the person losing weight*. He or she will find it and feel resentful.

⇨ *Do not threaten*. Behavior is best changed with a soft touch, not coercion, so be nice.

⇨ *Do not avoid social situations because of the person's weight*. This will batter the self-esteem of the family member losing weight and will breed resentment in the family.

⇨ *Do not expect perfection or 100 percent recovery*. Weight problems are something a person learns to control, not cure. There will be periods of misery, weight gain, and overeating. The individual's achievements should be appreciated and the setbacks met with compassion.

⇨ *Do not lecture, criticize, or reprimand*. These rarely help. The person needs to feel better, not worse.

⇨ *Do not play the role of victim or martyr*. Overweight has many causes, both psychological and physiological. It is unfair for the family to blame the overweight family member and to feel victimized. Support and encouragement will do more than guilt and shame.

Things the Family Can Do

⇨ *Keep a positive attitude*. This sounds trite, but can be very important. It is not easy to be upbeat and encouraging when a program grinds on for months and months. Extra effort from the family can make life much easier for the person losing weight.

⇨ *Talk with others in your situation*. Being in a family where a weight problem exists generates strong feelings in the family members. It can help to talk about these with others who deal with the same issues. Many good ideas can be generated from this process.

⇨ *Keep the home and family relaxed*. This will permit the person on a program to pay attention to the task at hand, changing eating and exercise habits.

⇨ *Learn to ignore and forgive lapses*. The family can react many ways to mistakes, bouts of weight gain, and binges. The person losing weight feels bad when these occur, so it is best for the family to adopt a hands-off policy and to forgive and forget.

⇨ *Ask the person losing weight how you can help*. The best way to learn how to help is to ask. Family members are sometimes surprised by what the individual wants.

⇨ *Exercise with the person on a program*. This is a wonderful and healthy way to spend time together. If only a daily walk, this provides time to talk and can help the person with the program.

⇨ *Develop new interests with the family member losing weight*. There are so many things in life to enjoy, and developing new interests can be good for everybody. Individuals losing weight sometimes feel they are embarking on a new life. New activities can involve the family in this process.

To summarize this section for the family, there are many ways the family can help the person losing weight. It begins with communication and proceeds to the things listed above. Both the family and the individual are responsible for making these happen.

Dealing with Pressures to Eat

A major challenge for individuals on weight loss programs is to cope with pressure to eat. Friends, relatives, and strangers—some well-meaning and some not—can make it difficult to lose weight by encouraging you to eat. There are a number of reasons for this.

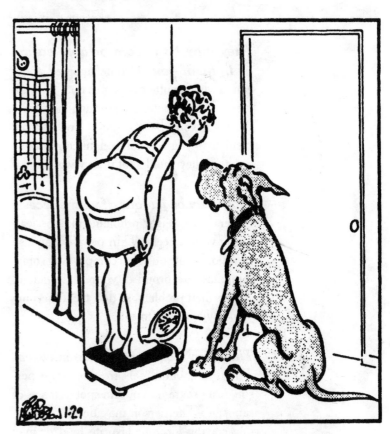

"It's all your fault. You stopped in front of the bakery store."

Pressures to Eat are Challenging

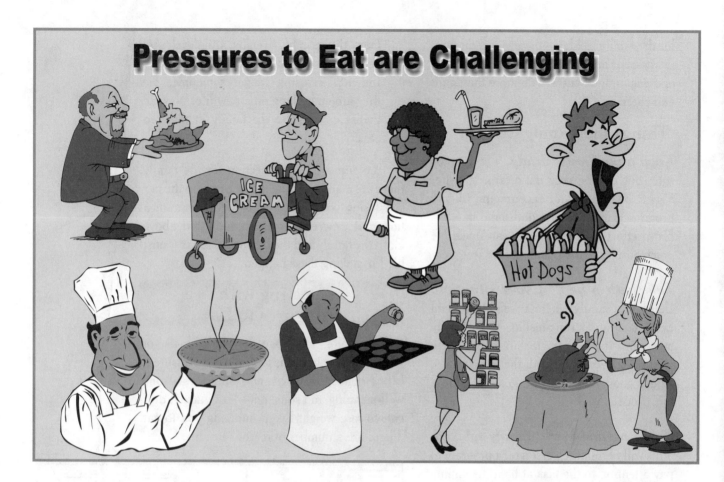

⇨ **They may be uncomfortable eating in front of you**. People agonize about eating when another person is not. They offer food to be polite, even though they know the offer won't be accepted. You can tell them that you do not feel uncomfortable and that they should eat if they wish.

⇨ **They may be jealous of your success**. Others with weight problems may be jealous of your success. Thin people may also be jealous that you are accomplishing something and are proud of your achievement. This is their problem, so don't let it become yours by agreeing to eat.

⇨ **They may not want you to succeed**. This is rare, but it spells trouble for the person on a program. You can spot it in acts of sabotage. The person may develop a sudden craving for your favorite food or may say demoralizing things like, "You have always failed before and will fail again."

There are several reasons why another person would act this way, but I do not want to launch into a lengthy psychological analysis. You are better off ignoring these comments. Confronting the person rarely helps and can make the situation worse. Again, this is their problem, so don't let it influence you. If they offer you food or encourage you to eat, refuse in a polite way, but be sure to refuse. The person will get the message and will quit trying.

⇨ **They think you are starving**. These people can imagine themselves in your shoes and are certain they would be ravenous. Because so many people associate food with love, encouraging you to eat is one way to show concern. Assure them that you are fine and that they can help by ignoring your diet and by not offering you food.

⇨ **They want to test your determination**. They may want to tease you or to see how serious you are about your program. It seems cruel, but it happens. Show them just how serious you can be.

Be Polite, but Be Firm

When you are pressured to eat, stand up for yourself and refuse. Avoid being aggressive or insulting, even if you suspect evil motives. The polite approach works best. After a few polite refusals, most people will learn that their pressures will not work and will quit pestering you.

If Aunt Irma offers you fudge, you might say, "Gee Irma, I love your fudge, but I'm not very hungry." If your husband stops to get ice cream with you in the car, say "I hope you enjoy it, but I really don't want the calories."

If you have trouble being assertive, try to predict the situations in which you might be pressured to eat. Plan a response, and practice it so you arrive prepared to be polite and firm.

Another Attitude Trap: Imperatives

TAPE 4
SECTION 3

Imperatives include words that imply urgency and no room for error. Examples of imperative words are "always," "must," and "never." If you are like most people, your vocabulary may be peppered with imperatives. Using these words can pave the path to trouble. Here are some examples from our clients.

"I will *never* eat more than 1200 calories."

"I *must never* eat cookie dough ice cream again."

"I will eat a salad for lunch *every* day."

"I will *always* say no when Vicki offers me coffee cake."

"I must *always* control my cravings for sweets."

"Chocolate is my downfall, so I will avoid it *always*."

"I will exercise *every* day."

"I must have *perfect* control of my eating."

"I will *always* control the moods that make me eat."

These thoughts can float around in your mind waiting to take pot shots at your control. If you exceed your calorie level some day, you can recover from the extra calories if your control stays intact. However, the imperatives can get a clean shot at you if your mind cranks out thoughts like, "I should never eat more than I'm told." When this happens, you may be a goner. Disappointment occurs, and one can lose sight of positive accomplishments because of a few mistakes.

Individuals who feel they should avoid certain foods are especially likely to fall prey to the imperatives. If you forbid yourself peanuts, you will be fine for a week or two. You may then start to crave peanuts, wonder how they would taste, and fantasize about a peanut feast when the program ends. Then you might eat some peanuts, either because you are offered some or you break down and buy them. Feeling like a failure might then weaken control even further

"Be on the lookout for those imperatives; they can derail your progress."

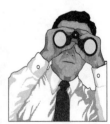

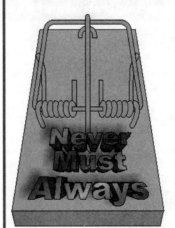

Another Attitude Trap: Imperatives

Never Must Always

"**I** *will* **never eat more than 1200 calories.**"

"**I** *must always* **control my carvings for sweets.**"

"**I** *must* **have** *perfect* **control of my eating.**"

"**I** *must* **never eat cookie dough ice cream again.**"

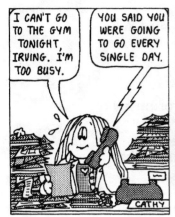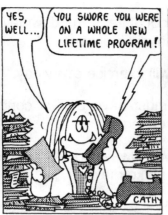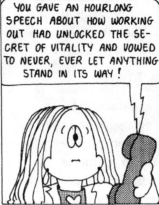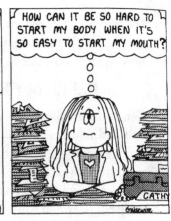

and dichotomous thinking (I'll discuss this later in Lesson Fourteen on page 220) can lead to *falling off* your program.

Try to find imperatives in your vocabulary. What do you expect of yourself, and how can you banish words like *never* and *always* from your internal conversations? Replace the imperatives with language that allows some room for error and flexibility. Remember, there is no such thing as a perfect person.

In the table below are some examples of common imperative statements and some methods to counter them. These may apply to you in one way or another, but if they do not, you can use them as examples to form your own methods of dealing with the imperatives. Once again, being prepared can make you ready to deal with most difficult situations.

The imperatives are habits just like other behaviors and attitudes. To develop a new habit, practice is the key. It seems funny to practice thinking a certain way, but it really works. Once you know what attitudes give you trouble, you can gradually weaken their ability to influence you by replacing them with positive approaches.

Stress and Eating

**TAPE 4
SECTION 2**

A very interesting (and unexplained) paradox is that stress makes some people eat more and some people eat less. Scientists are working to understand this, but one thing is clear—stress is often cited as a major issue for people who wish to lose weight.

When I discuss the complexity of weight loss with clients in my clinic, the issue of stress arises repeatedly. Some people point to a spe-

Imperative and Counter Statements (examples)	
Imperative Statement	**Counter Statement**
I will never eat candy bars.	I will do my best to eat fewer candy bars, but if I have one, it is a sign to increase my control, not to let down.
I will never get depressed because it makes me eat.	Everybody feels down at times. If I get depressed, I must think of reacting with something other than eating—walking may be a good choice.
I will exercise every day.	This is my goal, and I will do my best to reach it. When I can't, I will try harder the next day.

cific stressful event to explain why they gained weight in the first place. Others say that stress makes them want to eat all the time, so they nibble. Still others feel that stress threatens their ability to maintain weight loss and puts them at risk for relapse.

It is no surprise that stress exerts such an important effect on eating. There are clear links between stress and health. Health problems ranging from the common cold to chronic diseases like heart disease, diabetes, and asthma are thought to be affected by stress. It is reasonable to believe that reducing stress would make many people happier and healthier, and less stress would facilitate control over eating and weight in the process. Do you feel that stress influences your eating? Here are some questions to ask yourself:

❶ **When you feel pressure to accomplish something, do you feel pulled toward food or pushed away from it?**

❷ **If you were sitting at a desk working on a project that had to be done quickly, would you want to be eating something?**

❸ **Do you believe food is something you use to feel better when you are stressed?**

❹ **Does stress make you eat more?**

If you answered "yes" to any of these questions, stress and eating might be linked in important ways. The question then is, what to do about it?

There are two solutions. One is to respond to stress with activities other than eating. In Lesson Fourteen on page 218, I discusses means for developing alternative activities. With a list of such alternatives, you can use the urge to eat as a signal to engage in another activity. Hence, the same stimulus (stress) might exist, but you would not react by eating.

A second solution is to reduce stress. This is an appealing possibility, because stress reduction might affect not only your eating, but other areas of your life as well. It may be helpful, therefore, to learn stress management techniques. It would take another book the size of this to provide a complete stress management program, but I can provide a few details about stress and then refer you to materials or programs for more detailed information. At the end of this section I'll discuss an exciting new stress management program.

Stress is a fascinating interplay between body, mind, and environment. We each respond to situations in our environment in a unique way. Events that disturb one person mean nothing to another. Some people respond to stress with a racing heart and anger, while others respond with nausea and fear. What is certain is that the ways we think and act are key factors in how we handle stress. Therefore, there are a number of things a person can do to better manage stress. These are skills that you can learn, much as you are learning weight management skills in this program.

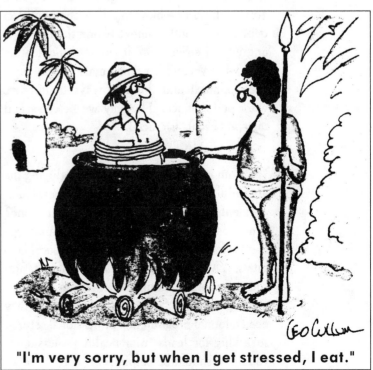

"I'm very sorry, but when I get stressed, I eat."

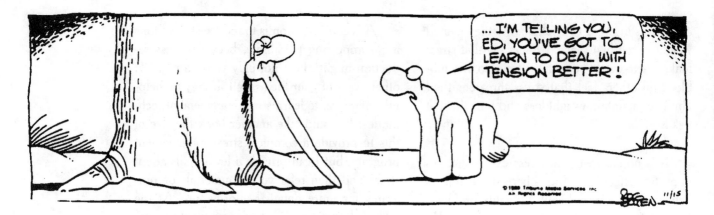

I will provide two examples here. The first is the use of relaxation training. Good stress management programs teach specific relaxation skills, so that when stress begins, a person has the ability to halt the process by countering a stress response with relaxation responses. Learning relaxation skills can be very helpful and can help an individual calm down before an undesirable action occurs (like overeating).

The second example deals with what scientists have called *appraisal*. When an event occurs in our lives, we appraise the situation and then respond. The appraisal determines the response. One person who receives a negative evaluation from a boss might have a negative appraisal, suffer a blow to self-esteem, and feel depressed. Another might blame the boss, get angry, and strike back in some self-defeating way, while yet another might make a more positive appraisal and think of ways to improve work performance. The way we perceive and interpret events is crucial.

Both relaxation training and modifying the appraisal process are part of most stress management programs. So, how do you find one? One possibility is to seek out stress management seminars or training programs. Local hospitals, YMCA's and YWCA's, colleges, and some corporate settings offer stress management programs. Some individuals find they need a formal program in a professional setting, so asking for leads from health professionals you know should be helpful.

Other people do not need a formal program and can use written materials in a very positive way. An excellent guide is a step-by-step manual by Drs. David Barlow, Ronald Rapee, and Leslie Reisner titled *Mastering Stress 2000—A LifeStyle Approach*. This program is part of the LEARN LifeStyle Program Series™ and is published by the American Health Publishing Company (the company that publishes *The LEARN Program for Weight Management 2000*). Information can be obtained by calling 1–888–LEARN–41 or by contacting The LifeStyle Company at the address provided in the Supplemental Resources and Ordering Information at the end of this manual on page 303.

Let's Consider Jogging and Cycling

What a change there has been in society's attitude about exercise, particularly running. As recently as the early 1970s, the longest race in most track meets was two miles, and most people had trouble believing that kooks actually raced for six miles in cross-country meets.

Jogging and Running

Now it seems routine for people to brag about doing their 3, 5, 10, or even more miles. The number of people who proclaim themselves runners is staggering. There are running magazines, running clubs, and even running software for computers. It is tempting to poke fun at this hysteria and to pass it off as a fad. That would, in my opinion, be a mistake.

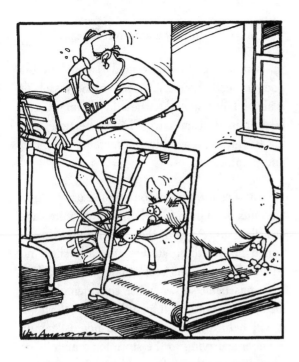

Before we discuss running in more detail, let me emphasize again the virtues of brisk walking. Running is fine, but for people who still have many pounds to lose, brisk walking is easier and brings nearly all the benefits. This section is designed to show that running can be helpful to some people, but walking is a fine alternative.

The benefits of running are indisputable. Many positive physical changes occur, as discussed in Lesson Two. However, the psychological advantages are often overlooked. I am not talking about the widely touted runner's high, but about a general sense of accomplishment, self-confidence, well-being, and good feelings.

This psychological advantage may come from running itself or may simply result from the mastery of something new. I lectured on the psychological benefits of exercise at a sports medicine conference in The Netherlands. Dr. John Garrow, an outstanding researcher from England, asked me a telling question. He asked if people would get the same positive effects from something unrelated to exercise, such as learning to play the cello.

Dr. Garrow was questioning whether something inherent to exercise would be beneficial or whether the effects were due to the excitement of improving at any activity. This is a difficult question to answer. From a practical standpoint, exercise is a good means for producing this mastery because it carries physical benefits as well. After all, it burns more calories than playing the cello!

Cycling

Cycling has the advantages of running and is more enjoyable for some people. Riding a stationary bicycle indoors or a traditional bike outdoors is good exercise. It spares the knees, ankles, and feet from the pounding they take when running and is nice for heavy people because weight is supported by the bike. It is an excellent method for burning calories.

If cycling outdoors is feasible for you, give it a try. Cycling to work is terrific when possible. If not, consider buying a stationary bicycle for your home. I have one and like to alternate between running, cycling, and playing tennis. The cycling is nice in bad weather, and you can do it while watching the news or listening to music.

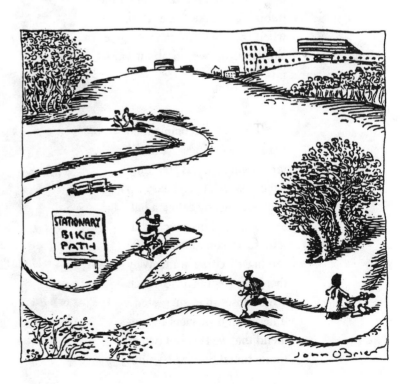

Running and cycling are not the only exercises, but they are good ones. These activities (along with walking and swimming) are top choices among my clients, so please give them a try. If you are doing something else regularly, stick with it. If you are sporadic in your habits or have not tried anything seriously, consider lacing up your shoes to hit the road or jumping on a bike to sail down the street.

More about Water Soluble Vitamins

In Lesson Eight on page 120, I introduced the topic of vitamins and discussed the difference between water soluble and fat soluble vitamins. Let's look closer at the water soluble vitamins.

Vitamin C: Good or Bad?

No matter what we hear, people continue to think that vitamin C helps to cure and prevent colds. It has been ascribed other wondrous qualities as well. I recently read reports of a study where vitamin C had been used with cancer patients, as the vitamin advocates recommend. It did no better than a placebo. The advocates claim that the dosage was faulty. It is difficult for the public to make wise decisions when the scientists cannot agree. So, what do we do about vitamin C?

The Recommended Daily Allowance (RDA) for vitamin C is 60 mg, which is relatively easy to consume just by eating a balanced diet. This much vitamin C is contained in one serving of citrus fruit. Why then, do people take much larger doses than suggested? The vitamin pushers recommend that we take not two or three times the RDA, but

100 or 1000 times the amount. Does it help?

Vitamin C (ascorbic acid) is used by the body for teeth, bones, cells, and blood vessels. It is absolutely essential for health. Vitamin C can be obtained from citrus fruits, berries, fruit juices, green vegetables, tomatoes, cabbage, and potatoes.

Studies have been done on the use of large amounts of vitamin C in hopes it will cure various illnesses. As with the cancer study I mentioned above, these studies typically show no advantage for taking more than recommended. This has been shown most convincingly with the common cold. Still, people cling to the hope it will help and may send the nearest family member scurrying to the store for orange juice when they get the sniffles.

Because so many people take so much vitamin C, there is reason to be concerned about possible dangers. Fortunately, vitamin C is water soluble. Excessive amounts, for the most part, are excreted through the urine, so your body only uses what it needs. However, there is some evidence that vitamin C can build up in body tissue when large doses are taken.

B-Complex Vitamins

The B-complex vitamins are also water soluble. This complex includes vitamin B_1 (thiamine), vitamin B_2 (riboflavin), niacin, vitamin B_6, and vitamin B_{12}. Each serves a different purpose and has different recommended amounts for healthy functioning.

Vitamin B_1 is necessary for the heart and nervous system because of its role in carbohydrate metabolism. It is available in enriched cereals, bread and other flour

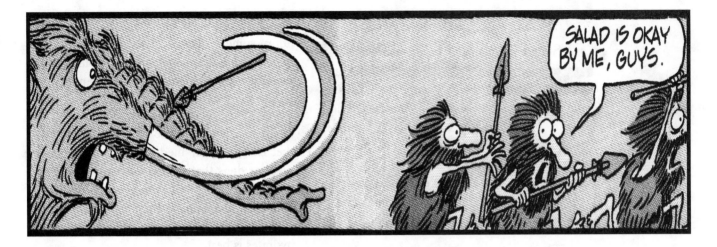

products, fish, meat, liver, milk, poultry, and whole-grain cereals. Vitamin B_2 is important in carbohydrate metabolism and tissue repair. It is necessary for the skin and prevents light sensitivity in the eyes. It is available in leafy green vegetables, lean meat, liver, milk, eggs, and dried yeast.

Niacin is important for the metabolism and absorption of carbohydrate, so it plays a key role in converting food to usable energy. It is available in enriched cereals and bread, eggs, lean meats, liver, and dried yeast.

Vitamins B_6 and B_{12} are becoming more popular in health food stores. Vitamin B_6 is used for metabolism of protein, carbohydrate, and fat, and is available in many foods, including chicken, fish, liver, whole grain cereals, and egg yolks. Vitamin B_{12} helps prevent anemia and aids in the work of the nervous system. It is found in lean meat, liver, kidney, milk, saltwater fish, and oysters.

As with vitamin C, the B-complex vitamins are being hawked in health food stores and nutrition centers for all sorts of ills. Most people get enough of the B vitamins from normal eating. There are some conditions for which additional B vitamins are needed, but these should be diagnosed by a physician, not a store clerk. Because these vitamins are water soluble, extra amounts will be excreted, so your money goes just where the extra vitamins end up.

What about Multiple Vitamins?

It is reasonable to take a well-formulated multiple vitamin if you are concerned about getting enough vitamins and minerals in your diet. Check the label to see what percentage of the RDA's they provide, and do not exceed 100 percent.

Don't be confused by the fancy sounding vitamins at your store. There is no advantage to natural vitamins (another health food ploy). The store-brand generic vitamins are as good as the more expensive brand names.

Buy a multiple vitamin, which should contain the basic vitamins and minerals you need. Also, be cautious of vitamins that are supposed to help with things like stress. If you think you have some specific vitamin deficiency, consult a dietitian or physician.

Carbohydrates and Your Diet

I promised earlier that I would discuss carbohydrates in this lesson. So, let's get to it. People like to blame carbohydrates for everything. Some people on weight loss programs say that carbohydrates excite the binge center in their brain, and parents blame sugar when their kids misbehave. There is much talk about simple and complex carbohydrates, carbohydrate craving, and low-carbohydrate diets. You may be puzzled by all this, so let's clear the air.

What are Carbohydrates?

Stated in technical terms, carbohydrates are a combination of hydrogen, oxygen, and carbon atoms, which join together to make simple sugars, complex sugars, or starches. These sugars provide energy to the body. Complex sugars must first be broken down by the body into simple sugars to be utilized. This is why simple sugars (like sucrose) enter the body's energy supply more quickly than the complex sugars or starches in vegetables or cereals.

There are many sources of the simple sugars and starches. Simple sugars consist mainly of sucrose (table sugar), fructose (in fruit and honey), and lactose (in milk). The starches are in foods like cereals, pasta, rice, breads, and vegetables.

Like protein, carbohydrate provides 4 calories per gram. In contrast, fat has more than twice the calories per gram. The major part of our diet is carbohydrate, and it is easy to eat too much. Many of the carbohydrate foods we eat are of poor nutritional value and contain only calories from sugar. They are a poor source of nutrition, hence the term *empty calories*. Foods like these are prime candidates for elimination or reduction for individuals trying to lose or maintain weight.

In order for the diet to provide an adequate balance of nutrients, an adult should have approximately 165–180 grams of carbohydrate per day (based on a diet of 1200 calories). This would total from 660–720 calories (140–150 grams at 4 calories per gram). Adults are advised to have 55–60 percent of their total calories in carbohydrates.

What does all this jargon mean? Carbohydrates are essential in the diet and are not necessarily bad. In fact, most people should increase their intake of complex carbohydrates. Starches should not have the bad rap they receive. People consider potatoes fattening because they are high in starch, yet potatoes are reasonable to eat because of their nutrition. The amount eaten is usually the problem, along with the goodies that adorn some of these foods. For example, sour cream and butter, which are mainly fat, rapidly increase the caloric intake of eating an innocent potato.

It is unwise to follow a low-carbohydrate diet except under medical supervision. Some popular diets that restrict carbohydrate to less than 100 grams per day make it very difficult to maintain adequate nutrition. A sensible plan with 55–60 percent of your calories from carbohydrates is best.

Try to be on the lookout for simple sugars in your diet. These tend to come from foods with many calories and little nutrition. Examples are crackers, doughnuts, pastries, soft drinks, candy, and so forth.

These simple sugars stimulate insulin release. Because insulin is related to hunger, you will feel hungry in less time with simple sugars than with complex sugars. Moving away from candy and other sweet foods, toward vegetables and other complex carbohydrates, is a wise decision.

Carbohydrates and Extra Calorie Burning

For many years, a simple statement ruled in the minds of experts—"A calorie is a calorie." The belief was that calories are handled in the same way by the body no matter where they came from. If you ate 3500 calories of oat bran and tofu, you would gain the same weight as you would by eating the same calories from a triple cheeseburger and onion rings. No longer.

The body has an easier time converting fat calories to body fat than it does converting carbohydrate calories. Between 20–25 percent more energy is required for the body to handle carbohydrate than to handle fat. As an example, let's say you eat 100 calories of a high-fat food like butter. On another day, you eat 100 calories of a food high in complex carbohydrates, like a whole grain cereal. Your body will use 20–25 percent more calories to metabolize the carbohydrate. Therefore, the calories from fat and carbohydrate are not equal once they enter your body.

This is good news. Foods high in complex carbohydrates are good to eat for health reasons, and you will burn more calories when you eat them. Many people report that it is much easier to lose weight when they cut back on fat and eat more fruits, vegetables, and grains. With this in mind, let's look at the Vegetable Group of the Food Guide Pyramid.

Vegetables in Your Diet

Do you remember your mother saying to you, "Eat your vegetables, they're good for you"? Mom was right, vegetables are good for you. In fact, both fruits and vegetables *are* so important in the diet that the Food Guide Pyramid breaks them into separate groups.

Vegetables are an excellent source of vitamins A, C, and folate. In addition, they provide minerals, including iron and magnesium, and as we mentioned earlier, they are an excellent source of carbohydrates. Vegetables are also naturally low in dietary fat. This is good news for people losing weight.

Most Americans fall short in their consumption of vegetables, perhaps because adding produce to their diet is inconvenient, time-consuming, or boring. Vegetables may not appeal to everyone's palate, especially in the ways they are usually prepared, but they are an important ingredient in a healthy and low-fat diet.

How Many Servings?

The suggested number of daily servings is three to five. This may sound like a lot, but it is actually less than you may think. For instance, just ½ cup of boiled green beans, one medium carrot, two stalks of celery, or half of a broccoli spear make one serving.

How Much Is a Serving?

As a general rule, the following will serve as a simple guide to help you include the right amount of vegetables in your daily diet:

1 cup of raw, leafy vegetables

½ cup of other vegetables, cooked or chopped raw

¾ cup of vegetable juice

The table on page 168 may help you better understand the portion size of a serving. The foods listed count as a single serving.

Serving Tips

There are a large variety of vegetables for you to choose from in our food supply. With a little creativity and planning, vegetables can become a fun and enjoyable part of your everyday diet. Here are some serving tips that you may find helpful:

Fresh vegetables make excellent snacks that you can easily take with you to work, school, or simply enjoy around the house. Celery, carrots, cauliflower, green peppers, cucumbers, and broccoli are good choices.

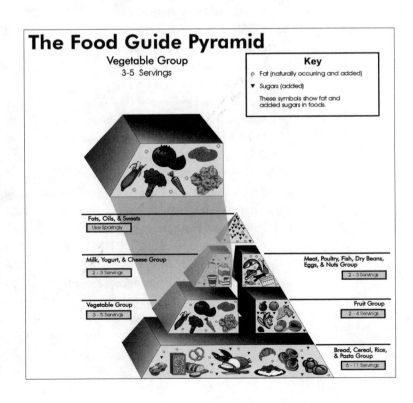

The Food Guide Pyramid

Vegetable Group
3-5 Servings

Key
- Fat (naturally occurring and added)
- ▼ Sugars (added)

These symbols show fat and added sugars in foods.

Fats, Oils, & Sweets
Use Sparingly

Milk, Yogurt, & Cheese Group
2 - 3 Servings

Meat, Poultry, Fish, Dry Beans, Eggs, & Nuts Group
2 - 3 Servings

Vegetable Group
3 - 5 Servings

Fruit Group
2 - 4 Servings

Bread, Cereal, Rice, & Pasta Group
6 - 11 Servings

167

Steaming vegetables also can be fun and can add variety to your meals. Best of all, it is easy to do and does not leave a big mess. While steaming the vegetables, you can add herbs or other seasonings to enhance flavor, or serve the steamed vegetables with a splash of lemon.

Think of creative ways to add vegetables to the foods you already eat and enjoy. Adding a slice of tomato, two large leaves of lettuce or spinach, and a pickle on the side turns a sandwich into a meal that includes one serving of vegetables.

When you eat fast food, be creative. Some fast food establishments now offer vegetable alternatives to french fries. Try a garden salad or baked potato next time. But be careful with dressings and toppings—make sure they are low fat. Remember to watch those *hidden* calories.

My Personal Goals for This Week

This is an excellent time to set goals related to relationships. The information for you and your family to read can be an excellent stimulus

Vegetables

Description	Calories	Protein (g)	Carbohydrate (g)	Fat (g)
Asparagus, boiled (½ cup)	22	2.3	4.0	.3
Beets, boiled (½ cup)	26	.9	5.7	.0
Broccoli, boiled (½ cup)	23	2.3	4.3	.2
Brussels Sprouts (½ cup)	30	2.0	6.8	.4
Cabbage, raw (1 cup)	16	.8	1.6	.2
Carrots, boiled (½ cup)	35	.9	8.2	.1
Cauliflower, boiled (½ cup)	15	1.2	2.9	.1
Celery, raw (½ cup diced)	11	.4	2.6	.1
Corn—yellow, boiled (½ cup)	89	2.7	20.6	1.1
Cucumber, raw (½ cup diced)	7	.3	1.5	.1
Eggplant, raw (½ cup pieces)	11	.5	2.6	.0
Green beans, boiled (½ cup)	22	1.2	4.9	.2
Lettuce, raw (1 cup)	10	.8	2.0	.2
Lima beans, boiled (½ cup)	109	7.4	21.2	.3
Mixed vegetables, canned (½ cup)	39	2.1	7.6	.2
Mushrooms, boiled (½ cup pieces)	21	1.7	4.0	.4
Okra, boiled (½ cup slices)	25	1.5	5.8	.1
Onion rings, frozen (7 rings)	285	3.7	26.7	18.7
Peas, green, boiled (½ cup)	67	4.6	12.5	.2
Potato, canned w/o skin (½ cup)	54	1.3	12.3	.2
Potato, French fried (10 pieces)	158	2.0	20.0	8.3
Potato, hash brown (½ cup)	163	1.9	16.6	10.9
Potato, mashed (½ cup)	111	2.0	17.5	4.4
Potato, scalloped (½ cup)	105	3.5	13.2	4.5
Squash—zucchini, boiled (½ cup)	14	.6	3.5	.1
Sweet potato, boiled (½ cup)	172	2.7	39.8	.5

Note: Each of the food items listed above counts as one serving. This table should be used as a guide for the foods listed. Since food values vary by brand name it is important to read the food labels for these foods.

for discussion. It can open the door for you to express how the family might be most helpful to you. Keep alert for imperatives finding their way into your vocabulary and remember that they leave no room for error. On the nutrition front, do your best to eat plenty of carbohydrates from the Vegetable Group of the Food Guide Pyramid. Try to become more aware of your stress level. How do you think stress and eating are related in your life? In addition, think about personal goals you can set based on your experience thus far in the program. Which behavior or attitude changes are most important for you? Be sure to continue to record your weight changes on the Weight Change Record on page 154 of Lesson Nine. Good luck this week!

T F 76. The Food Guide Pyramid suggests three to five servings each day from the Vegetable Group.

T F 77. Vitamin B_{12} is the only vitamin for which mega doses are recommended for weight loss.

T F 78. Because all vegetables have only small amounts of fats, it is not as important to count the amount of fat in these foods as it is to count the dietary fat from meat and dairy products.

(Answers in Appendix C, page 271)

My Self-Assessment

Lesson Ten

T F 71. It's not important to involve family members in your weight loss program because behavior changes are all up to you.

T F 72. Imperatives are words like always and never. They leave no room for error.

T F 73. There are many benefits to jogging and cycling. They are good forms of exercise for people trying to lose weight.

T F 74. Carbohydrates are not as important as other nutrients, and they should make up only about 30 percent of your daily diet.

T F 75. When someone offers you food, it is best to accept it as a sign of their friendship.

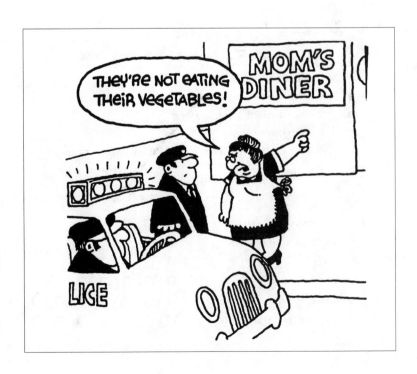

Monitoring Form—Lesson Ten   *Today's Date:* _____

TIME	FOOD AND AMOUNT	CALORIES
TOTAL DAILY CALORIES		

PERSONAL GOALS FOR THIS WEEK	MOST OF THE TIME	SOME-TIMES	RARELY
1. REFUSE OFFERS TO EAT			
2. BANISH IMPERATIVES			
3. TRY JOGGING OR CYCLING			
4. WATCH VITAMINS			
5. DAILY SERVINGS FROM THE VEGETABLE GROUP			
6. EAT LESS THAN _____ CALORIES PER DAY			

FOOD GROUPS FOR TODAY	PHYSICAL ACTIVITY	MINUTES OR STEPS
MILK, YOGURT, AND CHEESE ☐ ☐ ☐	(M)	
MEAT, POULTRY, ETC. ☐ ☐ ☐	(Tu)	
FRUITS ☐ ☐ ☐ ☐	(W)	
VEGETABLES ☐ ☐ ☐ ☐ ☐	(Th)	
BREADS, CEREALS, ETC. ☐ ☐ ☐ ☐ ☐ ☐ ☐ ☐	(F)	
SERVINGS OF WATER (8 OZ) ☐ ☐ ☐ ☐ ☐ ☐ ☐ ☐	(Sa)	
	(Su)	

I begin this lesson with a discussion of more good news about physical activity. The topic of aerobics is raised, and I'll then will cover ways to bring more pleasure to a program partnership. You will learn more about vitamins and I'll discuss the facts about dietary fiber. This week's lesson discusses the Fruit Group of the Food Guide Pyramid. Let's get started with a discussion about more exciting news about physical activity.

More Good News about Physical Activity

TAPE 3
SECTION 9

We have focused on lifestyle activity, programmed activity, and more vigorous types of exercise like running, jogging, and cycling. Most overweight people can start becoming more active by walking. By now, however, you may feel more comfortable with being physically active and may be ready for more. In Lesson Eight on page 126, I discussed programmed activity, and in the last lesson, we covered jogging, running, and cycling.

I expect that about half the people who read this manual will be ready for more rigorous activity than walking. The others can continue walking and lose more weight before taking on programmed activity. If you are in the second group, reread the section on Selecting and Starting a Programmed Activity on page 126,

and refer back to it when you are ready to increase your activity. In the meantime, continue to increase your walking by adding time or by increasing the speed at which you walk.

As I mentioned earlier, programmed activities include jogging, walking, aerobics, racquetball, swimming, cycling, or any regular activity. As I discussed in Lesson Eight, selecting the right activity is something of an art. Let's now address the issue of just how much exercise is necessary.

Great News about Activity

For many people, exercise is a major factor in their long-term prospects for weight management. It is true that many people lose weight without exercise, but for others, exercise makes an enormous difference. Do you remember the graph in Lesson Seven on page 109 that showed the difference between the maintainers and the regainers?

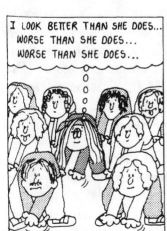

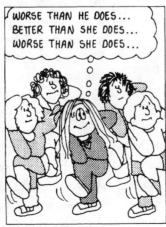

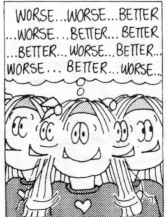

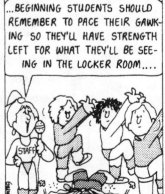

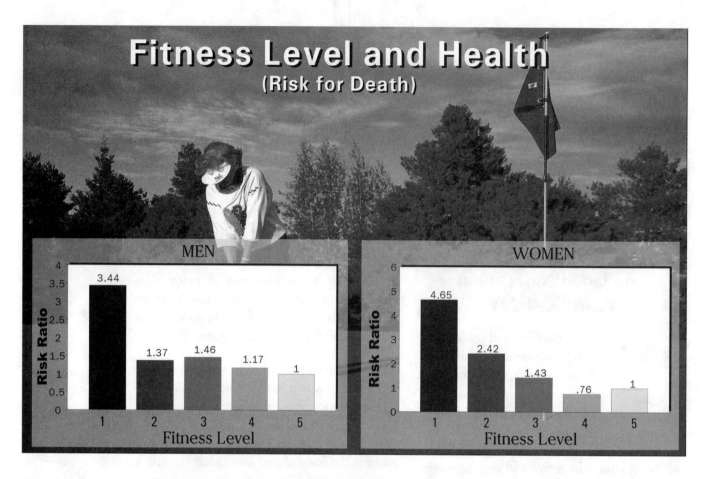

Fitness Level and Health
(Risk for Death)

MEN

Risk Ratio vs Fitness Level

- 1: 3.44
- 2: 1.37
- 3: 1.46
- 4: 1.17
- 5: 1

WOMEN

Risk Ratio vs Fitness Level

- 1: 4.65
- 2: 2.42
- 3: 1.43
- 4: .76
- 5: 1

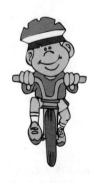

"People who exercise and are physically active live longer."

Exercise helps people lose weight for both physical and psychological reasons. It burns calories and may boost metabolic rate. Perhaps as important are the ways exercise makes us feel good. Each time we exercise, we are sending a signal to ourselves that we are making positive changes. The exercise may reduce stress and may give us more energy for life's other activities (like planning our weekly diet). Some people find exercise especially helpful by scheduling it at times they are most likely to eat.

One bit of very good news about exercise comes from work by Dr. Steven Blair and his colleagues at The Cooper Institute for Aerobics Research in Dallas, Texas. These researchers studied physical fitness and health in 10,224 men and 3120 women. Each person in the study underwent a detailed medical exam that included a maximal stress test on a treadmill. The people were grouped into categories of physical fitness based upon their performance

on the treadmill test. They were then followed for an average of eight years.

Dr. Blair and his colleagues placed these people into five categories of fitness, ranging from the very unfit (Fitness Level 1) to the very fit (Fitness Level 5). The graphs shown above give the risk ratio (which represents the death rate) for both men and women depending on their level of fitness. The risk for the most fit people is given a value of one, and then risks for the other categories are given in reference to that number. For instance, in the figure showing risk rates for men, the men in Fitness Level 5 (the most fit) have a risk factor of one. The risk increases to 1.17 (a 17 percent increase) for men in Fitness Level 4 and to 1.46 (a 46 percent increase) for men in Fitness Level 3.

There are several striking aspects to this study. First, it is yet another piece to the puzzle showing that people who exercise and are physically active live longer. For our purposes, however, the important news is that even modest levels of fitness are associated with greatly reduced risk. Look at the figure showing numbers for the men. Men in the lowest level of fitness (Fitness Level 1) have a risk ratio of 3.44 compared to a ratio of 1.37 in Fitness Level 2. There is a substantial decline in risk by moving from the least fit group to the next group. There are certainly gains made by increasing fitness further, but the big drop occurs as people go from being completely sedentary to moderately active. The figure for women shows much the same pattern.

The moral to this story is that you do not have to kill yourself to keep from dying. Even small amounts of exercise are likely to have a big impact on health and will certainly be helpful for weight loss. In the Blair study, one only had to do regular walking at a moderate pace to be fit enough to be in Level 2, which had about half the risk of the group who were least fit. How much exercise should you do? You should do as much as you can and still have fun. Don't worry so much about how much or what type, just try to do it regularly.

Remember, any type of activity should be considered exercise. If you take an extra flight of stairs, rake the leaves, walk an extra block, or chase the rabbits out of your vegetable garden, you have exercised and should say so in your own mind. You deserve to feel good about these activities and can feel confident that you are making progress.

Are Aerobics for You?

The answer is probably "No!"—or so you think. I used to feel the same way. I remember when coaches and teachers used calisthenics as punishment or as a way to build character. Push-ups, sit-ups, squat thrusts, and leg lifts ranked somewhere below staying after school on my list of favorite activities.

The situation is much different today. Calisthenics have been replaced with aerobics, slimnastics, low impact activities, and the like. This signals not only a change in terminology

but a change in the way exercise is viewed. In my opinion, the changes are positive.

When aerobic training became popular, using exercise to build strength took a back seat to improving the condition of the heart. This involves getting the heart rate up and keeping it there. Many different movements can accomplish this, hence the use of dance and other types of movement in aerobics classes. This makes exercise more interesting and more healthy than the calisthenics of old.

Aerobic activities require a large increase in the body's use of oxygen. This is best accomplished by use of large muscle groups, and it involves some form of vigorous and rhythmic movement. Running, cycling, swimming, and rope jumping are examples, but so are dancing to fast music and the other movements you associate with aerobics classes. As I mentioned before, these are the *only* types of exercise that will improve cardiovascular conditioning. They are *not* the only exercises that will help you lose weight, but they are certainly among the best.

Aerobics can be done in so many ways that they are suitable for almost everybody. If you want to do it alone, there are books, TV shows, videotapes, and records. Most of these workout approaches are aerobic in nature. If you would like company, aerobics classes are held at the

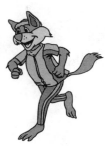

"Exercise is a key component in long-term weight management."

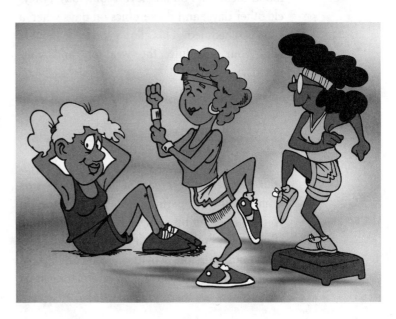

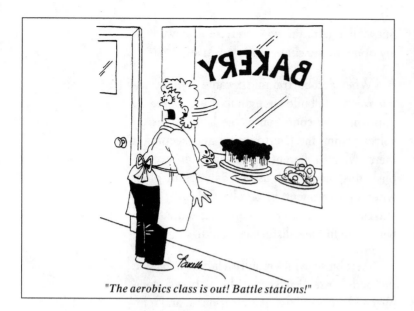

"The aerobics class is out! Battle stations!"

YMCA, YWCA, exercise centers, and in many companies, churches, and community centers. You can do aerobics at your own pace, even if you are with a group, so don't worry about the shape you're in. There are many excellent books on aerobic exercises. I suggest any of the books by Dr. Kenneth Cooper. These books are available in most bookstores. They discuss what to do, how much to do, and how to have fun doing it.

Many people losing weight use more than one form of exercise. This breaks monotony and gives you a chance to do whatever your mood dictates. You might run some days, bicycle other days, and do aerobics on days when a class is scheduled. This allows you to be flexible with your schedule, the weather, and your moods.

Pleasurable Partner Activities

There are many nice things you can do with your partner. These can be used as rewards from you to your partner, from your partner to you, or as a joint bit of pleasure to acknowledge efforts from both of you. The list on page 175 gives many possible activities. Some are appropriate for partners in romantic relationships while others are for any partnership.

Share these ideas with your partner and use them for special times. If you are working together as a team, it will be nice to have some fun in addition to the work. Remember that there are many nice partner activities not on the list, so be creative. Add as many ideas to the list as you can.

More about Fat Soluble Vitamins

In Lesson Ten, I discussed the water soluble vitamins. In this lesson, we will focus on the vitamins that are fat soluble. Vitamins A, D, E, and K are fat soluble. They are stored in fat tissue in the body if consumed in excess. This is why toxic doses are a more important issue with fat soluble than water soluble vitamins. You should be especially wary of people who promote large doses of these four vitamins. As with all vitamins, no more than the Recommended Daily Allowance (RDA) is suggested.

⇨ Vitamin A is used for growth of the skin, bones, and teeth and is important in vision. It is found in leafy green vegetables, yellow vegetables, milk, eggs, fortified margarine, liver, and kidney.

⇨ Vitamin D is crucial for development of bones and teeth, and helps the body use calcium and phosphorus. It is abundant in cod liver oil and is found in egg yolk, milk, tuna, and salmon.

⇨ Vitamin E is useful for the functioning of red blood cells, and helps the body use essential fatty acids. Vitamin E is present in wheat germ, egg yolks, vegetable oils, cereals, and lettuce.

⇨ Vitamin K is used by the liver in the production of prothrombin. It is found in liver, cabbage, spinach, and kale. The RDA has not been established for vitamin K.

⇨ Above all, watch out for bold claims. Taking extra amounts won't do a thing for weight loss and may damage your health.

Pleasurable Partner Activities

Take a romantic walk
Go to a concert
Plan a day at the park
Take a nature walk
Send flowers
Pick fresh fruit
Go bowling
Buy a nice wine
Play a new sport
See the city
Send a singing telegram
Plan a mystery weekend
See a movie
Buy cologne or perfume
Get gift certificates
Get a nice plant
Buy a tape or CD
Make Sunday breakfast

Ride bicycles
Go window shopping
Go on a picnic
Get a puppy or a kitten
Send a card
Go to a museum
Get a board game
Buy a new book
Buy a pedometer
Find a fair or festival
Visit a mutual friend
Do your partner's laundry
Write a thank you note
Plan a surprise party
Fix something broken
Balance the checkbook
Watch the sunset
Just sit and enjoy each other

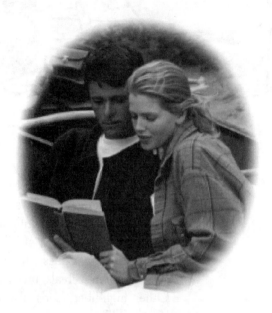

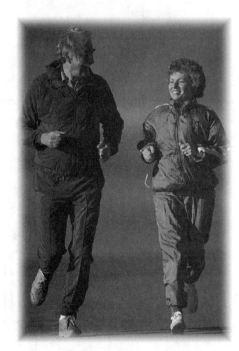

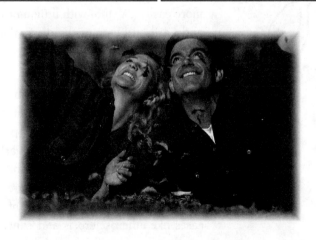

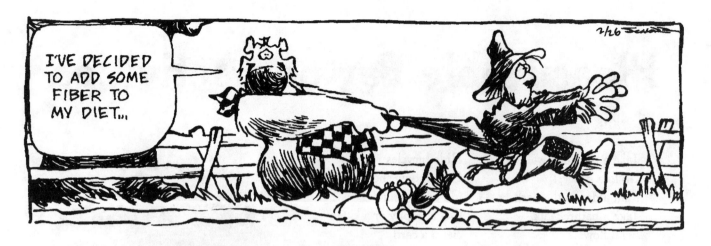

Facts, Fantasies, and Fiber

Over the years, many parents have implored their children to eat more roughage. This basic, good advice was about the only attention fiber received until the 1970s, when there was an explosion of interest in the topic. Books and magazines carried fiber diets, and sales of bran cereals increased dramatically. Other high-fiber foods also appeared in the stores. This is a positive development that I hope is not destined to pass with other food fads.

Dietary fiber comes primarily from the tough cell walls of plants. These materials include cellulose, hemicellulose, lignin, and pectin (which is used in home canning to turn fruit

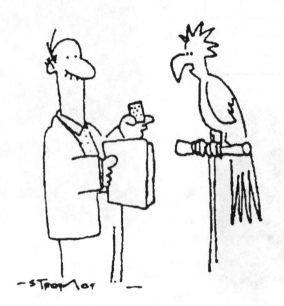

juice to jelly). Fiber is not broken down by digestion like other foods and retains its basic structure during transit through the digestive system. The strand-like quality of fiber maintains its rigid structure as it passes through the digestive tract.

Fiber absorbs water during the digestive process. This moisture helps with movement of waste products through the bowel. A brief lesson on digestion should clarify this process.

When you chew and swallow food, both the chewing and saliva begin to break down food into smaller nutrients. Stomach acid continues the process as food moves along, then more digestion continues in the small intestine. Toward the end of the line, waste products combine with water in the large intestine and are eliminated as stools. A stool with much water is larger and softer and moves through the colon more easily. A stool with little moisture is small and hard and creates the discomfort of constipation.

Much of the desirable moisture that facilitates movement of the stools comes from fiber. This is why increased fiber is prescribed for people with problems in the gastrointestinal tract such as diverticulitis, irritable bowel syndrome, and constipation. Some experts claim that fiber also reduces the risk of serious diseases like atherosclerosis and cancer of the colon.

High-Fiber Fruits, Vegetables, and Cereals

Fruits

Apples*	Cherries	Oranges	Pineapples
Apricots*	Dried fruit	Peaches*	Plums*
Bananas	Figs	Pears*	Prunes
Berries	Grapefruit		

*With peel

Vegetables

Asparagus	Corn	Mushrooms	Rhubarb
Beans	Eggplant	Okra	Sauerkraut
Broccoli	Endive	Onions	Spinach
Brussel sprouts	Green beans	Parsnips	Squash
Cabbage	Greens, all	Peas	Tomatoes
Carrots	Lettuce	Potatoes	Turnips
Cauliflower	Lima beans	Radishes	Watercress
Celery			

Cereals

Brans	Oatmeal	Shredded wheat
Brown rice	Puffed wheat	Whole wheat cereal

The study of fiber and health gained momentum with the discovery that Africans living in rural settings rarely get diverticulitis. This occurs when a bubble or mucous membrane pushes out from inside the intestine. The diet of these Africans averages 25 grams of fiber per day, compared to 6 grams per day for the typical American. Cancer of the colon follows a similar pattern—it occurs rarely in rural Africa but is common in industrialized countries. Furthermore, rates for these diseases have increased in the U.S. In the past century, fiber intake has decreased dramatically because of processed foods and less intake of fresh fruits and vegetables.

Of course, fiber in the diet is only one of many factors that distinguish the rural Africans from us. One such factor is fat in the diet, which also has been linked to disease. There are dozens of non-dietary factors (stress, etc.) that might be involved. What does this mean for our diet?

With the current state of science, it is not possible to say with absolute certainty that increased fiber in the diet protects against disease, but there are strong hints in this direction. The comparisons between rural and industrialized cultures have now been joined by laboratory studies, so that government agencies like the National Cancer Institute advocate increased fiber in the diet.

The average American should increase the fiber in his or her diet. Fiber comes from fruits, vegetables, and cereals. The table above shows high-fiber foods. The government has not yet established strict guidelines for daily intake of fiber. Most nutritionists suggest that a healthy goal is to aim for an average intake of 25 to 35 grams of fiber each day. Try to increase the number of these foods in your diet. They may help control your appetite because they add bulk. They may also have health benefits.

The Food Guide Pyramid

Fruit Group
2-4 Servings

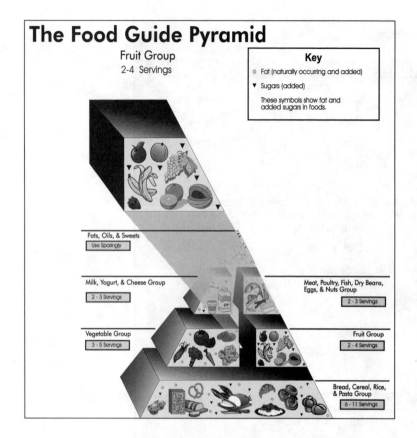

Key

○ Fat (naturally occurring and added)

▼ Sugars (added)

These symbols show fat and added sugars in foods.

Fats, Oils, & Sweets
Use Sparingly

Milk, Yogurt, & Cheese Group
2 - 3 Servings

Meat, Poultry, Fish, Dry Beans, Eggs, & Nuts Group
2 - 3 Servings

Vegetable Group
3 - 5 Servings

Fruit Group
2 - 4 Servings

Bread, Cereal, Rice, & Pasta Group
6 - 11 Servings

Fruit in Your Diet

Fruit and fruit juices are an important ingredient of a well-balanced diet. Fruits are naturally low in sodium and dietary fat, and they are an excellent source of fiber and carbohydrate. They provide generous amounts of vitamins A and C and potassium. Vitamin A is essential for the growth of teeth, skin, and bones, and it is important for good vision.

Increasing Fruit in Your Diet

Most Americans fall short in their daily consumption of fruits. This is particularly true of children and adolescents. When this happens, the body suffers from a lack of important vitamins, minerals, and fiber. Here are some tips that may help you add fruit to your diet.

Snacks

Fruit makes a good snack—whether in the morning, afternoon, or evening. Canned juices are also convenient and easy to take with you when you are on the go. Instead of a soda or cup of coffee, drink fruit juice. If you don't have fresh fruit available for a snack, canned fruit will do fine, but watch out for the heavy syrup and added sugars.

Breakfast

Breakfast is an important meal—one that should not be skipped. This is a good opportunity to have a serving of fruit. Six ounces of fruit juice is a good way to start the day. But be careful to make sure you are drinking 100 percent fruit juice. Many of the fruit drinks, aides, and punches on the market contain only a small percentage of actual fruit juice and have a lot of added sugar.

If you have cereal for breakfast, top it off with fresh fruit instead of sugar. Strawberries, blueberries, bananas, and grapes are smart choices and take little time to prepare. If you are in a rush, take the fruit with you. Keep fresh oranges, bananas, kiwi, apples, peaches, or pears available to take with you.

Lunch

If you take your lunch to work or school, include some fresh or canned fruit. Fruit is a healthy substitute for dessert. If you eat out, it is still possible to have some fruit. Many restaurants now offer fresh fruit as an appetizer or for dessert, but there are still some that do not offer fruit on the menu. If fruit is not available, ask for fruit juice.

Dinner

Dinner time is a good opportunity to review your fruit intake for the day. If you missed a serving or two during the day, add a glass of fruit juice to your evening menu. Fresh fruit also can be included with your meal (e.g., a fruit salad) or as a dessert.

How Many Servings?

The Food Guide Pyramid suggests two to four servings per day from the Fruit Group. This is less than you may think and should not be difficult to include in your daily diet.

Fruits

Description	Calories	Protein (g)	Carbohydrate (g)	Fat (g)	Fiber (g)
Apple, w/skin (1 med)	81	.3	21.1	.5	9.2
Apple juice (6 oz)	87	.15	21.8	.2	.4
Applesauce, sweetened (½ cup)	97	.2	25.5	.2	1.5
Apricots (4 med)	68	2.0	15.7	.5	1.9
Apricot nectar, canned (6 oz)	106	.7	27.1	.2	1.1
Banana (1 med)	105	1.2	26.7	.6	1.8
Blackberries, raw (1 cup)	74	1.0	18.4	.6	6.6
Blueberries, raw (1 cup)	82	1.0	20.5	.6	3.4
Cantaloupe, raw (1 cup)	57	1.4	13.4	.4	1.2
Casaba melon, raw (1 cup)	45	1.5	10.5	.2	.8
Cherries, raw (10 med)	49	.8	11.3	.7	.4
Dates, dried (10 med)	228	1.6	61.0	.4	4.2
Figs, raw (3 med)	111	1.2	28.8	.6	1.8
Fruit cocktail, in water (½ cup)	40	.5	10.4	.1	.5
Grapefruit, raw, pink (½ med)	37	.7	9.5	.1	.2
Grapefruit juice, fresh (6 oz)	72	.9	17.0	.2	n/a
Grapes, raw (½ cup)	29	.3	7.9	.2	.4
Grape juice (6 oz)	116	.8	28.4	.2	0.0
Honeydew melon, raw (1 cup)	66	1.6	15.4	.6	1.0
Kiwi, raw (1 med)	46	.8	11.3	.3	2.6
Mandarin oranges (½ cup)	46	.8	11.9	.0	.3
Mango, raw (1 med)	135	1.1	35.2	.6	2.2
Nectarine, raw (1 med)	67	1.3	16.0	.6	2.2
Orange, raw (1 med)	65	1.4	16.3	.1	3.1
Orange juice, fresh (6 oz)	83	1.3	19.4	.4	.2
Papaya, raw (1 med)	117	1.9	29.8	.4	5.4
Peach, raw (1 med)	37	.6	9.7	.1	1.4
Peach, in light syrup (½ cup)	68	.6	18.3	.1	1.0
Peach nectar (6 oz)	101	.5	26.0	.1	.3
Pear, raw (1 med)	98	.7	25.1	.7	4.2
Pear, canned in light syrup (½ cup)	72	.3	19.1	.1	1.0
Pear nectar (6 oz)	112	.2	29.6	.0	1.2
Pineapple, raw (½ cup pieces)	38	.3	9.6	.4	.9
Pineapple juice (6 oz)	103	.8	25.4	.2	.2
Raspberries, raw (1 cup)	61	1.1	14.2	.7	5.8
Strawberries, raw (1 cup)	45	.9	10.5	.6	3.8
Watermelon, raw (1 cup)	50	1.0	11.5	.7	.6

Note: Each of the food items listed above counts as one serving. This table should be used as a guide for the foods listed. Because food values vary by size and brand name, it is important to read the food labels for these foods.

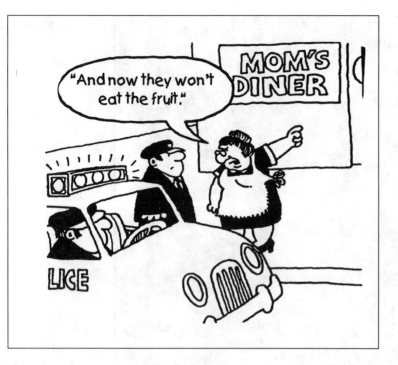

"And now they won't eat the fruit."

MOM'S DINER

LICE

How Much Is a Serving?

Servings from the Fruit Group are relatively easy to remember. The table on page 179 includes food items that count as a single serving. As a general rule, the following count as one serving:

1 medium apple, orange, banana, peach, or pear

½ cup of chopped, cooked, or canned fruit

1 cup of small berries

¾ cup or 6 oz of fruit juice

Selection Hints

In most parts of the country, certain fruits are seasonal, which makes it necessary to choose from a variety of different fruits. Variety is important because different fruits provide different amounts of important nutrients. The following tips may be helpful in your selection:

⇨ Choose citrus fruits, melons, and berries regularly—these are rich in Vitamin C.

⇨ Choose fresh fruits as often as you can—they do not have added sugars and other preservatives. Try to avoid fruits that are canned or frozen in heavy syrups and sweetened fruit juices—you'll save many unwanted calories this way.

⇨ Choose fruit juices that are pure fruit juice and do not contain large amounts of added water and sugars.

My Personal Goals for this Week

We began this lesson with a discussion of some additional benefits of physical activity. Try aerobic activities as part of your physical fitness routine and remember all the ways to do aerobic activities: on your own, at the YMCA or YWCA, and at spas, health clubs, community centers, and places of work. Use the suggestions for partner activities if you are using the partnership approach. Watch to see that you get the vitamins you need, but avoid falling victim to the vitamin hawkers who promise that large doses will cure nearly any ill. Think also of goals you have carried forward from other lessons. This week, focus on eating the appropriate number of servings from the Fruit Group of the Food Guide Pyramid. Record your weight change on the Weight Change Record in Lesson Nine on page 154.

My Self-Assessment

Eleven

T (F) 79. Fat soluble vitamins give you energy, but water soluble vitamins do not.

T (F) 80. Small bouts of exercise are of little value for weight management and overall health.

T (F) 81. Aerobic activities are designed to build strength in the shortest possible time.

(T) F 82. Fruits, vegetables, and cereals tend to be high in fiber.

T (F) 83. Most Americans eat plenty of fruits and should not worry about increasing their daily intake.

(T) F 84. A diet high in fiber may help protect against certain diseases.

(T) F 85. A healthy diet should contain between 25 and 35 grams of fiber each day.

T (F) 86. Exercise must be strenuous in order to be beneficial.

T (F) 87. The best kind of exercise is rigorous enough to build muscle, which in turn speeds up metabolism.

T (F) 88. The emphasis on fiber may be dangerous because fiber is indigestible material that can harm the intestinal system.

(Answers in Appendix C, page 271)

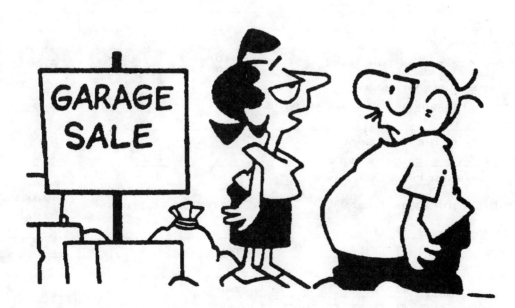

"Better lose weight, Stanley. Someone thought you were a beanbag chair and offered me $5 for you."

Monitoring Form—Lesson Eleven   *Today's Date:* _____

TIME	FOOD AND AMOUNT	CALORIES
	TOTAL DAILY CALORIES	

PERSONAL GOALS FOR THIS WEEK	MOST OF THE TIME	SOME-TIMES	RARELY
1. WATCH THE FAT SOLUBLE VITAMINS			
2. EXPERIMENT WITH PLEASURABLE PARTNER ACTIVITIES			
3. TRY AEROBIC ACTIVITY			
4. DAILY SERVINGS FROM THE FRUIT GROUP			
5. EAT LESS THAN _____ CALORIES PER DAY			
6. EAT _____ GRAMS OF FIBER EACH DAY			

FOOD GROUPS FOR TODAY	PHYSICAL ACTIVITY	MINUTES OR STEPS
MILK, YOGURT, AND CHEESE ☐ ☐ ☐	(M)	
MEAT, POULTRY, ETC. ☐ ☐ ☐	(TU)	
FRUITS ☐ ☐ ☐ ☐	(W)	
VEGETABLES ☐ ☐ ☐ ☐ ☐	(TH)	
BREADS, CEREALS, ETC. ☐ ☐ ☐ ☐ ☐ ☐ ☐ ☐	(F)	
SERVINGS OF WATER (8 OZ) ☐ ☐ ☐ ☐ ☐ ☐ ☐ ☐	(SA)	
	(SU)	

I begin this lesson with a discussion of lifestyle tips to help you with eating away from home. This discussion includes the infamous fast-food restaurants. In the exercise arena, we'll be working more on lifestyle activity. This lesson ushers in the last tier of the Food Guide Pyramid, so we'll be spending some time talking about breads, cereals, rice, and pasta. And finally, it is time to review your quality of life. I hope you are pleased with your progress and that you take the credit for all the hard work you have put into this program.

Eating Away from Home

Trips to restaurants can be a mine field of temptation. The best intentions can crumble when you are enjoying yourself with people who feast on delicious foods. Two aspects of this concern me. The first is how much you eat, but there are methods for keeping eating under control. The second is to control your response to the event.

One trip to a restaurant never torpedoed any weight management program with its calo-

ries alone. An extraordinary meal of 5000 calories could bring only 1½ pounds of weight. The *response* to those calories, however, could lead to trouble. Your attitudes during and after these events are as important as what you eat.

Eating at Restaurants

It is hard to be virtuous at restaurants. This is a real problem for people in business or those whose lifestyle includes eating away from home.

What should you do when dessert comes with the meal? What about a waitress who

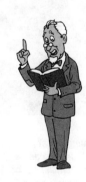

"Trips to restaurants can be a mine field of temptation."

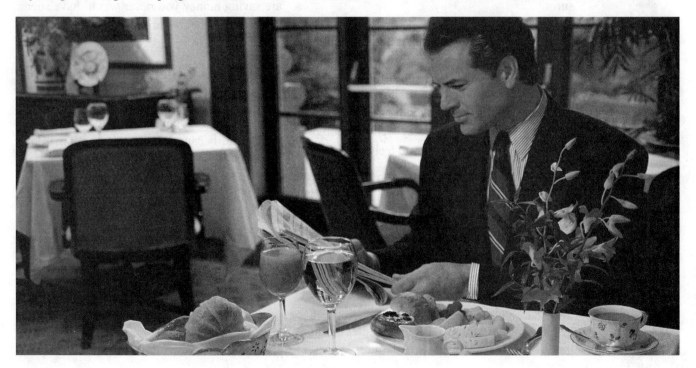

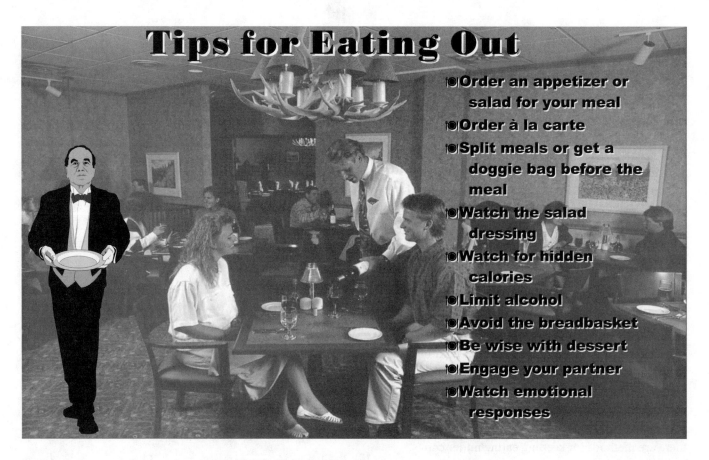

Tips for Eating Out

- ⦿ Order an appetizer or salad for your meal
- ⦿ Order à la carte
- ⦿ Split meals or get a doggie bag before the meal
- ⦿ Watch the salad dressing
- ⦿ Watch for hidden calories
- ⦿ Limit alcohol
- ⦿ Avoid the breadbasket
- ⦿ Be wise with dessert
- ⦿ Engage your partner
- ⦿ Watch emotional responses

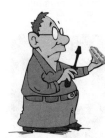

"Eating out at restaurants can be a real challenge for weight managers."

pours 14 gallons of dressing on your salad? How do you deal with a hot loaf of bread the waiter delivers before the meal even begins? How can you refuse when the dessert cart rolls up like a Brink's truck ready to unload its treasures?

Order from the appetizer or salad section of the menu

If you find something healthy among the appetizers, or find a salad you like, try ordering this for your meal. There may well be enough food to fill you up and make you feel like you are having a nice meal out.

Order à la carte meals

You may be inclined to order full meals because the cost is less than for the sum of its parts. This group plan is a booby trap because you order more than you need simply because the price seems attractive. The "value" meals at fast-food restaurants are classic examples of this problem. However, the logic is faulty.

The regular price for a roast beef sandwich might be $5, but for $6 you could get french fries and cole slaw that would normally cost $1 each. The package deal makes sense only if you wanted the other two items anyway. If not, you are saving money you never would have spent. Most of these extras are high-calorie foods like french fries. Order just what you want.

Split meals or get a doggie bag before the meal

Splitting a meal with someone can be a great idea, because often there is enough food for two. This is worthwhile even if the restaurant charges you for the extra plate. And, getting a doggie bag before the meal and putting in a portion of the food when it's served insures that it's out of sight and won't tempt you.

Watch the salad dressing

Because salad dressing is high in fat (oil), eating more than you need really boosts the calories. Ask for salad dressing on the side so you are not at the mercy of a heavy-handed server.

Better yet, leave the salad dressing off completely.

If you need dressing, consider bringing your own bottle of low-fat dressing. Many people do this, and unless you're at the White House for an awards banquet, you shouldn't be embarrassed. I usually order dressing on the side and then dip my fork in the dressing before putting a bite of salad on my folk. It's amazing how little dressing this uses and how much of the good taste you can still have.

Watch for hidden calories

Many foods contain calories that are added in subtle ways. These hidden calories are important to consider. Think about rich sauces added to meats and vegetables in French restaurants, oils added in Italian restaurants, and things breaded and fried in any restaurant. If you cannot guess what is in a dish, ask the waiter or waitress.

Watch the Alcohol

As I will discuss later in Lesson Fourteen on page 223, alcohol is loaded with calories, and it is easy to consume more than you want in the spirit of being social. This is a real temptation when you sit in the bar area waiting for a table in the restaurant.

When you order alcohol, avoid the hard liquor and sweetened drinks. A jigger of whiskey has 110 calories and a Tom Collins has 180 calories. White wine is a better choice, and better yet is a white wine spritzer. You could also order club soda or tomato juice.

Alcohol generally has *empty* calories. Its sugar brings calories with little or no nutrition. You can estimate the calories in alcohol by remembering that the following drinks have about 100 calories:

12 oz of light beer

8 oz of regular beer

3½ oz of wine

1 shot of liquor

You may want to refer to the table on page 224 as a reminder of calories in alcohol.

Beware of the Breadbasket

Keep an eye out for that wondrous basket. It comes when you are hungry and excited about being at the restaurant. You can refuse the breadbasket, but if one arrives against your will, let it rest across the table. If you are still tempted, imagine there is a mousetrap under the napkin that covers the bread!

There are some people who actually benefit from the breadbasket. They are the ones who use a piece of bread (without butter) to take the edge off their hunger, so that they will eat less higher-calorie foods later in the meal. You might try this approach, but don't use it as an excuse to eat lots of bread and then eat what you would anyway.

Bread does *not* have empty calories. It is an important part of your diet— breads and cereals comprise the largest of the five food groups of the Food Guide Pyramid. The purpose of watching the breadbasket is not to cut down on bread, but to avoid eating lots of bread just because it's there.

Be wise with dessert

Do you deserve dessert when you eat out? After all, you don't get special desserts often, so why not enjoy yourself? Ignore this rationalization and get dessert under two conditions: you

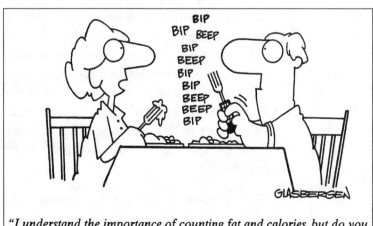

"I understand the importance of counting fat and calories, but do you really need a fork with a built-in calculator?"

My Plans for Dining Out

My Challenge	My Technique
_____	_____
_____	_____
_____	_____
_____	_____
_____	_____
_____	_____
_____	_____

are still hungry, or you have planned it in your day's calories. Think about fresh fruit or gelatin. Both taste good and have far fewer calories than traditional choices.

Engage your partner

Restaurants are a place where your partner can help. This can begin before you arrive for the meal. Some individuals decide with their partners what to order in advance, before their restraint is weakened by the smells and atmosphere of a nice restaurant. Some even have their partner order for them. At the restaurant, the partner can keep the breadbasket in a safe place and can help by not pushing drinks or desserts.

Watch your emotional response

If you eat more than you plan, be careful not to consider it a catastrophe. We have been working to avoid the attitude traps, such as considering some foods _illegal_ and setting unrealistic goals of never overeating. If you feel guilty, reread the earlier material, and be prepared to rebound from a bout of overeating by eating less, not more. Do _not_ use this as a rationalization to overdo it, but keep these events in perspective and use them as a sign that you can do better the next meal or the next day.

These are techniques that people use to control their eating in restaurants. You may think of others yourself. For example, you might drink extra water to help fill up before the meal comes. I have provided a worksheet above for you to list your challenges and techniques that will be helpful for you when dining out. Take a few minutes now to complete the worksheet. Feel free to make a copy and carry it with you. When you find yourself eating out, take out your chart and review it before going into the restaurant. Also, if you discover additional difficulties, write down techniques that may be helpful in the future. Have fun, but keep control!

Exercise—The Many Points of Light

The topic of physical activity is something I discuss time and time again. Because this manual is about weight management, I have focused on the effects of activity on weight loss and weight maintenance. There is more, much more.

Being physically active has many beneficial effects beyond weight management. The diagram on page 188 shows just how broad these effects can be. This diagram comes from an article by Bonnie Liebman in the *Nutrition Action Healthletter*, an excellent publication from the Center for Science in the Public Interest. Information on subscribing can be obtained by calling 202–332–9110 or logging on to the Internet at www.cspinet.org.

Using the Stairs

Climbing stairs is a handy way to increase your exercise. It is an ideal way to work extra activity into your lifestyle. It is an efficient way of burning calories. As you may know, climbing stairs burns more calories per minute than almost any activity. Its major virtue, however, is its ready availability. Most of us have several opportunities each day to use stairs. Stairs may be in our home, at work, and in stores. Let's see if you can exploit this opportunity.

People are willing to increase their use of stairs, but rarely think of it. This was shown in a study I did with several colleagues at the University of Pennsylvania. I had observers measure the use of stairs in three public places where stairs and escalators were adjacent: a shopping mall in Philadelphia called the Gallery, a commuter-train station, and a bus termi-

nal. The observers patiently recorded whether 40,000 people used the stairs or escalators.

The results were quite informative. Only 5 percent of people used the stairs. For every five normal-weight people who used the stairs, only one heavy person did, which meant that only 1 percent of heavy people used the stairs. People would avoid the stairs even when they had to wait in a crowd to go up the escalator.

We then stationed a sign encouraging people to use the stairs at the base of the stairs and escalators. The sign carried the figure shown here and was designed for us by Tony Auth, the Pulitzer Prize winning political cartoonist of the *Philadelphia Inquirer*. The sign made a big impact. It nearly tripled the number of people using the stairs and increased the number of overweight people using the stairs by sevenfold. Apparently, people were willing to use the stairs if reminded to do so.

Here is a bit more encouragement. Studies in England and the U.S. were done to investigate the link between exercise and life span (longevity). People who exercised regularly lived longer than those who were sedentary. The U.S. study, done by Dr. Ralph Paffenbarger from Stanford University, found

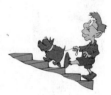

"Climbing stairs burns more calories per minute than almost any activity. Find ways to exploit this opportunity."

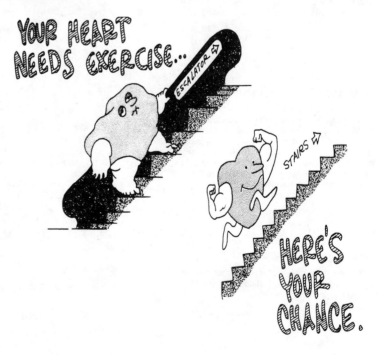

A Dozen *Other* Reasons to Exercise

The promise of thinner thighs or a slimmer midsection is what gets most people off the couch. And exercise can help you lose fat, preserve muscle, and keep off the excess weight you manage to lose. But if that's your only reason for moving, your're missing a lot. Here are a dozen others, including some concrete findings from selected studies. For more information, check out the 1996 Surgeon General's Report on Physical Activity and Health at www.cdc.gov/nccdphp/sgr/sgr.htm

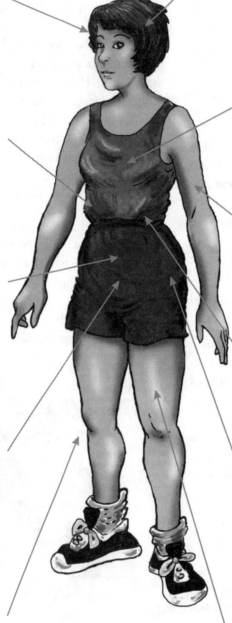

Sleep

A 16-week exercise program (30 to 40 minutes of brisk walking or low-impact aerobics four times a week) improved the quality, duration, and ease of falling asleep in healthy older adults.[1] Exercise may improve sleep by relaxing muscles, reducing stress, or warming the body.

[1]*J. Amer. Med. Assoc. 277:* 32, 1997.

Gallstones

Active women are 30 percent less likely to have gallstone surgery than sedentary women. In one study, women who spent more than 60 hours a week sitting at work or driving were twice as likely to have gallstone surgery as women who sat for less than 40 hours a week.[1]

[1]*N. Eng. J. Med. 341:* 777, 1999.

Colon Cancer

The most active people have a lower risk of colon cancer—in two studies half the risk—compared to the least active people.[1,2] Exercise may lower levels of prostaglandins that accelerate colon cell proliferation and raise levels of protaglandins that increase intestinal motility. Increased motility may speed the movement of carcinogens through the colon.

[1]*J. Nat. Cancer Inst. 89:* 948, 1997.
[2]*Ann. Intern. Med. 122:* 327, 1995.

Diverticular Disease

In one of the few studies that have been done, the most active men had a 37 percent lower risk of symptomatic diverticular disease than the least active men.[1] Most of the protection against diverticular disease—pockets the wall of the colon that can become inflamed—was due to vigorous activities like jogging and running, rather than moderate activities like walking.

[1]*Gut 36:* 276, 1995.

Arthritis

Regular moderate exercise, whether aerobic or strength-training, can reduce joint swelling and pain in people with arthritis.[1]

[1]*J. Amer. Med. Assoc. 277:* 25, 1997.

Anxiety & Depression

Getting people with anxiety or depression to do aerobic exercises like brisk walking or running curbs their symptoms, possibly by releasing natural opiates.[1,2]

[1]*J. Psychosom. Res. 33:* 537, 1989.
[2]*Arch. Intern. Med. 159:* 2349, 1999.

Heart Disease

In one study, men with low fitness who become fit had a lower risk of heart disease than men who stayed unfit.[1] In another, women who walked the equivalent of three or more hours per week at a brisk pace had a 35 percent lower risk of heart disease than women who walked infrequently.[2] Exercise boosts the supply of oxygen to the heart muscle by expanding existing arteries and creating tiny new blood vessels. It may also prevent blood clots or promote their breakdown.

[1]*J. Amer. Med. Assoc. 273:* 1093, 1995.
[2]*N. Eng. J. Med. 341:* 650, 1999.

Blood Pressure

If your blood pressure is already high or high-normal, low- or moderate-intensity aerobic exercise—three times a week—can lower it.[1] If your blood pressure isn't high, regular exercise helps keep it that way.

[1]*J. Clin. Epidem. 45:* 439, 1992.

Diabetes

The more you move, the lower your risk of diabetes, especially if you're already at risk because of excess weight, high blood pressure, or parents with diabetes. In one study, women who walked at least three hours a week had about a 40 percent lower risk of diabetes than sedentary women.[1]

[1]*J. Am. Med. Assoc 282:* 1433, 1999.

Falls & Fractures

Older women assigned to a home-based (strength- and balance-training) exercise program had fewer falls than women who didn't exercise.[1] Exercise may prevent falls and broken bones by improving muscle strength, gait, balance, and reaction time.

[1]*Brit. Med. J. 315:* 1065, 1997.

Enlarged Prostate *(men only)*

In one study, men who walked two to three hours a week had 25 percent lower risk of benign prostatic hyperplasia (enlarged prostate) than men who seldom walked.[1]

[1]*Arch. Intern. Med. 158:* 2349, 1998.

Osteoporosis

Exercise, especially strength-training, can increase bone density in middle-aged and older people.[1] Bonus: postmenopausal women who take estrogen gain more bone density if they exercise.

[1]*J. Bone Min. Res. 11:* 218, 1996.

that people who climbed only 50 stairs (not flights) or more each day had reduced risk of heart attack.

The value of using the stairs is not well known, but some people are regular stair climbers and are proud of it. The study with the stairs and escalators was reported in many newspapers because of a wire service article. I received letters from all over the country from people who had been climbing the stairs for years for their exercise program. Some even reported running in a race that is up the stairs of the Empire State Building! This is way beyond what I have in mind for people losing weight, so let's examine ways to use the stairs sensibly.

There are many clever ways to use stairs. At work, try the bathroom and water cooler on another floor. This will add several trips. Use the stairs at a mall in lieu of an escalator. If you work on the 9th floor of a building, take the elevator part way up and walk the remaining flights. Walk down all the flights. Use the stairs whenever possible at home. Walk to a different floor to make a phone call or to use the bathroom. Whatever you can do will add up.

Fast Food

Fast-food restaurants are part of the American landscape. In 1970, there were 30,000 fast food outlets, rising to 140,000 by 1980. In 1997, there were 23,132 McDonald's alone, with three new McDonald's opening every day. Within a 15-minute drive of where I live in Connecticut, I bet I could find 25 fast-food restaurants, and an ocean occupies half of the available space! In addition to McDonald's, I would find other restaurants, such as Burger King, Kentucky Fried Chicken, Wendy's, Popeye's, and heaven knows what else. And with 24-hour service, breakfast, and drive-through windows, convenience has reached new levels. If you can believe it, 7 percent of the American population eat at McDonald's every day.

The world of fast food has undergone many interesting, and in a few cases, positive changes. Chicken has found its way onto the menu, but in some cases, in better form than others (broiled chicken vs. chicken nuggets). Healthier oils are being used to cook french fries in some places, yet people are consuming fries (and, therefore, fat and calories) in record amounts. Some developments, such as drive-through windows and package deals ("value meals"), very likely increase the number of customers and amount eaten per customer.

Fast foods vary widely in their nutritional value. *The LEARN Healthy Eating and Calorie Guide* includes a complete section on fast-food restaurants. Foods from these restaurants can be high in saturated fat, sodium, cholesterol, and calories, and low in calcium, vitamins A and D, and fiber. The news is not all bad, however. One can walk into some fast food chains and escape with a reasonable meal.

Some places have a salad bar or prepared salads so you can load up with vegetables (ask for low-fat dressing). Grilled chicken sandwiches are better than fried ones, and you can save yourself calories and fat by not having cheese and sauces. You also can control portion sizes. If you have a hankering for fries, get the

Believe it or not; 7 percent of the American population eat at McDonald's every day."

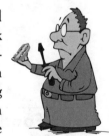

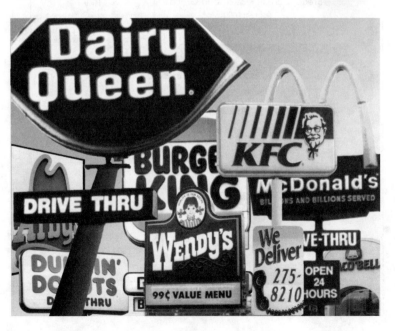

small size. A hamburger or cheeseburger will have fewer calories than a bacon double cheeseburger, a quarter pounder, or the deluxe burger that requires a forklift. And, if you are used to regular soft drinks, switch to diet drinks, have skim milk or juice, or drink water. Most soft drinks have no nutrition and loads of calories, especially the large sizes.

Breads, Cereals, Rice, and Pasta in Your Diet

Here we are, at the last tier of the Food Guide Pyramid. Over the last few weeks we have covered a lot of material on nutrition and on helping improve your diet. By now, you should feel very familiar with the Food Guide Pyramid.

Foods from this group of the pyramid are good sources of complex carbohydrates. These foods are good sources of low-fat energy and provide essential vitamins, minerals, and fiber. Foods from this group should make up the largest part of your daily diet. It is important, however, to watch out for the hidden fats and calories in some of these foods. Bread, cookies, and pastries, for example, typically include sugar and butter, oil, or margarine. Remember,

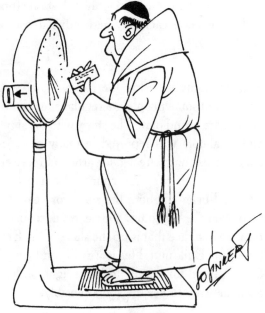

"Easy on the daily bread."

it is easy to eat many calories from this food group and not get good nutrition. Making wise food choices from this group is important.

Selection Hints

The following guidelines will help you to make good choices from the Bread, Cereal, Rice, and Pasta Group:

⇨ Dietary fiber is important for good health, and foods from this food group are good sources of fiber. Choose several servings a day from whole grains, which are found in whole wheat breads and whole-grain cereals.

⇨ Foods that contain low amounts of fat and simple sugars are the best choices for a healthful diet. Choose foods made with small amounts of sugars and fats. These food items include bread, English muffins, rice, and pasta.

⇨ Some foods from this group that are made from flour are typically high in fat and sugars. These include cookies, pastries, croissants, doughnuts, and cakes. Keep these foods to a minimum and use fat and sugar substitutes when possible.

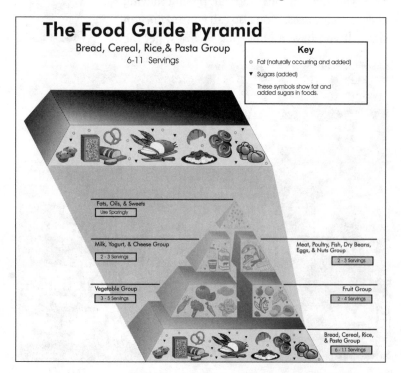

The Food Guide Pyramid

Bread, Cereal, Rice,& Pasta Group
6-11 Servings

Key
○ Fat (naturally occurring and added)
▼ Sugars (added)

These symbols show fat and added sugars in foods.

Fats, Oils, & Sweets
Use Sparingly

Milk, Yogurt, & Cheese Group
2 - 3 Servings

Meat, Poultry, Fish, Dry Beans, Eggs, & Nuts Group
2 - 3 Servings

Vegetable Group
3 - 5 Servings

Fruit Group
2 - 4 Servings

Bread, Cereal, Rice, & Pasta Group
6 - 11 Servings

Bread, Cereal, Rice, and Pasta

Description	Calories	Protein (g)	Carbohydrate (g)	Fat (g)
Bread, wheat (1 slice)	61	2.3	11.3	1.0
Bread, white (1 slice)	64	2.0	11.7	.9
Bagel (½)	82	3.0	15.5	.7
Cereal, cheerios (1 oz or ⅓ cup)	111	1.4	19.6	1.8
Cereal, corn flakes (1 oz or 1 cup)	110	2.0	25.0	1.0
Cookies, chocolate chip (2 med)	99	1.1	14.6	4.4
Cookies, oatmeal (2 med)	124	1.6	17.8	5.2
Danish, 1 small (1 oz)	161	2.6	18.8	8.8
English muffin, plain (½)	68	2.3	13.1	.6
Pancakes, 4 in. diameter (1)	62	1.9	9.2	1.9
Pasta, enriched cooked (½ cup)	100	3.3	18.7	1.2
Pie, fruit, 2—crust, 8 in. (1/12 piece)	116	.9	18.3	4.6
Rice, enriched cooked (½ cup)	141	4.1	49.6	.2

⇨ Spreads and toppings can add many unwanted calories to the foods in this group while providing little nutrition. The best advice is to leave these items off or to at least use low-calorie or low-fat toppings, spreads, and sauces.

⇨ Most pasta stuffings and sauces use butter or margarine. Use only half of the recipe amount. If milk or cream is called for, use low-fat milk.

⇨ If pasta sauces or stuffings call for meat, use lean meat. Trim away any visible fat before cooking, and drain all oil before including in your sauce or stuffing.

How Much Is a Serving?

Servings from this group are simple to remember. As a general rule, the following count as a single serving:

1 slice of bread

1 oz of ready-to-eat cereal

½ cup of cooked cereal, rice, or pasta

How Many Servings?

The Food Guide Pyramid suggests 6 to 11 servings each day from the Bread, Cereal, Rice, and Pasta Group. While this may sound like a lot, remember that foods from this group should be the largest part of your daily diet. The table above includes foods that count as a single serving.

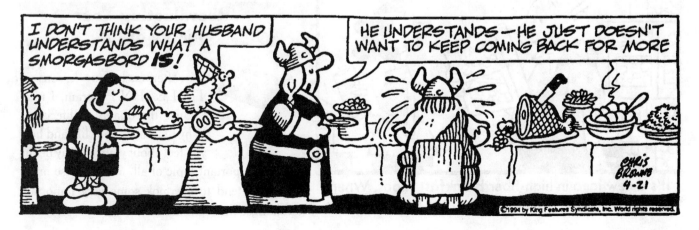

Breakfast Cereal: The Good, the Bad, the Sugar Coated

Most of us grew up eating cereals for breakfast. The experience included not only the cereal, but reading the box, twisting and tilting the box in all directions to beat our brothers and sisters to the free prize, and saving box tops and proof-of-purchase symbols for the wonderful toys we could buy.

Today's marketing of breakfast cereals is clever indeed. Cereals are associated with cartoon characters and sports figures. The manufacturers are sensitive to our nutrition-conscious culture and to the bad rap given to sugar-coated cereals. Witness, for example, how some old favorites have changed names. *Sugar Smacks* are now *Honey Smacks*, *Super Sugar Crisp* is now *Super Golden Crisp*, and *Sugar Frosted Flakes* are now simply *Frosted Flakes*. Some cereals of questionable nutritional value are advertised on television as "part of a nutritious breakfast." The nutritious breakfast they show includes foods like juice, milk, muffins, fruit, and the like, so I suppose one could replace the cereal with a rock and make the same claim.

Breakfast plays an important role in your daily diet. One characteristic common to overweight individuals is that they seldom eat breakfast. As they lose weight, many resume eating breakfast. Because cereal is part of the usual breakfast picture, the listing in the cereal table on page 193 may be helpful in choosing a cereal with both calories and healthful eating in mind. The ratings have been adapted from an article in *Consumer Reports* magazine published in October, 1996. If you are interested in even more information, I urge you to read the article yourself.

Cereals can be good sources of fiber and other nutrients, because the basic grains from which cereals are made (oats, wheat, corn, etc.) contain many nutrients for the calories. However, cereals differ greatly in nutritional value. Some have as much as 16 grams (3 teaspoons) of sugar in every serving, so more than half the weight of the cereal is sugar.

The article in *Consumer Reports* points to cereals as "best choices" if each serving has 5 grams or more of fiber, 5 grams or less of sugar, and 3 grams or less of fat. The authors point out that some cereals that sound healthy may have fat and sugar in surprisingly high amounts. *Raisin Nut Bran*, *Quaker 100% Natural Oats*, and *Blueberry Morning* cereals have more than 3 grams of fat per serving, and *Cracklin' Oat Bran* has a whopping 8 grams of fat per serving, including 3 grams of saturated fat. Some cereals have less than 1 gram of fiber per serving and 10 grams or more of sugar (e.g., *Cocoa Puffs*, *Cocoa Pebbles*, *Trix*, *Frosted Flakes*, *Fruity Pebbles*). It pays to look at the labels, not the name of the cereal.

Reevaluating Your Quality of Life

After each four lessons in The LEARN Program, I reintroduce the quality of life issue. Why? Because your life and how you feel about yourself may be the most important topic of all, and because many people tend to overlook some very important changes they have made.

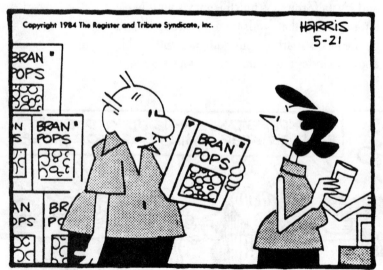

"It's a new idea in high-fiber breakfast foods. When the cereal is gone, you eat the box!"

A Nutrition Scorecard for Cereals

The cereals below represent nutritious and not-as-nutritious choices based on the *Consumer Reports* comparison of more than 100 top-sellers. All are national brands; similar store brands should have similar nutrition. Note that cereal ingredients change fairly often. If you're concerned about nutrition, check a cereal's label before buying.

Best Choices
High Fiber, Very Low Sugar, Low Fat

(A serving from this list has 5 grams or more of fiber, 5 grams or less of sugar, and 3 grams or less of fat.)

General Mills Fiber One

Kellogg's All-Bran Extra Fiber

Kellogg's All-Bran Original

Nabisco Shredded Wheat (regular, spoon-size, and wheat 'n bran)

Ralston Wheat Chex

Other Choices
Very Low Sugar, Low Fat

(A serving from this list has 5 grams or less of sugar, 3 grams or less of fat, and 0 to 4 grams of fiber.)

General Mills Kix

General Mills Cheerios

General Mills Total Corn Flakes

General Mills Total Whole Grain

General Mills Wheaties

Health Valley Honey Clusters & Flakes with Apples & Cinnamon

Kellogg's Corn Flakes

Kellogg's Crispix

Kellogg's Rice Krispies

Kellogg's Product 19

Kellogg's Special K

Ralston Rice Chex

Ralston Corn Chex

Other Choices
High Fiber, Low Fat

(A serving from this list has 5 grams or more of fiber, 3 grams or less of fat, and 6 to 20 grams of sugar.)

Familia Original Recipe Swiss Muesli

Kellogg's Bran Buds

Kellogg's Complete Bran Flakes

Kellogg's Frosted Mini-Wheats

Healthy Choice Multi-Grain Squares

Healthy Choice Raisin Squares

Nabisco Frosted Wheat Bites and 100% Bran

Post Fruit & Fiber Dates, Raisins, Walnuts

Post Grape-Nuts

Post Premium Bran Flakes

Ralston Multi Bran Chex

Raisin Brans (from various manufacturers)

Plenty of Fat

(A serving has more than 3 grams of fat.)

General Mills Cinnamon Toast Crunch

General Mills Raisin Nut Bran

Kellogg's Cracklin Oat Bran

Post Banana Nut Crunch

Kellogg's Blueberry Morning

Kellogg's Great Grains Raisin, Date, Pecan

Quaker 100% Natural Oats, Honey & Raisins

Little Fiber, Plenty of Sugar

(A serving has less than a gram of fiber and at least 10 grams [2 teaspoons] of sugar.)

General Mills Cocoa Puffs

General Mills Reese's Peanut Butter Puffs

General Mills Trix

Kellogg's Cocoa Krispies

Kellogg's Frosted Flakes

Kellogg's Pop-Tarts

Post Cocoa Pebbles

Post Fruity Pebbles

Post Honey-Comb

Post Waffle Crisp

Ralston Cookie-Crisp Chocolate Chip

Quality of Life Self-Assessment

Please use the following scale to rate how satisfied you feel now about different aspects of your daily life. Choose any number from this list (1 to 9) and indicate your choice on the questions below.

1 = **Extremely Dissatisfied**	6 = **Somewhat Satisfied**
2 = **Very Dissatisfied**	7 = **Moderately Satisfied**
3 = **Moderately Dissatisfied**	8 = **Very Satisfied**
4 = **Somewhat Dissatisfied**	9 = **Extremely Satisfied**
5 = **Neutral**	

1. _____ Mood (feelings of sadness, worry, happiness, etc.)

2. _____ Self-esteem

3. _____ Confidence, self-assurance, and comfort in social situations

4. _____ Energy and feeling healthy

5. _____ Health problems (diabetes, high blood pressure, etc.)

6. _____ General appearance

7. _____ Social life

8. _____ Leisure and recreational activities

9. _____ Physical mobility and physical activity

10. _____ Eating habits

11. _____ Body image

12. _____ Overall quality of life

Let's take self-esteem as an example. Is there any greater gift than self-esteem? If you are feeling better about yourself, feel like you have more control over your destiny, and feel that you are conquering some problems you thought would get the best of you, you have made great progress. It is my pleasurable task to help point this out to you and to be certain you don't let the occasion slip by without celebrating.

Once again, I provide the Quality of Life Self-Assessment above. Complete the form, and use the Review of Quality of Life Self-Assessments worksheet on page 195 to compare your responses from the beginning of the program on page 9 in the Introduction and Orientation Lesson. I hope you are pleased with your progress.

My Personal Goals for This Week

Much of this lesson focused on developing strategies for eating away from home. If you eat away from home this week, set a goal of developing strategies that help you keep within your calorie goal for the day. For your exercise, see if there are ways to work extra stair climbing into your lifestyle. Watch the foods from the fast-food restaurants. Continue monitoring your intake of the recommended number of servings from the Bread, Cereal, Rice, and Pasta Group of the Food Guide Pyramid. Read the food labels on your cereal boxes and try to improve the quality of the cereal that you eat.

As has been the case in previous lessons, I urge you to select goals that are specific to you. Goals that you have learned from experience motivate you in important areas should be a constant part of your weight management landscape. Finally, remember to record your weight change on your Weight Change Record in Lesson Nine on page 154.

My Self-Assessment

Lesson Twelve

(T) F 89. Alcohol can be a problem when eating out because it contains many calories and weakens dietary restraint.

(T) F 90. Ordering à la carte meals at restaurants helps avoid unwanted calories that come in package meals.

(T) F 91. Using stairs is a convenient and accessible way for many people to increase activity.

(T) F 92. Foods from the Bread, Cereal, Rice, and Pasta Group are a good source of complex carbohydrates buy may contain hidden fat.

(T) F 93. One characteristic common to overweight persons is that they seldom eat breakfast.

(Answers in Appendix C, page 271)

Review of Quality of Life Self-Assessments

(a) Category	(b) Score from Introduction and Orientation Lesson	(c) Score from this Lesson	(d) Change in Scores (column c minus column b)
1. Mood (feelings of sadness, worry, happiness, etc.)			
2. Self-esteem			
3. Confidence, self-assurance, and comfort in social situations			
4. Energy and feeling healthy			
5. Health problems (diabetes, high blood pressure, etc.)			
6. General appearance			
7. Social life			
8. Leisure and recreational activities			
9. Physical mobility and physical activity			
10. Eating habits			
11. Body image			
12. Overall quality of life			

Monitoring Form—Lesson Twelve

Today's Date:_____

TIME	FOOD AND AMOUNT	CALORIES
TOTAL DAILY CALORIES		

PERSONAL GOALS FOR THIS WEEK	MOST OF THE TIME	SOME-TIMES	RARELY
1. PRACTICE TECHNIQUES FOR DINING OUT			
2. INCREASE USE OF STAIRS			
3. WATCH THE CALORIES IN FAST FOODS AND CEREALS			
4. DAILY SERVINGS FROM THE BREAD GROUP			
5. EAT LESS THAN _____ CALORIES PER DAY			
6. EAT LESS THAN _____ GRAMS OF FAT EACH DAY			

FOOD GROUPS FOR TODAY	PHYSICAL ACTIVITY	MINUTES OR STEPS
MILK, YOGURT, AND CHEESE ☐ ☐ ☐	(M)	
MEAT, POULTRY, ETC. ☐ ☐ ☐	(Tu)	
FRUITS ☐ ☐ ☐ ☐	(W)	
VEGETABLES ☐ ☐ ☐ ☐ ☐	(Th)	
BREADS, CEREALS, ETC. ☐ ☐ ☐ ☐ ☐ ☐ ☐ ☐	(F)	
SERVINGS OF WATER (8 OZ) ☐ ☐ ☐ ☐ ☐ ☐ ☐ ☐	(Sa)	
	(Su)	

196

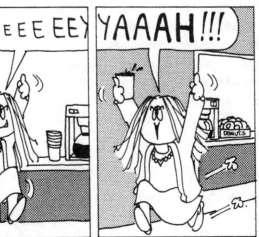

LESSON THIRTEEN

e are at a point where it makes sense to take stock of where you stand and to make a plan for launching into the next phase of your program. We will look back over the important issues that have been covered thus far, gaze into the future, and think about ways to make changes that can be truly permanent. To do this, you will learn about the Behavior Chain. This gives you a system for deciding which of many techniques to use in a given situation. I consider this extremely important. I'll give you a method for taking your pulse for positive feedback on your activity program, discuss poultry in more detail, and introduce the topic of a "toxic" food environment. We have much to cover, so let's begin.

Taking Stock of Your Progress

TAPE 3
SECTION 7

If you have been reading one lesson each week, you are almost four months into the program. This is an important landmark. Four months is a long time, so you deserve credit for working hard this long. Many people give up before this point; you may have done so in the past yourself. So, persistence pays off.

What also pays off is being a student of your life circumstances. If you understand the circumstances that prompt you to eat well and be active, and the circumstances that make you eat more and be inactive, you are poised to act.

Acting means having a plan so that you place yourself in the circumstances where you can cope in a constructive way. Let's take stock of where you are with each part of The LEARN Program.

Your Lifestyle Achievements

A key concept I introduced in Lesson Four dealt with the ABC's (Antecedents, Behaviors, and Consequences). This is a scheme for thinking about the events that occur before, during, and after eating. This is a great time to re-apply that scheme to your eating and activity patterns.

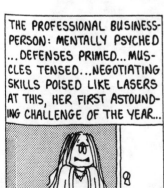

THE PROFESSIONAL BUSINESS-
PERSON: MENTALLY PSYCHED
...DEFENSES PRIMED...MUS-
CLES TENSED...NEGOTIATING
SKILLS POISED LIKE LASERS
AT THIS, HER FIRST ASTOUND-
ING CHALLENGE OF THE YEAR...

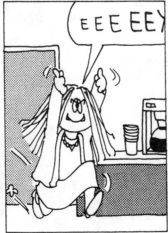

EEE EEY YAAAH!!!

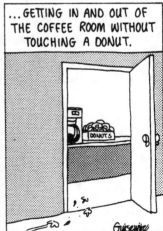

...GETTING IN AND OUT OF
THE COFFEE ROOM WITHOUT
TOUCHING A DONUT.

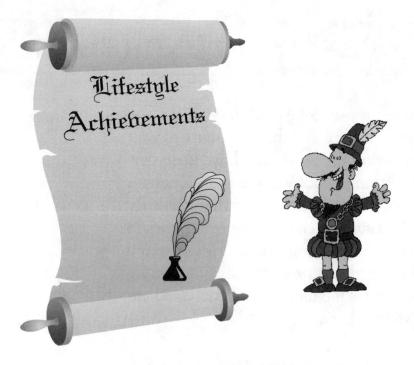

Lifestyle Achievements

You have confronted many situations in which you were and were not successful at sticking with your program. Can you think about what precedes situations in which you have trouble (the antecedents)? For many people, negative feelings such as anger, loneliness, depression, or jealousy make a person want to eat. The time of day might matter or whether other people are eating in your presence. Can you develop a plan to change the situations that promote eating? Think also about changing the behavior itself (your eating) or the consequences (such as your reaction to making a mistake). Then you can implement the ABC plan to its fullest.

Which lifestyle changes are most important to you? Is it eating slowly, sticking with an eating schedule, keeping tempting foods out of the home, keeping a food diary, or one of the other techniques we discussed? If it works, use it. But go beyond this to understand why it works. Then you can develop additional means for remaining in charge.

Your Exercise Achievements

A great deal has been said about physical activity thus far in the program. Let's review a few of the key points.

⇨ Being physically active is one of the strongest predictors of long-term success at weight management.

⇨ Physical activity has benefits far beyond weight management. It is associated with reduced risk of a number of serious diseases, including heart disease. People who are active live longer than those who are not.

⇨ We now know that rigorous activity is not necessary to derive health benefits from physical activity.

⇨ Several bouts of activity during the day are as good as one long bout.

⇨ The best type of activity is something you enjoy and, hence, will continue doing over the long term.

⇨ Anything you do to be active, no matter how small, should "count" in your mind as

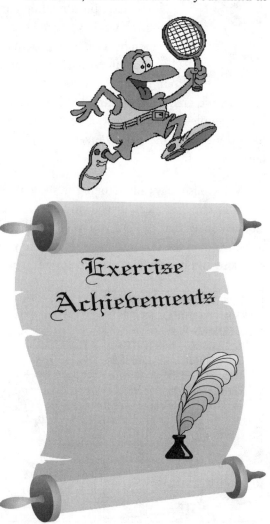

Exercise Achievements

My Commitment to Be Physically Active

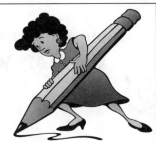

1. I will _____

2. I will _____

3. I will _____

4. I will _____

5. I will _____

activity. This makes you feel like an "exerciser" and increases your opportunity to feel like you are making progress.

I have spoken thus far about why activity is linked to weight management (Lesson Two, page 34), starting an activity program (Lesson One, page 19), fine-tuning a walking program (Lesson Five, page 78), continuing your walking and lifestyle activity (Lesson Seven, page 110), how you can increase activities in your day-to-day routine and make physical activity count (Lesson Six, page 91), how to select a programmed activity (Lesson Eight, page, 126), and more. Reread this material to help get inspired, and then find ways in your day-to-day routine to be more active, along with ways you can schedule activity to occur on a regular basis. Declare in the space above what you intend to do.

Your Attitude Achievements

It comes as no accident that the A (Attitudes) is at the center of LEARN. How we think is central to who we are as people. How we think affects how we feel, and our thoughts and feelings are key drivers of our behavior. Eating and exercising are behaviors, so thinking right goes a long way toward acting right.

If you accept the proposition that attitudes are key, then you are in a good position to spot helpful and unhelpful thoughts and to develop ways to think positively. By thinking positively, I do not mean you should love everyone, expect world peace, and write smiley faces when you sign your name. I mean interpreting your progress in a realistic way; having positive, but real-

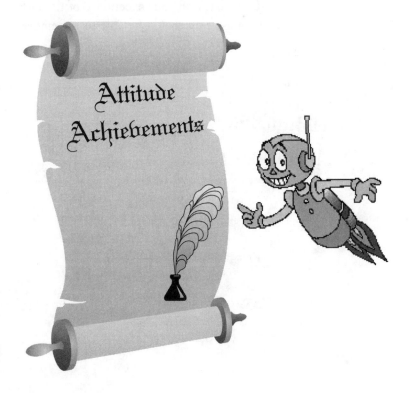

Some Thoughts that Get in My Way	Some Better Thoughts that Will Help Me
_____	_____
_____	_____
_____	_____
_____	_____
_____	_____
_____	_____

istic expectations; recovering from lapses; and thinking about your weight, your eating, and your body in a constructive way.

Think back on your experience of the last few months. You should be able to remember

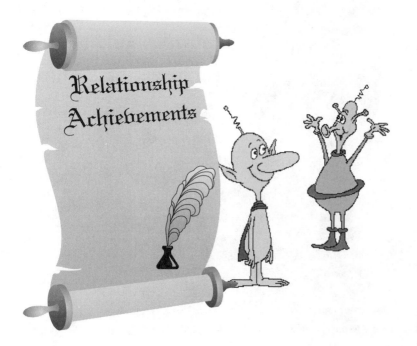

thoughts that have hurt or helped your cause. They might relate to how you thought about your rate of weight loss, how you felt when you had setbacks, or how much confidence you had in coping with difficult situations. Write down, in the space above, some positive and negative thoughts. When you have identified the helpful, positive thoughts, practice them. The negative thoughts have probably occurred many hundreds of times over many years, so you will have to work to counter them. The more you repeat the new thoughts to yourself, the more real they will become, even if the process seems artificial at first.

Your Relationship Achievements

Support from others can be a real asset. Not everyone wants or needs this support, but if used the right way, it can make a real difference for some people. In Lesson Five on page 79, I discussed how to decide whether you would benefit from support (remember the distinction between social and solo changers?).

You may want go back and read the information on Relationships in Lessons Six (page 89), Nine (page 143), and Ten (page 155) to ask again whether you are the type of person who would benefit from support, and if so, what you can do to get and keep support from others. Also, it's not an all-or-none matter. You may not need support under ordinary circumstances but may want to call for it in a pinch. Let's say you start to slip off the program, or you feel your control is threatened because of some upsetting events in your life. Support can often be used as crisis intervention.

There are formal ways to get support, if you feel they might help. Overeaters Anonymous provides a great deal of support, to the point where you can have a sponsor you can call day or night. Other programs can provide support from group meetings or from a leader or counselor, and of course, support can come from a professional like a psychologist or dietitian.

Your Nutrition Achievements

As with the other LEARN components, awareness in the nutrition area is important. You can go a long way toward correct nutrition if you use common sense, eat a variety of foods, and follow some plan like the Food Guide Pyramid. The two key issues to remember are a balanced diet and calorie control. And remember, the key to calorie control is to accurately measure serving sizes and record them on your monitoring form.

Calorie control is necessary for weight loss and maintenance. By now you should know the calories in most foods and should be pretty good at estimating portion sizes. If the calories you take in are less than what your body burns, you will lose weight. If you eat more than you need, you will gain. Eat the exact amount the body needs, and your weight will be stable. It sounds simple, and it is.

Eating a balanced diet is necessary for good health. You could have a low calorie intake and lose weight, but still eat a terrible diet. The

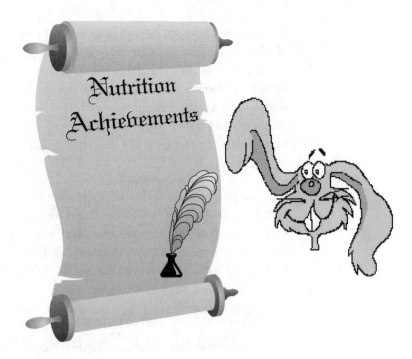

weight loss is gratifying, but you will pay a price in energy level and the general condition of your body. You can eat a balanced diet *and* keep the calories low. This satisfies your need for both weight management and good health.

There is no magic in nutrition. I can offer an iron-clad guarantee you will continue to see diet books, magazine articles, and the like that promise some new discovery. Some will tell you to eat lots of certain nutrients (like protein or carbohydrate) and little of others. Others will say that the time at which you eat foods makes a difference, or that certain foods have special fat-burning qualities. Many of these are old diet plans packaged by a new huckster with new hype.

What is common to most of these is that they promise what people want to hear—a new solution and something that sounds like magic. They may spin a rationale that sounds good, talking about insulin, hormones, brain chemicals, and things like food addiction and carbohydrate craving. When you get lucky, you will find a plan that won't hurt you. Some might hurt you. Think of how many such plans you have read or heard about in your lifetime. How many could you name? Where are they now?

How much would you be willing to bet that any of those that are popular now will still be around in a year or two? If they worked, they'd be around forever, and everyone in the world would want a copy. Few have been tested, and if they ever get tested, my guess is that none will be superior to something like the Food Guide Pyramid.

Are you eating a balanced diet? Are you able to keep your calories where you'd like on most days? You can expect better and worse days, so remember that what counts is how these balance out and how you do over a longer period, such as a week or a month.

Bringing it All Together: The Behavior Chain

TAPE 4
SECTION 4

We need to organize the information in this program into a logical picture. I have covered ways to identify problem situations, along with techniques (more than 70 by now) to help you control eating and increase exercise. You are still left with an important challenge.

What each person needs is a mental card file or computer database to summon the right technique at the right time in a given situation. For example, if playing a card game (let's say bridge) with your friends is a high-risk situation, you could look in your file under "Playing Bridge" for a list of techniques. The card in

your file would list different aspects of this situation that would determine its degree of risk. These aspects might be who the friends are, whether they serve food, how hungry you are, how well your program has been going, and so forth. Then when a situation arises, perhaps the arrival of potato chips and dip, your card would list several responses.

The Behavior Chain is the path to this process. It is a method for breaking eating episodes into discrete parts. When you examine each part, ideas emerge for stopping an episode in its tracks. The ideas that follow can truly increase your understanding of eating.

A Chain and its Links

We can view eating as a chain of events that contains many links. The links string together like an ordinary chain. We can use a familiar phrase: *A chain is only as strong as its weakest link*. The good news is that you want to break this chain, so attacking at the weakest link is ideal.

If we return to the example of playing bridge with friends, eating the potato chips resides at the end of a long chain. Preceding it were links like having the chips available, going to the card game hungry, having friends offer the food, and so forth. The chain could be broken at any of these points.

Each act of eating can be viewed with the chain in mind. Once you identify the links in

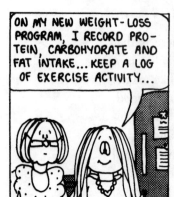
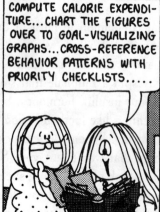
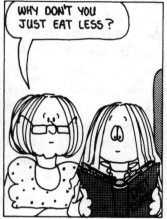
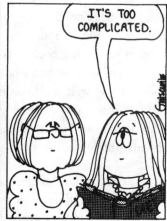

your chain, you can spot the best link to break and how to break it. The more links you break, and the earlier in the chain you break them, the easier it will be to control eating.

A Sample Behavior Chain

Let's illustrate the chain concept with the example of Laura. In her chain, Laura ate 10 cookies, felt guilty, and then ate even more. Laura's eating occurred in a chain that included many links before the eating and several links after the eating. We could help Laura control her cookie intake by analyzing this chain. Remember that this is an example to illustrate the *principle of a chain. Think about how this concept applies to your situation.*

Laura's chain began when she bought the cookies. She was home on Saturday afternoon and was tired and bored. She got the urge to eat and then ate the 10 cookies while watching TV. She felt guilty and ate more cookies later. We can find 12 links in Laura's chain. These are shown in the figure displayed on page 204.

These are the 12 steps to Laura's dilemma. It started when (1) Laura bought the cookies. She then (2) left the cookies on the counter where they were plainly visible. She was (3) home on Saturday afternoon, which she knows from experience is a high-risk time and place for overeating.

She was (4) tired and bored. She (5) felt an urge to eat and (6) went to the kitchen. She (7) took the cookies to the den and (8) ate them while watching TV. She (9) ate rapidly until she felt full, then (10) felt guilty and like a failure. This (11) weakened her restraint further until (12) she ate even more cookies.

Is Laura an innocent victim of an inevitable chain, or can she do something to interrupt it at a critical point? As you probably guessed, Laura has many options for interrupting the chain. Before we discuss these, think of your own lifestyle and the eating habits you have.

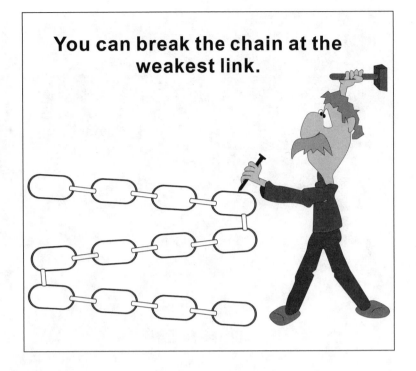

You can break the chain at the weakest link.

How do they exist as chains, and what are the links in the chains?

Take some time now to form a picture of an eating chain that applies to you. Use the blank chain provided on page 206 to fill in the details. You can use Laura's chain as an example, but make the situation specific to you. Pick a high-risk situation that really gives you trouble. Examples might be arriving home from work, watching television in the evening, feeling depressed or lonely, etc.

Your chain can contain fewer links or more than the blank chain permits, but try to include each important detail. You will see how the links are inextricably tied together to form a sequence of events that is hard to stop once it gets started. If you come armed with techniques for dismantling the chain, you will increase your control.

Interrupting the Chain

Your mind was probably buzzing with ideas as we were discussing Laura's eating chain and as you were writing your own chain. We can use Laura's chain for an example of how a chain might be broken. Some of the pos-

Sample Behavior Chain

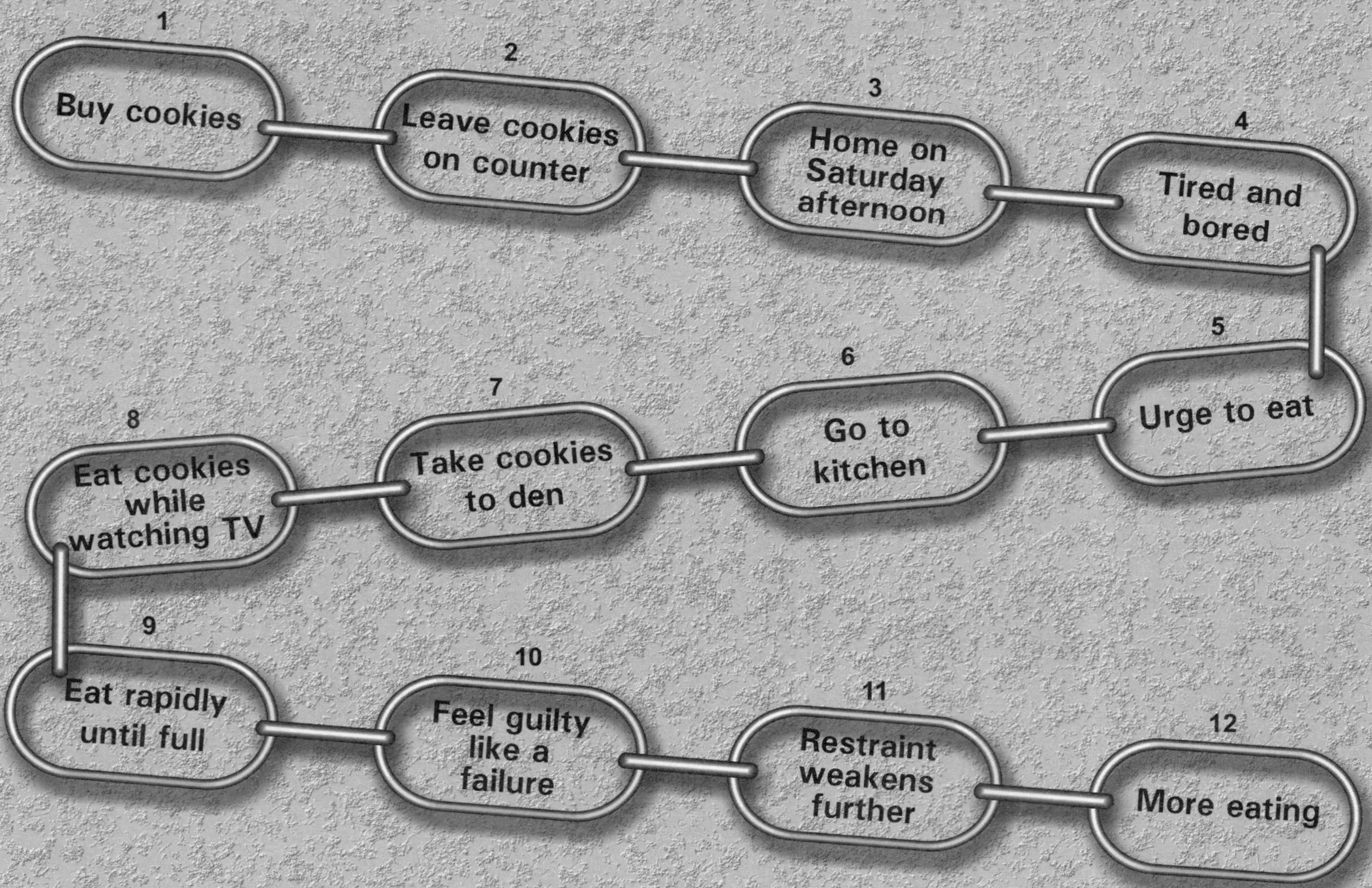

1 Buy cookies

2 Leave cookies on counter

3 Home on Saturday afternoon

4 Tired and bored

5 Urge to eat

6 Go to kitchen

7 Take cookies to den

8 Eat cookies while watching TV

9 Eat rapidly until full

10 Feel guilty like a failure

11 Restraint weakens further

12 More eating

Breaking the Links in
Laura's Behavior Chain

Link	Link-Breaking Techniques
Buy cookies	Shop from a list Shop on a full stomach Shop with a partner Have a partner do your shopping Buy cookie mix (needs baking)
Cookies on counter	Store in opaque container Freeze cookies Store in inaccessible place
Home during high-risk time	Go shopping Schedule programmed activity Plan an enjoyable activity
Tired and bored	Exercise Get more sleep
Urge to eat	List of alternatives to eating Wait five minutes; urge may pass Separate hunger from cravings
Go to kitchen	Use alternative activities Get some exercise Leave house Low-calorie foods available
Take cookies to den	Eat in one place
Eat while watching TV	Do nothing else while eating
Eat rapidly until full	Put food down between bites Pause during eating Serve one cookie at a time Stop automatic eating
Feel guilty, like a failure	Watch dichotomous thinking Banish imperatives Set realistic goals Plan adaptive response
Restraint weakens	Resolve to increase control Read LEARN Manual for ideas
More eating	Examine chain, use techniques Watch attitude traps

My Behavior Chain

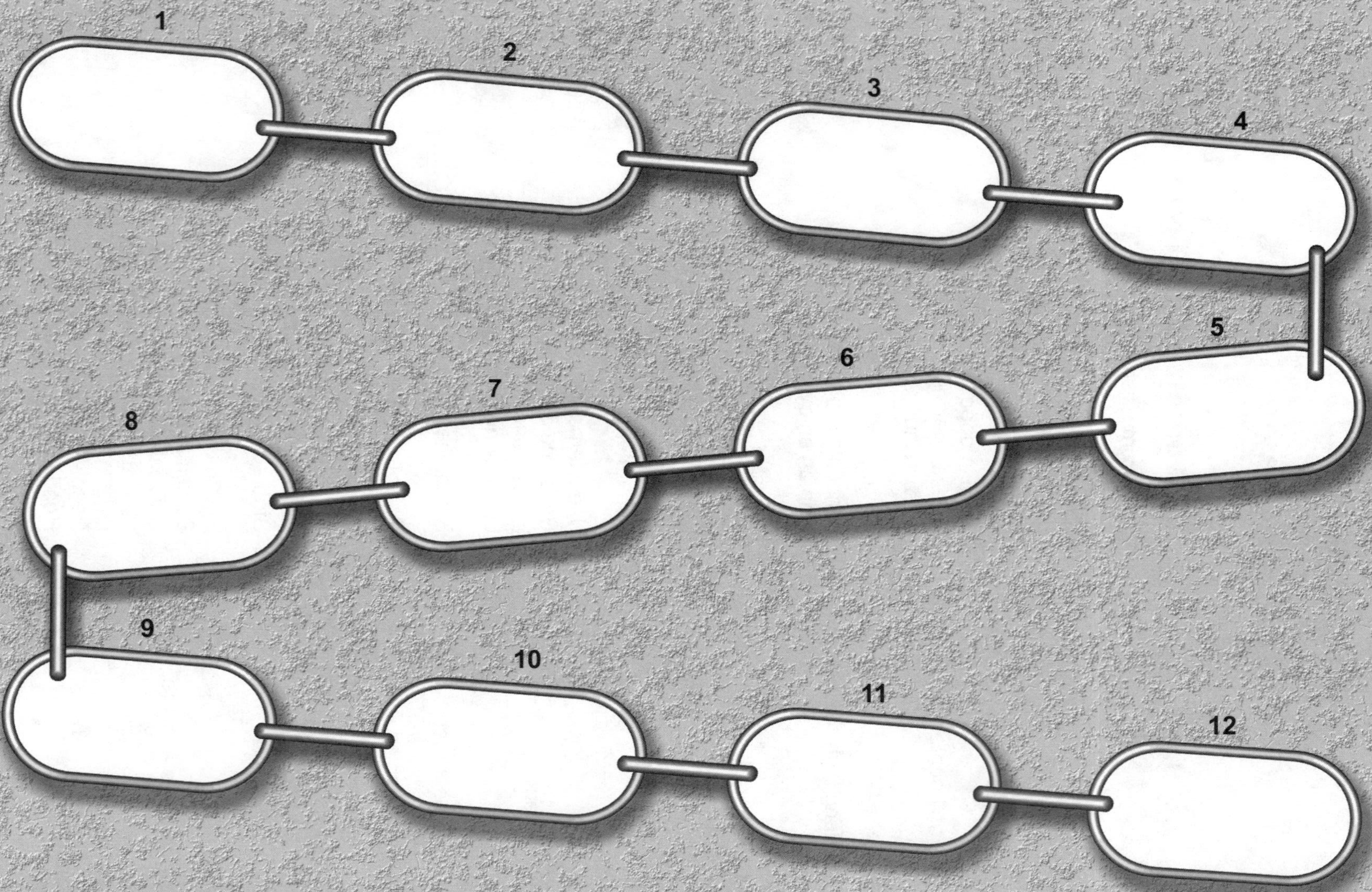

1

2

3

4

5

6

7

8

9

10

11

12

206

sible ways Laura might interrupt her chain are shown in the table page 205.

Analyzing Your Eating Chain

This chain concept could be a key part of your program. If you can analyze your eating according to the chain notion, you can devise many ways to get control. Contrast this with the common approach that relies solely on willpower once the chain is advanced and food beckons.

Now we can go to work on *your* chain. Look at each of the links in the chain and write down at least two ways the chain could be broken at each link. With Laura's chain, we listed 34 ways to break at least one link. Use the information you have learned in the program to think of *link-breaking techniques*. You might refresh your memory on techniques by referring back to the Monitoring Forms from previous weeks.

There are several things to remember when listing these techniques. The first is to concentrate on the weakest links. For instance, if eating ice cream is the final link in your chain, it might be easier to avoid buying the ice cream initially than to count on willpower when confronted by

the food. This leads to the second point, which is to interrupt the chain as early as possible. This does not diminish the importance of interrupting the steps late in the chain, but starting early in the chain gives you more links to work with.

We know what happens when we read things where the author asks us to fill something out. We usually think it's not worth the effort, and we read ahead. You may feel that you need not go through this exercise, and you might be correct. Remember, however, that the act of writing these things down will make you think and analyze your high-risk situations like never before.

A Pulse Test for Positive Feedback

The Pulse Test is a simple means of feedback on your progress with exercise. The directions on the following page explain how to take your pulse and how to estimate your heart rate. Doing this every few weeks can reveal one important physical change due to exercise—a lower heart rate.

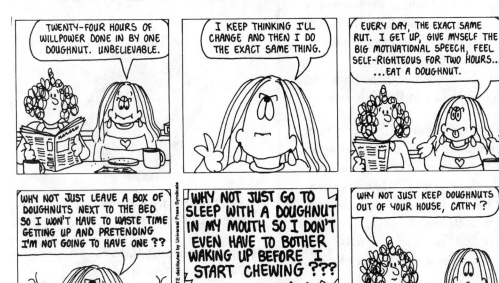
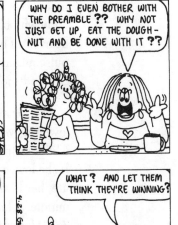

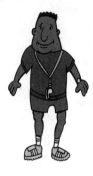

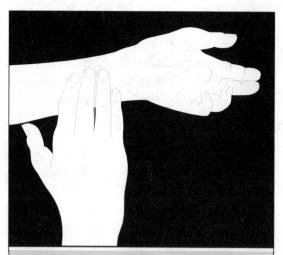

Steps for Taking Your Pulse

❶ **Select either wrist.**

❷ **Place the fingers of one hand on the back of the other wrist as illustrated.**

❸ **Press the index and middle fingers on the upturned wrist until you feel the regular pulsing of the blood through the vessel.**

❹ **Count the number of beats (pulses) in exactly 15 seconds.**

❺ **Multiply the number by four to calculate your beats per minute.**

Your pulse, or heart rate, is the number of times your heart beats per minute to supply the body with blood. A high pulse means that your heart must beat many times to do its job. A low pulse means the heart is in better condition and can do its job with less effort (fewer beats).

An example can illustrate the benefits of lowering your heart rate. Consider a woman whose resting heart rate is 75 beats per minute. If she lowers her heart rate to 70 beats per minute, her heart has five fewer beats to make each minute. This is 300 fewer beats per hour and 7200 fewer per day! By taking your pulse periodically, you can estimate the positive changes you make.

Before we move on to the actual Pulse Test, a few facts are important to mention. First, this is not a sophisticated exercise fitness evaluation that a cardiologist or exercise specialist would do. The numbers you estimate for your heart rate cannot be used to judge your overall fitness or your cardiovascular condition.

Second, some people improve their fitness in leaps and bounds but show no change in heart rate. This is particularly true of people who exercise regularly and/or have low heart rates. Beta-blocker drugs, which are prescribed for hypertension, lower heart rate so only small changes may be possible with exercise. Do not get discouraged if you walk like a real trooper and your pulse stays the same. You will be able to feel your improvement in many other ways. For most people, however, the Pulse Test will detect changes in heart rate as their condition improves.

Steps for Taking Your Pulse

There are two times to take your pulse. The first is when you are at rest. Be still for at least five minutes, then take your pulse. The second time is during exercise. Do this during your walking program. Walk for at least three to four minutes at a comfortable pace. Stop walking,

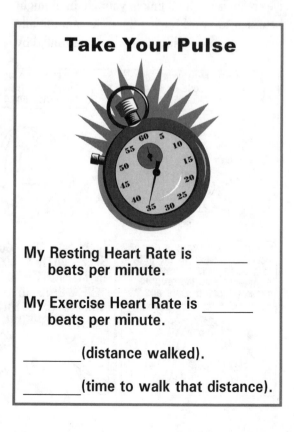

Take Your Pulse

My Resting Heart Rate is _____ beats per minute.

My Exercise Heart Rate is _____ beats per minute.

_____(distance walked).

_____(time to walk that distance).

and take your pulse immediately. How rapidly your heart rate recovers to its resting level is one index of fitness. In the space provided on page 208, write down the distance you walked, how long it took, and record your pulse rate.

Follow the Steps for Taking Your Pulse illustrated on page 208. Take your resting and exercise pulse rates as soon as possible, and write them in the spaces provided. You can refer back to these figures as your condition improves. For the exercise figures, you should find improvements in the time it takes to walk a given distance, in heart rate, or both. Take your pulse and write it down every two weeks. This will show your improvement over time.

Bracing Yourself Against a Toxic Environment

TAPE 3
SECTION 5

People with weight problems face a difficult, even toxic environment. The temptations to eat are constant, powerful, and compelling. If you pause for a moment to think, you might be surprised by how we accept this without the slightest protest.

Think of the number of fast food restaurants you find within a 15-minute drive of your home. In addition to the national chains like McDonald's, Burger King, Wendy's, and Kentucky Fried Chicken, there are local and regional restaurants. Most now have drive-thru windows, that make it easier and faster to get loads of calories and fat. Many also now serve breakfast, and some are open 24 hours. Nearly every service station has been closed and remodeled to contain a mini-market, and almost every mall has a food court. There are vending machines everywhere, and fast-food chains like McDonald's are showing up in airports, airplanes, and even hospital lobbies!

Let's take another example. Many of the fast-food restaurants offer package meals called value meals. More unhealthy food for less money—some value, eh? They also offer, at a seemingly good price, the opportunity to get ex-

tra large drinks and fries, when you "supersize it." This is so much a part of our landscape that the word "supersize" has become a verb in our vocabulary.

The value meals and the supersize portions are a powerful and effective means companies use to market their foods.

Food advertising is also a problem. Madison Avenue's brightest minds set to work to convince us that we should eat foods that often can be very high in calories, fat, and sugar. The average American child sees 10,000 food commercials each year, 95 percent of which are for fast foods, sugared cereals, candy, and soft drinks.

It is not stretching the language to say that we are exposed to a toxic food environment. We are exposed to and are encouraged to consume things that can cause deadly diseases such as heart disease and cancer. We rail against the tobacco companies for exposing us to temptations to smoke (especially when the inducements are aimed at children), but we remain remarkably quiet when the same thing happens with unhealthy food. I expect that over time the public

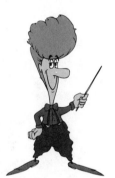

"You must find creative ways to resist the environmental pressures to buy unhealthy foods."

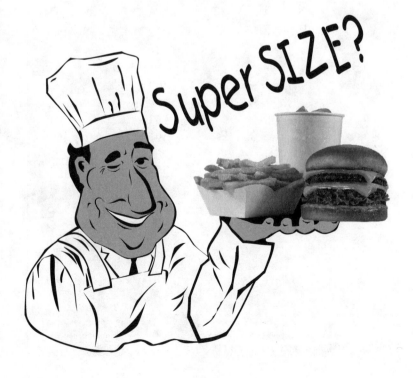

will begin to develop a more militant attitude toward this.

What does this mean for you? It means that you must find creative ways to resist the environmental pressures to buy unhealthy foods. Part of this lies in developing an attitude, in some cases an angry one. When you see the drive-thru sign, remember that it is designed to make it easier for you to spend your money on products that can harm you. When you see the junk food stores in the food court, remember that they are in business to feed their high-fat food to as many people as possible. When you fill your car with gas, remember that there is an industry that sells chips, pastries, ice cream, and soft drinks that wants you to succumb. Get mad, and resist!

The other way to deal with this pressure is be aware of it and avoid exposure as much as possible. When you can, avoid going around these places. If at the mall, stay away from the food court. Use a credit card to pay for gas at the pump rather than go inside where the food is. Try not to drive by the fast-food places when you are hungry. Most of all, keep alert to these inducements to eat and see that you—not a multi-billion dollar food industry—are in charge of your eating and your health.

Poultry: Better than Red Meat?

An article by Bonnie Liebman in the *Nutrition Action Healthletter* provided some interesting facts about poultry. In only 20 years, the intake of chicken in the U.S. has doubled and turkey has risen by two-thirds. This is a positive development because poultry can be helpful in reducing the intake of saturated fat.

The fact that poultry consumption increased so dramatically was not lost on the beef and pork industries, and for obvious reasons, both are attempting to convince the public that their product is like chicken. You may hear ads stating that beef has no more cholesterol than chicken. This is not novel news, because beef is not particularly high in cholesterol. It does, however, have much more saturated fat than chicken, and saturated fat is reported to be a worse culprit than dietary cholesterol in raising blood cholesterol. The YGSN (You've Got Some Nerve) award has to go to the campaign by the pork industry to characterize pork as the *other white meat*. This seems to me a direct attempt to make pork seem like chicken (pork can have twice the saturated fat of chicken and turkey) and to distance pork from *red meat* (pork can have as much fat as beef).

Birds differ in the amount of fat they provide. The leanest poultry is turkey. After poultry is cooked and skinned, chicken has double or triple the fat of turkey, and duck and goose have 50 percent more fat than chicken. The calories and amount of fat in various forms of poultry are in the table at the left. As Liebman points out in her article, averages can be deceiv-

Calories and Fat in Poultry

(per 4 oz roasted portion)

Type of Poultry	Calories	Fat (g)
Duck, with skin	384	36.5
Duck, without skin	229	14.5
Goose, with skin	348	28.5
Goose, without skin	271	16.5
Turkey, light, with skin	187	6.0
Turkey, light, without skin	160	1.5
Chicken, light, with skin	253	14.0
Chicken, light, without skin	197	6.0
Chicken, dark, with skin	288	20.5
Chicken, dark, without skin	234	12.5
Ground turkey (3 oz)	191	12.5
Chicken hot dog	116	10.0
Turkey bologna (2 oz)	114	9.0

Note: Figures in table abstracted from Liebman, B. CSPI's Poultry Primer. *Nutrition Action Healthletter*, November 1986. Their source for calorie and fat information was USDA Handbook #8-5, #8-10, #8-13.

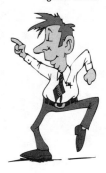

Office Calories

Activity	Calories
Throwing in the towel	0
Beating around the bush	35
Bending over backwards	75
Hitting the nail on the head	75
Dragging your heels	90
Tooting your own horn	100
Flirting at the water cooler	150
Avoiding the boss	175
Jumping to conclusions	200
Passing the buck	300
Making mountains out of molehills	400
Running around in circles	450
Climbing the walls	500

ing, because some cuts of red meat and some parts of poultry can have more or less fat than the average. In general, however, turkey breast without the skin has relatively little fat, and chicken has about half the fat of lean red meats.

When preparing poultry, several factors should be considered. First, removing the skin reduces fat by about 50 percent. Second, fat intake is increased greatly when chicken is battered and fried, because the batter soaks up fat. A fried chicken breast from Kentucky Fried Chicken can have two or three times the fat of a roasted breast (even with the skin on). Finally, think of creative ways to use turkey and chicken in salads with fruits, pasta, and other foods. This can make for some innovative dishes. The cookbooks listed in Lesson Seven provide many ideas for making interesting dishes using poultry.

Hard Work at the Office

Most people think that working in an office is the perfect setting for getting flabby. Wrong! Certain office activities require great effort. The table above shows just how strenuous life in the office can be.

My Personal Goals for This Week

Much of this lesson focused on reviewing your progress in the program and the Behavior Chain. Be sure to fill out the blank chain in this lesson and devise plans to break as many links as possible. Use this idea of the Behavior Chain in analyzing your high-risk situations and in planning in advance for countering pressures to eat. You may find it useful to draw out more than one chain to help with your most difficult situations. Take your pulse this week using the information you learned in this lesson. Be aware of the toxic environment that lurks about, drawing you in to thwart your weight management efforts. Be strong, and don't give in to the high-pressure marketing tactics.

As you think back over the three months you have been in the program, take a moment to review the changes you feel are most important. What are the keys to your success? Use these to establish your personal goals. I have left the first two lines of the Monitoring Form in this lesson blank for you to complete with your own personal goals for this week. Remember also, to record your weight change on the Weight Change Record in Lesson Nine on page 154. Good luck with this week's lesson.

My Self-Assessment

Lesson Thirteen

(T) F 94. Being a student of your own life circumstances is important for making and maintaining positive lifestyle changes.

(T) F 95. A Behavior Chain, like any chain, is only as strong as its weakest links.

T (F) 96. Once the eating chain begins, it is not possible to stop because the links are so strong.

T (F) 97. It is best to interrupt an eating chain at one of its last links when you know what foods confront you.

T (F) 98. Your resting pulse will increase as you lose weight and get in better condition.

T (F) 99. Exercise is not a good predictor of who will keep weight off over the long run, but the health benefits are reason enough to be active.

(T) F 100. It can be helpful to develop a militant attitude about the "toxic food environment" we face.

(T) F 101. It is important to know the fat content of poultry meats because of the wide variation in fat content.

(Answers in Appendix C, page 271)

Monitoring Form—Lesson Thirteen   *Today's Date:* _____

TIME	FOOD AND AMOUNT	CALORIES
TOTAL DAILY CALORIES		

PERSONAL GOALS FOR THIS WEEK	MOST OF THE TIME	SOME-TIMES	RARELY
1.			
2.			
3. SKETCH YOUR BEHAVIOR CHAINS			
4. BE AWARE OF THE TOXIC ENVIRONMENT			
5. EAT DAILY SERVINGS FROM THE FIVE FOOD GROUPS			
6. EAT LESS THAN _____ CALORIES PER DAY			

FOOD GROUPS FOR TODAY		PHYSICAL ACTIVITY	MINUTES OR STEPS
MILK, YOGURT, AND CHEESE	❑ ❑ ❑	(M)	
MEAT, POULTRY, ETC.	❑ ❑ ❑	(Tu)	
FRUITS	❑ ❑ ❑ ❑	(W)	
VEGETABLES	❑ ❑ ❑ ❑ ❑	(Th)	
BREADS, CEREALS, ETC.	❑ ❑ ❑ ❑ ❑ ❑ ❑ ❑	(F)	
SERVINGS OF WATER (8 OZ)	❑ ❑ ❑ ❑ ❑ ❑ ❑ ❑	(Sa)	
		(Su)	

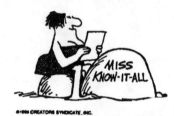

Dear Miss know-it-all,

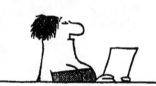

what's the quickest way to lose fifty pounds in a hurry?

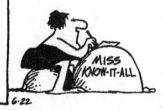

GO TO AN ENGLISH GAMBLING CASINO.

LESSON FOURTEEN

his lesson begins the last three of the program. In many ways, these last lessons together may be our most important because we turn our attention to permanent maintenance of weight loss. Central to this notion are three terms: *lapse, relapse,* and *collapse.* These will be discussed in this lesson. I also will introduce the last of the five categories of problem thinking—dichotomous (light bulb) thinking. Finally, you will learn about the role of cholesterol in your diet. Let's begin.

Preventing Lapse, Relapse, and Collapse

TAPE 4
SECTION 6

Far too often, a minor slip propels a person to misery. The guilt from a slip makes a person susceptible to more slips and can ultimately lead to loss of all control. This is a gloomy picture, but good news is around the corner! There *are* ways to turn the tables.

Maintenance of weight loss may be the greatest challenge facing overweight persons. Losing weight is difficult enough, but keeping it off ranks up there in difficulty with winning the lottery and finding a compassionate auditor from the Internal Revenue Service. Most overweight people have lost and regained weight many times, so something must be done to interrupt these cycles. The trick is to prevent slips

from occurring and to respond constructively when they do occur.

Everyone makes mistakes. Some bounce back and use the slip as a signal to increase control. It is common, however, for the slip to cause a negative emotional reaction (guilt and despair) that builds until all control is lost.

There are two paths to success. The first is to avoid or prevent slips and mistakes and the second is to respond to slips with coping techniques that put *you* in control. I will cover each path separately. In this lesson, we will work on preventing slips, and in Lesson Fifteen, I will emphasize recovering from slips.

Much of our discussion on this topic is drawn from the excellent work of Dr. G. Alan Marlatt and Dr. Judith Gordon, both psychologists from the University of Washington. They

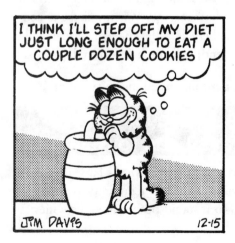

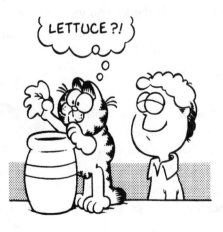

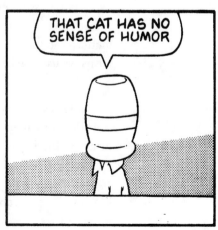

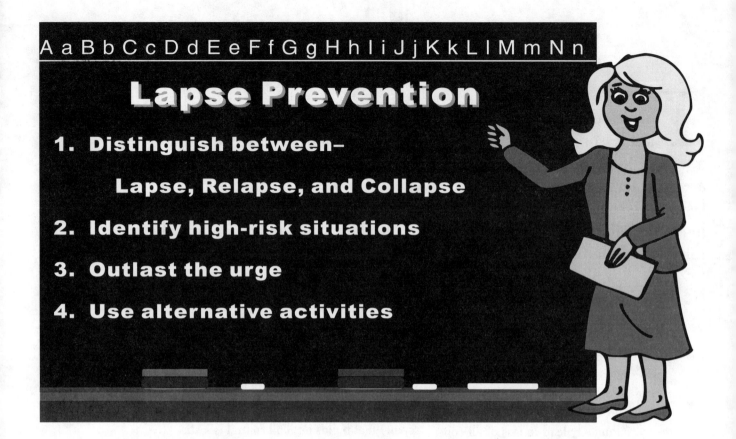

Lapse Prevention

1. Distinguish between–

   Lapse, Relapse, and Collapse

2. Identify high-risk situations

3. Outlast the urge

4. Use alternative activities

have studied the situations associated with relapse in overweight persons, alcoholics, smokers, drug addicts, and compulsive gamblers. They have also proposed methods for preventing relapse.

Distinguishing Lapse, Relapse, and Collapse

I have used several terms to describe deviating from your weight management plan: mistake, lapse, slip, error, etc. Relapse implies something different and collapse is yet another matter. We fuss with these words because the terms we use can be important.

In recovering alcoholics, one slip or lapse is considered by many to be a relapse (i.e., "one drink, a drunk"). Some think the same is true for people who stop smoking. Having a single cigarette begins an inevitable path to relapse. However, there is abundant evidence that this is not true.

Many recovering alcoholics have had at least one drink since their reformation, and it is a rare ex-smoker who has not had a cigarette. Yet, they recover from their lapses and prevent a relapse. The same is unquestionably true with overweight individuals.

A *lapse* is a slight error or slip, the first instance of backsliding. It is a discrete event like eating a forbidden food, exceeding a calorie level, or gaining weight. *Relapse* occurs when lapses string together and the person returns to his or her former state. When relapse is complete and there is little hope of reversing the negative trend, *collapse* has occurred.

The most important message is that

A Lapse Must Not Always Lead to Relapse.

The person who can view a lapse for what it is, an unfortunate but temporary problem, is prepared to respond positively to life's inevitable setbacks.

Identifying Urges and High-Risk Situations

The concepts of *urges* and *high-risk situations* were introduced earlier in the program. Distinguishing cravings (urges) from hunger was discussed in Lesson Three, conquering cravings was also covered in Lesson Four, and the behavior chain was introduced in Lesson Thirteen. These were all leading to the point we face now, the need to spot trouble before it occurs. Urges can now become a signal for corrective action.

Let's look back over what you have learned. You know much more about your eating than before, so let's take advantage of that information. Think carefully about when you are most likely to find your eating threatened. Is it when you have certain feelings, like loneliness or frustration? Is it when you have to deal with some person? Is it when you feel bad about your life and your weight? Is it when someone offers you food? Look back over your Monitoring Forms and your weight loss experience to identify these situations.

Now that you are a pro at identifying urges and high-risk situations, let's plan ahead. We will learn a technique called *outlasting the urges* and will learn to use alternatives to eating when the high-risk situations arise. These become our armor when we are barraged with temptation.

Outlasting the Urges

It is possible to prevent a lapse by dealing with urges. I title this section *Outlasting the Urges* because an urge will usually go away if you just wait it out. This is easier said than done sometimes, but the rewards are high when you succeed.

Dr. G. Alan Marlatt, the psychologist mentioned previously, feels that an urge can be compared to a wave building in the ocean and then breaking on the beach. Conquering the urges is like surfing. A wave begins small, builds to a crest, breaks, and then subsides. Urges follow a similar course. They usually build gently to their strongest point, weaken, and then gradually fade away.

The wave analogy is much different than the way people usually think about urges. Some people feel that an urge builds and builds and will create havoc unless it is gratified by eating. Actually, gratifying an urge by eating makes urges stronger and more frequent. In contrast, letting the urge pass, like the wave rolling in, will weaken it. If you can outlast enough of the urges, they will fade to obscurity.

The image of *urge surfing* is a good one. Pretend you are learning to surf. As the wave rolls in, you can battle it and be wiped out, or you can maintain your balance and ride the wave until it subsides.

Being a good urge surfer involves identifying the urges early in their development and then readying your skills to ride the wave. If the wave is upon you at full strength before you recognize it, you may wipe out no matter how well you surf. If you recognize the wave early, but

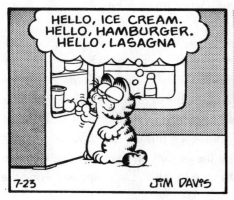
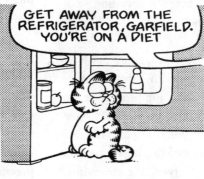
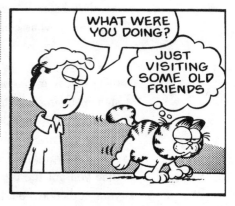

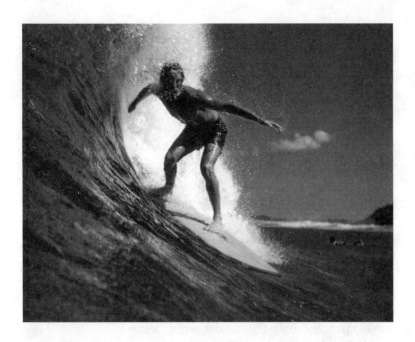

This same approach can work with eating. One cannot play the tuba and eat, so tuba practice would be a good alternative to eating. You might think of more practical methods that would involve activities you enjoy.

Making a List, Checking it Twice

Make a list of activities you could use when you are tempted to eat. The list should contain more than one activity so you have several choices. If you vow to consult the list when you want to eat, your control can improve. Make certain the list contains enjoyable activities so you will actually do them in lieu of eating.

The list provided on page 219 contains ideas for activities incompatible with eating. Some can be done at home, others take you out of the house. Some take little time while others are more involved. Many are examples from my clients. Do they give you more ideas?

Now that you have ideas from the list, it is time to establish your own list. Write out the activities that would make good alternatives for you in the space provided on the worksheet on page 219. Add as many activities as you can. They should be both enjoyable and feasible. Some may require planning and the right timing, like going to a movie. Others should be available at a moment's notice so you can spring into action when an urge hits.

Try consulting the list when you get the urge to eat. If you can distract yourself for even a few minutes, the urge to eat can fade and your control can increase. Studies show that hunger comes and goes during the day, so not succumbing the instant an urge hits can give you precious time to think. Do your best to ride the wave!

"Don't be wiped out by the urge to eat—you can ride it out!"

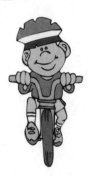

cannot surf, you will also wipe out. Therefore, both parts are important—early recognition and skills to cope with the urges.

Simply waiting for the urge to pass can be all you'll need, but not always. Some urges and high-risk situations are stronger than others, so techniques other than waiting are necessary. One such technique is the use of alternative activities.

Using Alternative Activities

The principle of using alternative activities is simple. When you get the urge, do something else. If you use urges as a signal for positive activity, eating will become less rewarding and the old associations between urges and eating will diminish. When you see food, think about food, or feel hungry because you are lonely, eating is simply a habit created by an association. You can make new associations.

When you recognize urges, think of an activity that is incompatible with eating. For instance, typing a letter and jumping rope are incompatible—both cannot be done at once, unless you are Rubber Man. If you were addicted to typing and agreed to jump rope each time you got the urge to type, the strength of your addiction would fade.

Activities Incompatible with Eating

Walk the Dog

File Coupons

Go to a Movie

Call a Friend

Shop for Plants

Take a Shower

Listen to Music

Take a Drive

Read a Romantic Book

Read a Mystery Book

Go to the Zoo

Buy a New Magazine

Kiss Somebody

Wash the Car

Kiss Somebody Again

Write a Letter

Get Some Exercise

Look at Photo Album

Play a Board Game

Ride a Bike

Brush Your Teeth

Read This Manual!

Frame Some Pictures

Refinish Furniture

Play Music

Knit a Sweater

Work in a Garden

Visit a Museum

Buy a Gift

Plan a Vacation

Paint a Picture

Buy Tickets

Work on a Hobby

Visit a Neighbor

Donate to Charity

Imagine Being More Fit

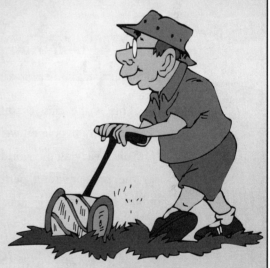

My Alternatives to Eating

1. _____

2. _____

3. _____

4. _____

5. _____

6. _____

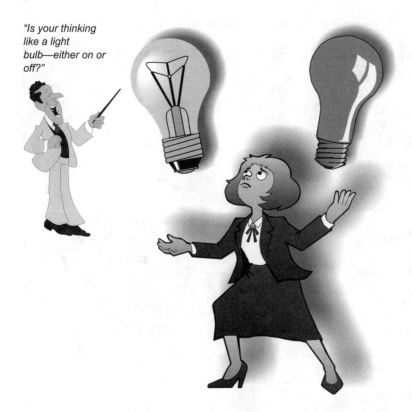

"Is your thinking like a light bulb—either on or off?"

Here are some examples. You might have six straight days in which you meet your calorie level and then splurge the seventh day by eating cake and boosting your calorie total to 2000. The common response would be "I really blew it now. I am off my program."

Notice the phrase "off my program." This is the dichotomous view that you are either perfect or terrible, that you are either on or off a program. This is where the term *Light Bulb Thinking* was born, because a light bulb is either on or off.

The danger is the despair that you feel about making inevitable mistakes. Having 2000 calories is insignificant in your total calories for a week, month, or year. However, your *reaction* to those calories can be devastating. If you feel guilty and depressed, the likely response to soothe the feelings is eating.

Another example is the tendency for people to classify foods as good or bad, dietetic or fattening, and legal or illegal. The specific foods that are good or bad vary from person to person. For you, ice cream might be the illegal food, but for another person it might be corn chips, beer, donuts, potato chips, or fast food. Dichotomous thinking occurs when you slip and feel you have blown the program. A slight transgression can send you into a tailspin.

Dichotomous (Light Bulb) Thinking

This is the classic attitude problem that plagues many people on weight loss programs. It involves viewing the world and losing weight as either right or wrong, perfect or terrible, good or bad, friend or foe, legal or illegal. I see this in nearly every client I work with.

Countering Dichotomous (Light Bulb) Thinking	
MY FAT THOUGHTS	MY COUNTER STATEMENTS
1.	
2.	
3.	
4.	
5.	
6.	
7.	
8.	

It is essential that you be aware of your dichotomous thoughts. Have you made internal rules about foods that you can and cannot eat, a calorie level you *must* maintain, things you must do to stay "on the program," or what constitutes proper dietary behavior? Notice how you feel when you violate the rules. Negative feelings usually indicate dichotomous thinking.

You can contend with dichotomous thinking by talking back to yourself. You realize how illogical it is to feel terrible about one slip or to make rules where eating some food throws you off your program.

Please realize that attitudes are habits just like any other. Simply reading this material and knowing that attitudes might be hindering your progress is not enough. It will help to practice the new thinking and then to practice again. Try not to be a passive recipient of my advice. Be active and search for these thoughts, and be poised to counter them when they occur.

In the spaces on page 220, write down your most common dichotomous thoughts and write a counter statement for each. You can then be prepared in advance when the fat thoughts occur.

Cholesterol

Cholesterol is a waxy substance necessary for the body's functioning. It can be manufactured by the body or can be eaten in food. High blood levels of cholesterol are related to risk for heart disease, and the blood level of cholesterol is determined in part by what you eat.

Cholesterol is carried in the bloodstream by something called lipoproteins. Some of the cholesterol is deposited on the walls of the arteries as fatty streaks. When these deposits build, they form a fibrous plaque that makes the wall of the artery less able to adjust to blood flow. If the artery narrows enough to stop or seriously restrict the flow of blood, vital tissue can be deprived and die. The result is a heart attack if the coronary arteries are involved, or a stroke if the blocked arteries supply blood to the brain.

Knowing your own cholesterol level can be important. The National Cholesterol Education Program, a nationwide effort of the National Institutes of Health, suggests that the desirable level of blood cholesterol is below 200 mg/dl. The range from 200–239 mg/dl is considered borderline, and a level above 240 mg/dl is considered high. Where you fall in these categories will indicate how often your blood cholesterol should be checked, the degree to which your diet should be changed, and whether special advice from your physician is necessary. Therefore, you should have your cholesterol level checked.

You may have heard talk about different types of cholesterol, particularly HDL (high density lipoprotein) cholesterol and LDL (low density lipoprotein) cholesterol. HDL is thought to protect against heart disease, so higher levels are better. LDL has the opposite effect, so lower levels are better. Scientists are learning more about how diet and exercise can be used to raise HDL and lower LDL. The same methods used to lower total cholesterol appear to have beneficial effects on HDL and LDL.

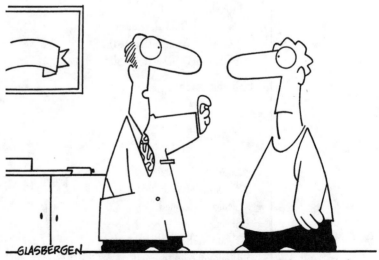

"To prevent a heart attack, take one aspirin every day. Take it out for a jog, then take it to the gym, then take it for a bike ride...."

Cholesterol Content of Common Foods

Food	Quantity	Cholesterol (mg)
Dairy Products		
American cheese	1 oz	41
Butter	1T (0.5 oz)	29–35
Buttermilk from skim	1 cup (8.6 oz)	5
Cheese, cheddar	1 oz	28
Cheese, cream	1 oz	31
Cheese, Swiss	1 oz	28
Cream, half & half	1T (0.5 oz)	6
Cream, whole (whipping)	1T (0.5 oz)	20
Ice milk, soft serve	1 cup (6.2 oz)	35
Ice cream, (16% fat)	1 cup (5.2 oz)	84
Low-fat cottage cheese	4 oz	6
Low-fat yogurt, vanilla/plain	8 oz	11–18
Milk, skim	1 cup (8.6 oz)	5
Milk (1% fat)	1 cup (8.6 oz)	15
Milk, whole (4%)	1 cup (8.7 oz)	34
Meats and Poultry		
Bacon, fried and drained	2 slices (0.8 oz)	12
Beef, ground, broiled	4 oz	107
Beef or calf liver, fried	4 oz	297
Beef pot roast, lean only	4 oz	103
Beef, sirloin steak, lean only	4 oz	103
Bologna	1 slice (1.3 oz)	14
Chicken, fried	4 oz fried in veg. oil	90–103
Chicken liver, simmered	4 oz	846
Egg, large, poached	1 (1.7 oz)	242
Egg, scrambled in veg. oil	1 (2.3 oz)	263
Ham, boiled	1 oz	15
Ham roast, lean only	4 oz	100
Hog dog	1 (1.6 oz)	29
Pork chop, broiled, lean	4 oz	100
Turkey, dark meat (roasted)	4 oz	115
Turkey, light meat (roasted)	4 oz	87
Fish and Seafood		
Clams, raw	4 (3 oz)	42
Cod	4 oz	57
Crab, canned	4 oz	116
Halibut steak, broiled	4 oz	68
Lobster	4 oz	96
Salmon, canned	4 oz	40
Scallops, steamed	4 oz	60
Shrimp	4 oz	170
Trout, fresh rainbow	4 oz	62
Tuna, oil pack, canned	4 oz	63

Note: Figures adapted from *The Dictionary of Sodium, Fats, and Cholesterol* by Barbara Kraus, New York: Putnam, 1974.

To help control blood cholesterol, it is important to limit the amount of fat and cholesterol ingested, and to be sensitive to the type of fat you eat. Saturated fat from animal sources (fats from beef, lamb, pork, ham, butter, cream, whole milk, cheese) and saturated fat from vegetable sources (coconut oil, palm oil, cocoa butter) should be limited. Try to limit saturated fats and replace them with polyunsaturated fats, which usually come from vegetable oils. Physical activity is also a powerful way for some people to control their cholesterol.

The table on page 222 may be helpful in guiding you in choosing foods low in cholesterol. It is important to remember that reducing saturated fat in the diet can have an even more powerful effect in lowering blood cholesterol than can reducing dietary cholesterol. Information on fat is provided in earlier lessons.

Warning: Alcohol and Calories

As you will see from the table provided on page 224, alcohol is packed with calories. A can of light beer will have 100 calories; the count for regular beer is 150 calories, about the same as a can of Coke or Pepsi. Mixed drinks and cordials are higher yet. Think of a daiquiri with more than 200 calories and a pina colada over 250.

Some people can have a pretty successful time with weight loss simply by eliminating or greatly reducing their alcohol intake. Many just decide the pleasure they derive from the drinks does not justify all the calories.

Remember that you get plenty of calories and no nutrition with alcohol. This is why the calories from alcohol are often referred to as "empty calories." So, if you use up part of your day's allotment of calories with alcoholic drinks, there will not be much room in the remaining calories to pack in the nutrients you need for healthy living. If the drinks are important to you, use the skills you are learning to help keep the amount under control. Pour small amounts,

taste every bit (calories should be tasted, not wasted), and be certain to drink only things that are special to you. Don't drink out of habit, and don't continue taking in calories just because you have done so in the past.

One other factor to be alert for is the "disinhibiting" effect of alcohol. Alcohol releases inhibitions in some people, and they do things they might not do when not drinking. You are working to inhibit your calorie intake, and drinking may make you vulnerable to the "what the heck" phenomenon in which you relax your guard and eat more than you might like.

My Personal Goals for This Week

There are several activities for you to use in setting personal goals for this week. The first is to distinguish lapses from a relapse, and the second is to identify high-risk situations. This information forms the basis for the next two parts of your weekly goal—to outlast the urges and to use alternative activities to eating, Try to avoid dichotomous thinking and be aware of the cholesterol in your food. Finally, if you drink alcohol, watch out for the calories

As I recommend in each lesson, you can supplement the goals I have listed above with goals that are personal to you. These could include any technique I have recommended, or something I have not discussed but you feel is important. The key is that the goal is meaningful for you. Remember to record your weight change on the Weight Change Record in Lesson Nine on page 154.

Calorie Costs of Alcohol

Beverage	Serving Size (oz)	Calories
Beer or ale	12	140–160
Beer, light	12	100
Bloody Mary	5	116
Bourbon and soda	4	105
Brandy or cognac	1	65–80
Champagne	4	90
Coffee-flavored creme liqueur	1.5	154
Cold Duck	4	120
Cordials and liqueurs, 34 to 72 proof	1	102–125
Creme de Menthe	1.5	186
Daiquiri (with lime)	4	222
Distilled spirits:		
Gin, vodka, rum, whiskey; 80 to 100 proof	1.5	95–124
Gin and tonic	7.5	171
Manhattan	2	128
Martini	2.5	156
Pina colada (canned)	4.5	346
Screwdriver	7	174
Sherry	3	125
Tequila sunrise	5.5	89
Tom Collins	7.5	121
Vermouth, dry	1	32
Vermouth, sweet	1	45
Wine, dry white	4	79
Wine, red	4	85
Wine, dessert (sweet)	4	181
Wine, light	4	52
Wine, nonalcoholic	6	60
Wine cooler	12	220

Note: The calorie values here are approximations only and may vary depending on a drink's proof, specific sweetness, age, and amount of ice used.

Lesson Fourteen

T (F) 102. When a person lapses, relapse is close behind because nothing can interrupt the negative cycle of lapses and out-of-control eating.

(T) F 103. If you can outlast enough of the urges, they will fade into obscurity.

T (F) 104. Light bulb or dichotomous thinking refers to your own bright ideas about losing weight.

(T) F 105. For controlling your blood cholesterol, it is important to limit your intake of saturated fat.

(T) F 106. It helps to have a list of alternatives to eating for use when urges strike.

(Answers in Appendix C, page 271)

Monitoring Form—Lesson Fourteen   *Today's Date:* _____

TIME	FOOD AND AMOUNT	CALORIES
TOTAL DAILY CALORIES		

PERSONAL GOALS FOR THIS WEEK	MOST OF THE TIME	SOME-TIMES	RARELY
1.			
2.			
3. OUTLAST URGES TO EAT			
4. AVOID DICHOTOMOUS THINKING			
5. IF YOU DRINK, WATCH CALORIES IN ALCOHOL			
6. EAT LESS THAN _____ CALORIES PER DAY			

FOOD GROUPS FOR TODAY	PHYSICAL ACTIVITY	MINUTES OR STEPS
MILK, YOGURT, AND CHEESE ❑ ❑ ❑	(M)	
MEAT, POULTRY, ETC. ❑ ❑ ❑	(TU)	
FRUITS ❑ ❑ ❑ ❑	(W)	
VEGETABLES ❑ ❑ ❑ ❑ ❑	(TH)	
BREADS, CEREALS, ETC. ❑ ❑ ❑ ❑ ❑ ❑ ❑ ❑	(F)	
SERVINGS OF WATER (8 OZ) ❑ ❑ ❑ ❑ ❑ ❑ ❑ ❑	(SA)	
	(SU)	

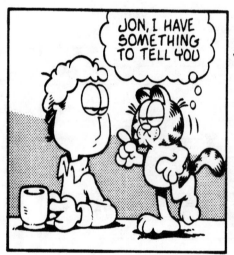
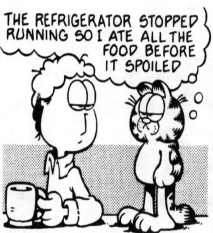
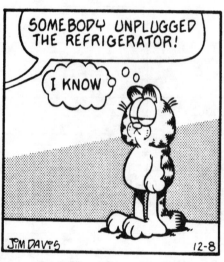

I hope you had a great week. Two lessons remain in The LEARN Program, yet we still have important areas to cover. In the last lesson, I noted two ways to keep the reins on urges and discussed techniques to prevent the common journey from lapse to relapse to collapse. One path, preventing lapses, can be attained by avoiding high-risk situations and by using alternative activities to short circuit the urges. This lesson focuses on the second path—coping with lapses once they occur. In the Nutrition area, I'll discuss why nutrition is so important and we'll look at more information about minerals. I'll give you some tips for handling holidays, parties, and special events. We'll conclude this lesson with a note about breakfast.

Coping with Lapse and Preventing Relapse

TAPE 4
SECTION 8

Lapses are inevitable. By this point in the program, most people losing weight have experienced peaks of joy and valleys of distress. It is the rare person who has not eaten some high-calorie foods, overeaten at a special event or holiday gathering, or resorted to favorite foods when times got tough. The issue is not so much *whether* the lapses occur, but the person's *reaction after they occur*.

An example might elucidate this. Two friends, Judy and Joan, were both on a weight loss program and attended a wedding. Both overate at the buffet, to the tune of 2000 calories. Judy did it on shrimp and steak, whereas Joan fixed her attention on bread and desserts. The extra 2000 calories should not sink their weight loss efforts because the calories amount to less than a pound of weight. Judy and Joan, however, reacted quite differently to the 2000-calorie lapse.

Judy felt guilty about the wedding episode and told herself, "I blew my eating plan." She then thought, "What the heck, I blew it already. I might as well enjoy myself." She ate more when she got home, felt guilty the next day, and continued the overeating for five days. Joan, on the other hand, felt bad about the 2000-calorie

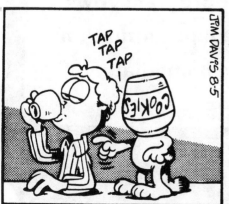

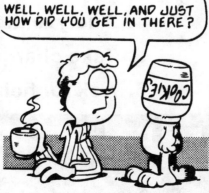

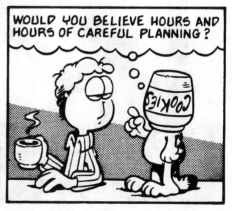

lapse, but responded in a more constructive manner. She reflected on what happened and planned accordingly. She increased her walking an extra 15 minutes for the next four days and cut back on her calorie intake.

Six Steps to Gaining Control

How can we learn from Joan and master our lapses? Following six specific steps can be a big help. These are adapted from the work of Dr. G. Alan Marlatt mentioned in Lesson Fourteen.

⇨ **Step 1: Stop, look, and listen**. A lapse is a signal of impending danger, like a train signal at the crossing gates. Stop what you are doing, especially if the lapse has started, and examine the situation. What is occurring? Why is a lapse in progress? Consider removing yourself to a safe location where you won't be tempted and where you can think in a rational manner.

⇨ **Step 2: Stay calm.** If you get anxious or blame yourself for the lapse, the situation may get worse. You may conclude that you are a hopeless binge eater and that control is impossible. Coming to these conclusions

is easy when you get all worked up. Try to separate yourself from the situation and view it as an objective observer would—that one lapse does not prove failure. Keeping a cool head makes the following steps easier.

⇨ **Step 3: Renew your weight loss vows.** Take a minute to remind yourself of how far you have come, the progress you have made, and how sad it would be if one lapse canceled out all your hard work. Restate your program goals and renew the vows you made when you began your program.

⇨ **Step 4: Analyze the lapse situation.** Instead of blaming yourself for letting go, use the situation to learn what places you at risk. Do certain feelings create the risk? Is it the presence of food, others eating, other activities, etc.? Did you do anything to defend against the urge? Did it work? Why or why not? What thoughts did you have?

⇨ **Step 5: Take charge immediately.** Leap into action with your planned techniques. Leave the house, feed the remain-

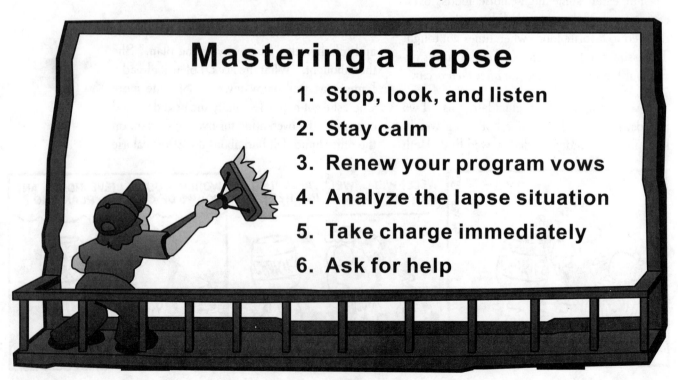

Mastering a Lapse

1. **Stop, look, and listen**
2. **Stay calm**
3. **Renew your program vows**
4. **Analyze the lapse situation**
5. **Take charge immediately**
6. **Ask for help**

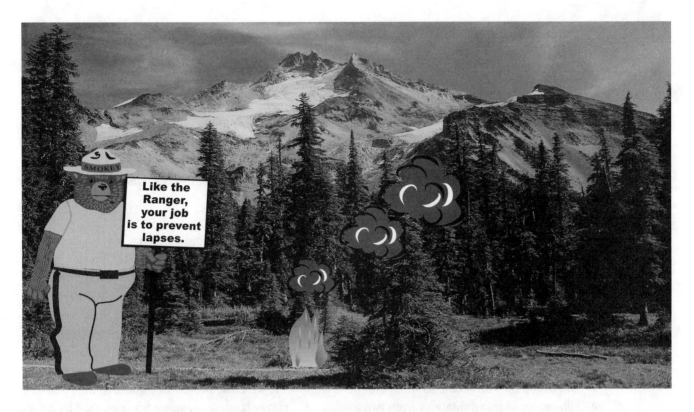

Like the Ranger, your job is to prevent lapses.

ing food to the disposal, or do whatever works for you. The alternative activities you listed in Lesson Fourteen on page 219 will be a good place to start. Don't wait; be decisive. Waiting is an excuse for letting go even more. Jump on that lapse like a dog on a bone! Remember that it is usually easier to get control if you leave the situation.

⇨ **Step 6: Ask for help.** Partners, friends, coworkers, and others can be a real source of support. You might review the material on Relationships from earlier lessons where we discussed who to ask for help, how to ask, and how to respond if help is given. If you could really use support during lapses, don't be shy about asking for help.

These six steps are easy to remember. You can even write them on a small card to keep in your wallet or purse. Using them, however, will require some effort.

Becoming a Forest Ranger

Consider yourself a forest ranger on the lookout for fires. Your job is to prevent fires and to put them out quickly if they start. Your lapses are like the fires. You will try to prevent them, but when they do flare up, extinguish them immediately. Occasionally a fire may seem out of control, but don't lose the forest!!

Let's develop this idea of the forest ranger a bit further. Your job is to take control over your eating, exercise, and weight. The ranger's job is to keep control over the forest. The ranger must do everything possible to prevent fires from breaking out. Because fires may be difficult to control once they start, the ranger believes in "an ounce of prevention . . ." Prevention is also important for you. You have learned dozens of ways to take control of your eating so that lapses will not occur. As you know, the key is to be prepared for high-risk situations, to plan in advance, and to keep the right attitude.

The forest ranger's second task is to stop the spread of fires once they do occur. The ranger's ability to do this will determine whether the forest is spared or destroyed. A lapse in your eating is like the fire that breaks out. Whether you bounce back and continue your progress, or let the mistake destroy your progress (lapse, relapse, then collapse) depends on your ability to use the techniques described here.

Please remember the dual tasks that confront both you and the forest ranger. You are concerned with both prevention and with crisis management. Identify the situations where you are most likely to confront problems. Then plan to use both your prevention techniques and the constructive methods you have learned to deal with lapses.

These are the ways to prevent lapses and to stop lapses dead in their tracks. The information here and in Lesson Fourteen, in my opinion, is crucial for long-term success. Please refer back to these lessons if you find yourself in trouble. This dual approach of preventing problems and of coping with problems when they do arise allows you to hit temptations from two angles.

Life on Chutes and Ladders

There is a well-known children's board game called "Chutes and Ladders," known formerly as "Snakes and Ladders." Many adults remember the game from their own childhood or from playing with their children. The basic idea behind the game provides a good moral to remember as we discuss lapse, relapse, and collapse.

In Chutes and Ladders, players use a spinner to advance over the 100 spaces on the board. At some points there are ladders that advance a player by many spaces. At other points, there are chutes that can send the player back many spaces. For example, a player who lands on space nine is shown cutting the lawn for his parents. For his effort, he can advance to space 31, which shows the boy going to the circus. A player landing on space 95 is greeted by a pic-

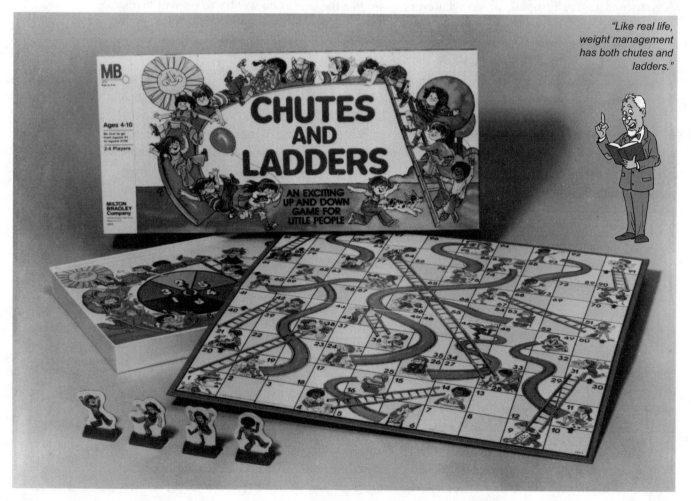

"Like real life, weight management has both chutes and ladders."

ture of a boy who hits a baseball through a window. His transgression sends him back to space 75 where he is emptying his piggy bank.

Sometimes playing Chutes and Ladders goes without a hitch. You land on the ladders and avoid the chutes. Other times the chutes seem to draw you like a magnet. However, even under the worst of circumstances, a player can reach the top of the board and win the game.

Let's say that the Milton Bradley Company made Chutes and Ladders relevant to the situations faced by individuals controlling their weight. One might advance up a ladder by eating under control at a buffet, but might slide down a chute by eating 400 peanuts during happy hour. Jogging would qualify one for a ladder and would speed the person toward the ultimate goal. Eating 15 of Cousin Clara's Cocoa Creme Balls would definitely hasten one's descent down a chute.

There are several points to remember from our hypothetical game of Chutes and Ladders. The first is that making progress up the ladders can always be interrupted by a chute. Even a program that goes smoothly for weeks can be stymied by setbacks. However, even the longest fall down a chute can be remedied by heading back up the board, hopefully with the aid of a few ladders. If you have the skills and the motivation to control eating and increase exercise, you will be poised to take advantage of the ladders and will advance more quickly.

Weight management, like life, has both chutes and ladders. Being prepared for this fact is half the battle. The other half is having the right attitude and behaviors to remain optimistic when trouble occurs and having the skills in hand to rebound from lapses.

Think now of the situations that can send you down a chute and plan some prevention strategies. Think also of the situations that can propel you up a ladder, then make them happen!

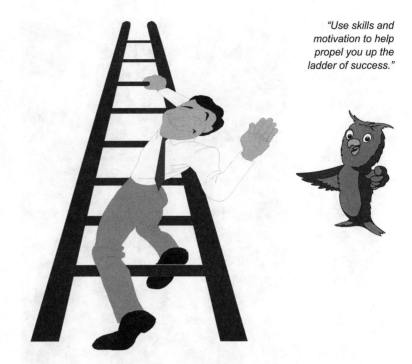

"Use skills and motivation to help propel you up the ladder of success."

When children play Chutes and Ladders, landing on a chute can be discouraging. He or she may want to quit playing because the immediate setback overwhelms the knowledge that things might get better (there might be a ladder ahead). The immediate bad feelings created by a dietary mistake can make individuals want to quit. It is crucial to remember that life has its chutes, particularly when you're working hard to control your weight. Look ahead for the ladder and, by all means, keep playing the game.

Holidays, Parties, and Special Events

Do you get stuffed more than the turkey on Thanksgiving? Do you love the salted nuts people offer at parties? Do you feel obligated to eat when a host or hostess prepares an elegant meal? There are several ways to deal with these special occasions.

Holidays, parties, and special events can be a problem because eating is encouraged. Not only does temptation abound, but everyone else is eating, the food is good, there may be social pressure to "try some of this," and it is natural to let go when celebrating. The trick is to be prepared and to avoid the anxiety that comes

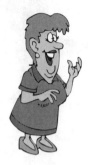

"Be prepared to deal with special events, and avoid the anxiety that comes from trying to diet and celebrate at the same time."

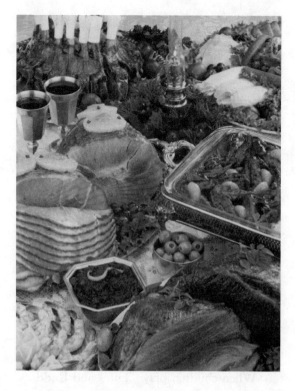

from trying to diet and celebrate at the same time.

One common mistake is for individuals on weight management programs to vow to eat nothing at the event. This is a real setup, because they either feel guilty when they eat or feel deprived when they don't. You can enjoy yourself and still watch what you eat. Here are six methods for having fun and keeping the reins on uncontrolled eating.

❶ *Plan ahead.* Think about the event before you go. Try to anticipate both the food you will face and the actions of other people. Think about your own desires to eat and the external pressures from others. Have a general idea of what you will eat. You can call ahead and ask what will be served. You can make a tentative list of what you will eat and add up the calories. How does it fit with your day's calorie goal?

❷ *Eat something before you go.* Don't go to a special event starved. Everything will look good, and you will forget that you only want to sample special foods. Have a salad, carrot sticks, cauliflower, or other low-calorie food before you go.

❸ *Eat only special foods.* Stay away from the potato chips, crackers, dip, nuts, bread and other foods that you can have any time. Use the chance to try new foods or foods you rarely have. Remember to make the best use of your calories.

❹ *Be the slowest eater.* Keep your eye on others and be the slowest eater at the event. Be the last to start and the last to finish. You will enjoy the food more and will feel satisfied with less. Pay attention to the texture, smell, and subtleties of taste. This will halt the rapid and automatic eating that brings so many calories.

❺ *Avoid alcohol.* Alcohol can make the calories in a meal really add up. Use other beverages if you're thirsty, and if you really want a drink, have just a little.

❻ *Keep a proper perspective.* If you do eat more than you intend, keep a positive attitude. Don't turn an event into more than it really is—just another day with meals and calories. In

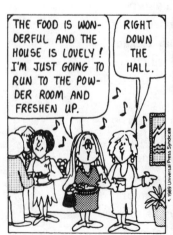

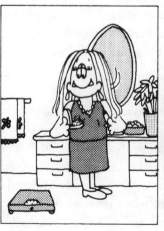

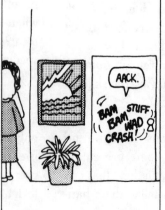

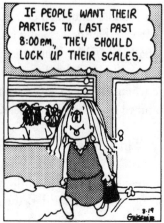

the scheme of a month or year's worth of eating, what can one day mean? One day's indiscretion should not ruin any program. There are plenty of formerly heavy people who occasionally overdo it. Their trick is to bounce back. As I stated before, your reaction to the eating is more important than the eating itself. Your attitudes are central to your ability to control your eating both during and after the event.

Why Is Nutrition So Important to Me?

Here's why. I am writing this section aboard an airplane bound from Spain to Germany. On this trip, I went from the U.S. to England, Ireland, and Spain, and then after Germany, I will arrive back in the U.S. The morning after I return, I am playing in a tennis match, and the next day I will run in a five-mile road race that is held on Father's Day in my town each year. All this requires me to be alert and fit—to have a healthy mind and a healthy body. If I eat a poor diet, even if I keep my calories low, I won't be fit.

My week-to-week existence does not involve so many activities and so much travel, and I only do the road races once in a while, but I still need to be healthy to be at my best. No matter what occupies your time, you'll be more effective if your body gets the fuel it needs. Feeling better about your body and your health helps you perform better at most everything and makes you feel better psychologically. When you climb stairs, walk somewhere, get up in the morning, or even do something as simple as get-

ting up out of a chair, you're reminded about your progress, because everything is easier. This gives you lots of opportunities to feel positive about your changes.

More on Minerals

The body contains some 60 different minerals, about 22 of which are essential for life. There are great differences in the amounts of various minerals in the body. The book *Introductory Nutrition* by Dr. Helen Guthrie, from which much of this discussion on minerals is drawn, gives two examples, cobalt and calcium. As mentioned earlier, a deficiency in cobalt (only two parts per trillion of body weight) can be more damaging than a deficiency of calcium (fully 2 percent—two parts per hundred of body weight). The essential minerals are listed in Lesson Eight on page 120.

Minerals serve to maintain the acid-base balance in the cells, to facilitate many biological reactions, to maintain water balance (sodium and potassium are the key minerals here), to form parts of essential body compounds, to regulate muscle contraction, to transmit nerve impulses, and to aid in growth of body tissue. It is important to consume sufficient amounts of minerals, but excessive amounts can be dangerous.

I will discuss three minerals of particular interest: calcium, sodium, and iron. These are the most frequently discussed minerals and have important implications for health. For a more

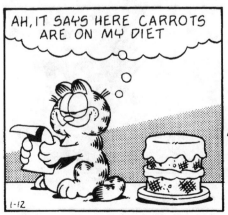
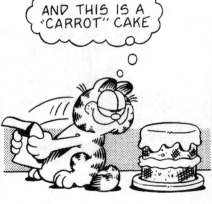
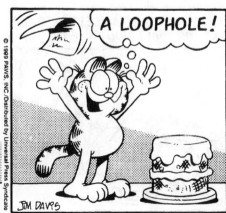

detailed discussion of these and the other minerals, refer to the book by Dr. Helen Guthrie mentioned above.

Calcium

Most people think of calcium for its role in formation of bones and teeth. It does play this role, but so do other minerals. Also, this is not the only function of calcium. Approximately 2 percent of the body is calcium, almost all of which is in teeth or bones. An infant's bones are soft and incapable of sustaining much weight. Calcium helps the bones harden, a process called calcification or ossification.

Calcium is necessary throughout life to sustain bone strength, but the amount actually needed by the body is often misunderstood. Inadequate calcium early in life makes one more susceptible to osteoporosis (a serious bone disease) in later years. However, there is dispute about how much calcium is needed. Different amounts are necessary during infancy, childhood, pregnancy, adult life, and the later years. The figures range from 540 mg/day for infants to 1200 mg/day for adults. The general RDA for calcium is 1 gram (1000 mg) per day.

Milk and milk products form the greatest supply of calcium in our diet. People who drink milk and eat milk products usually receive adequate calcium; males are more likely to do this than females. For people who avoid milk products, it is almost impossible to consume enough calcium from other foods to meet dietary standards. In addition to milk products, calcium is available in cereals, beans, some meats, poultry, fish, eggs, fruits, and vegetables.

The two conditions most commonly associated with calcium problems are kidney stones and osteoporosis. The issue of kidney stones is an easy one; there is no evidence that calcium intake is associated with the formation of stones. Osteoporosis is a different matter.

Osteoporosis is the condition of diminished bone mass. It occurs mainly in middle-aged and elderly women and can cause shortened stature, susceptibility to bone fractures, and pain in the lower back. There are multiple causes, but in many cases, calcium and sometimes fluoride supplementation can arrest this destructive process. This is a condition for a physician to monitor, so if you suspect this is an issue for you, speak with a doctor.

Sodium

Sodium is an important mineral which is present mainly in body fluids. It helps regulate fluid balance. Typical intake of sodium is between 3000 and 7000 mg per day, in the form of 7.5 to 18 grams of salt per day. A teaspoon of table salt provides 2000 mg of sodium, so to consume the three to seven grams of sodium daily means eating 1.5 to 4 teaspoons of salt. This seems like a lot, but the average person does it every day!

The suggested *safe and adequate* intake of sodium is 1100 to 3000 mg per day (½ to 1½

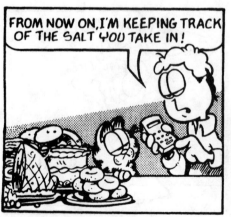
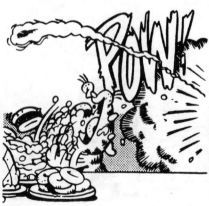
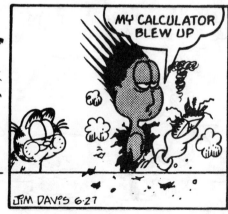

Sodium Content of Foods

Description	mg	Description	mg
Milk, Yogurt, and Cheese		**Fruits**	
Milk, 1 cup	120	Fruit, fresh, frozen, canned, ½ cup	Trace
Natural cheeses, 1½ oz	110–450	**Bread, Cereal, Rice, and Pasta**	
Processed cheeses, 2 oz	800	Bread, 1 slice	110–175
Yogurt, 8 oz	160	Cooked cereal, rice, pasta, unsalted, ½ cup	Trace
Meat, Poultry, Fish, etc.		Ready-to-eat cereal, 1 oz	100–360
Bologna, 2 oz	580	**Miscellaneous**	
Fresh meat, poultry, fish, 3 oz	Less than 90	Corn chips, salted, 1 oz	235
Ham, lean, roasted, 3 oz	1,020	Dill pickle, 1 medium	930
Tuna, canned, water pack, 3 oz	300	Salad dressing, 1T	75–220
Vegetables		Ketchup, mustard, steak sauce, 1T	130–230
Tomato juice, canned, ¾ cup	660	Peanuts, roasted in oil, salted, 1 oz	120
Vegetables, canned or frozen with sauce, ½ cup	140–460	Potato chips, salted, 1 oz	130
Vegetables, fresh, or frozen (cooked), ½ cup	Less than 70	Salt, 1t	2000
Vegetable soup, canned, 1 cup	820	Soy sauce, 1T	1030

teaspoons per day). You can see that this is far below the average intake, so over consumption of sodium is more a problem than under-consumption.

The sodium we consume comes from two sources: the salt naturally present in foods, and salt added during preparation and serving of food. Some foods, like bacon, are naturally high in sodium. Some foods have salt added in processing, as with some soups. Other foods usually have salt added after preparation (like french fries).

An example of having salt added is the case of potato chips. A potato has only 1 mg of sodium per 100 grams, while the same weight of potato chips has 340–1000 mg of sodium. The table above shows the sodium content of some common foods. The table was adapted from the *Home and Garden Bulletin, Number 252.*

Sodium has been implicated in hypertension. This is the reason that individuals with high blood pressure are often prescribed a low-sodium diet. Research has recently shown that increased potassium can lower blood pressure, so a combination of sodium restriction and potassium supplementation may be beneficial for blood pressure control.

Sodium intake can be reduced to about 3500 mg per day by limiting the use of table salt and by avoiding foods high in salt. To reduce the level further, to the 2000 mg or so recommended for blood pressure control, a strict diet of foods naturally low in sodium is necessary. This means eating very little of foods like canned soups, broth, canned vegetables, olives, cured foods, pickles, and salted foods like potato chips and crackers.

Iron

Compared to calcium and sodium, iron exists in rather small amounts in the body. It is still essential. Iron is found mainly in the blood, but some iron is present in every cell. Its primary function is to facilitate the transfer of oxygen and carbon dioxide among body tissues.

The need for iron varies according to age and sex. For instance, an adult man needs 0.9 to 1.2 mg of iron per day. Adult women require almost twice as much (1.4–2.2 mg/day), and adolescent girls need even more (1.9–3.7 mg/day). Liver is the only food that provides appreciable iron, so adding iron to the diet is often necessary. Much of this is done with food products that are fortified or enriched. Some 30 states require that flour be enriched, so additional iron is available in bread products.

Iron deficiency is not common, but can be serious when it does occur. It can result in anemia, which is a deficiency in the number or quality of red blood cells. Iron supplementation can usually remedy this problem.

Most people receive adequate iron in the diet and do not need supplements to prevent pseudo ailments like *iron-poor blood*. People who suspect an iron problem should consult a physician or dietitian.

What does all this information on minerals mean? As with vitamins, most people receive adequate minerals if they eat a carefully chosen, balanced diet. However, there are special groups of people who require mineral supplements. Examples are needs for calcium in elderly women and iron in teenage girls. It is best to get specific advice from someone trained in nutrition.

A Note about Breakfast

I mentioned in an earlier lesson that many overweight people skip breakfast. This happens because they may not feel hungry in the morning, they are in a hurry, or they feel that skipping breakfast is a good way to start off the day by saving calories. Most people who successfully lose weight resume eating breakfast as they lose weight. This prevents the situation where you find yourself famished later in the day.

Eating breakfast is consistent with the prevailing wisdom among health experts. There are some recent research findings that further support this view. Researchers at the University of Minnesota gave subjects one of five cereals varying in fiber content, plus milk and orange juice, for breakfast at 7:30 a.m. At 11:00 a.m., the subjects were given a buffet lunch, and the amount eaten was carefully recorded. The subjects who had the high-fiber cereals ate fewer calories at lunch than did the people eating the low-fiber cereals. Especially important is that the people eating the high-fiber cereals ate fewer total calories (combining breakfast and lunch) than the subjects with the low-fiber cereals.

Starting the day with breakfast, especially a breakfast high in fiber, may help control calorie intake the rest of the day. In the research study I just described, subjects who ate the high-fiber cereals ate less at lunch even when they felt just as hungry as subjects having the other cereals. So, beginning the day with breakfast will probably help you control your weight. The guide to breakfast cereals in Lesson Twelve on page 193 will give you some guidance about the calorie and fiber content of various cereals. In addition to helping you eat less, the fiber may have positive health consequences.

Indeed, breakfast could be the foundation to developing overall healthy eating habits. This is especially true for children, since many habits learned as children carry over into adulthood. There are many creative ways to make

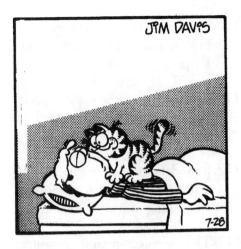
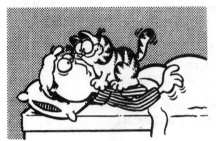
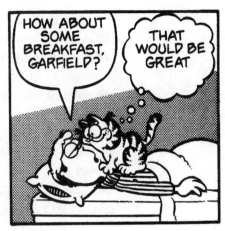

breakfast fun, fast, and easy; it just takes a little planning and dedication. If you are a breakfast-skipper, the breakfast tips that follow may help you incorporate breakfast as an important part of your day. If you are still not convinced, try it for a couple of weeks. The benefits may surprise you.

⇨ **No time?** Try getting up a few minutes earlier—10 minutes will do fine; once you are up and going, you will not miss the time. This is plenty of time to have a glass of juice, a bowl of cereal, and some fruit.

⇨ **Still no time?** Plan breakfast around foods that are ready to eat or take little time to prepare. Examples include canned or fresh fruit, juices, milk, instant-breakfast mixes, ready-to-eat cold cereals, yogurt, cheese, bagels, or toast.

⇨ **Take it to go**. If you still find yourself short on time, pack yourself a breakfast-to-go the night before and eat it the following morning when you have a few extra minutes. Try celery stuffed with cheese, fresh or dried fruits, packaged juice or milk, breakfast bars, a bagel, or English muffin.

⇨ **Be creative**. Top cereals with fresh fruit; add jelly or jam to toast, biscuits, or rolls; and add chopped nuts to hot cereals.

⇨ **Not hungry?** Drink some juice, and take something with you for a snack later in the morning. Bread or crackers will do fine. You may wish to add some cheese or fruit. Then drink some milk or water.

⇨ **Plan your breakfast the night before**. Make as much advanced preparation as possible. This way you are not confronted with the decision of what to prepare, and much of your meal can be ready and waiting for you when you wake up.

⇨ **Start a breakfast partnership**. Enjoy the company of your spouse, a child, or a friend. Take turns making healthy breakfast choices. You also can take turns preparing breakfast with a breakfast partner.

I cannot overstate the importance of a good breakfast. If you are a breakfast skipper, think of ways to overcome this behavior.

My Personal Goals for This Week

The main priority for this lesson is to use the six steps to deal with lapses. It is easy to remember the steps if you write them down on a card and keep them handy, perhaps in your wallet or purse. This way you will be prepared, so if trouble comes your way, you can whip out the card, and put the breaks on any temptations. Also, set a goal of being like the forest ranger and keep a look out for small problem areas. Snuff these out before they consume your weight management program.

Plan ahead for holidays, parties, and special events. When you see a special event on the horizon, whip out this manual and make your plans ahead of time. This will help you keep your weight management program on track. Keep your focus on good nutrition and be aware of the minerals in your diet. Remember to record your weight change on the Weight change Record in Lesson Nine on page 154.

My Self-Assessment

Lesson Fifteen

T (F) 107. Certain techniques are essential for all individuals controlling their weight.

(T) (F) 108. Getting nervous or anxious during a lapse is helpful because anxiety interferes with appetite and allows you to remove yourself from temptation.

(T) F 109. When dealing with a lapse, it is best to move quickly and decisively before control erodes even further.

T (F) 110. The best way to prevent relapse is to make sure that you *never* fall into a lapse.

(T) F 111. Controlling your eating at a special event is easier if you eat something before you go.

T (F) 112. Iron deficiency is common, and many people need to supplement their eating with additional iron.

(T) F 113. The average person consumes more than twice the safe and adequate intake of salt (sodium) each day.

(T) F 114. Calcium is necessary throughout life to sustain bone strength.

(Answers in Appendix C, page 271)

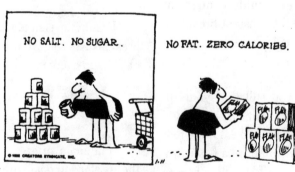

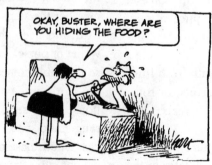

Monitoring Form—Lesson Fifteen   *Today's Date:*_____

TIME	FOOD AND AMOUNT	CALORIES
TOTAL DAILY CALORIES		

PERSONAL GOALS FOR THIS WEEK	MOST OF THE TIME	SOME-TIMES	RARELY
1.			
2. USE THE SIX STEPS TO COPE WITH LAPSES			
3. PLAN AHEAD FOR SPECIAL EVENTS			
4. BE A FOREST RANGER			
5. EAT LESS THAN _____ CALORIES PER DAY			
6. EAT LESS THAN _____ GRAMS OF FAT EACH DAY			

FOOD GROUPS FOR TODAY	PHYSICAL ACTIVITY	MINUTES OR STEPS
MILK, YOGURT, AND CHEESE ❑ ❑ ❑	(M)	
MEAT, POULTRY, ETC. ❑ ❑ ❑	(Tu)	
FRUITS ❑ ❑ ❑ ❑	(W)	
VEGETABLES ❑ ❑ ❑ ❑ ❑	(Th)	
BREADS, CEREALS, ETC. ❑ ❑ ❑ ❑ ❑ ❑ ❑ ❑	(F)	
SERVINGS OF WATER (8 OZ) ❑ ❑ ❑ ❑ ❑ ❑ ❑ ❑	(Sa)	
	(Su)	

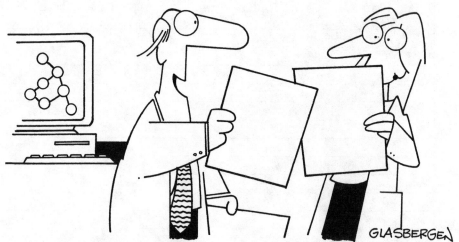

"Our new synthetic fat substitute is made
entirely from wool. With our product,
dieters will shrink when they get wet!"

Here we are now with only two lessons remaining in The LEARN Program, this one and the graduation (Commencement) Lesson. Important topics are yet to be covered. In this lesson, I will discuss material in the lifestyle and nutrition areas. Also, I will introduce a lifestyle factor of major importance, the Master Monitoring Form. Let's forge ahead!

The Master Monitoring Form

There has been a Food Diary or Monitoring Form for each lesson in this program. You have recorded food intake and changes in the five LEARN areas (Lifestyle, Exercise, Attitudes, Relationships, and Nutrition). This sets the stage for the Master Monitoring Form.

The Master Monitoring Form is similar to the forms you have seen throughout the program. It is unusual, in that it has blank spaces where techniques have been listed in other lessons. The aim is for you to list the techniques that best suit *your* needs. The new form is on page 250 of this lesson.

Keeping records is usually rated as one of the most important aspects of the program. Many clients continue to keep the records for years. Whether you do this or not depends on how long it takes for your new habits to become permanent. I strongly recommend that you complete the records, in some form, for at least

eight more weeks. If you have stopped keeping the forms, you might start again to see if the process is still helpful.

The Master Monitoring Form contains the same standard sections for recording eating and physical activity (on the left side and the bottom right side, respectively). The top right part, where the techniques to help you achieve your personal goals have been listed, is blank. You can complete this part of the form with the techniques you consider most important in achieving your personal goals.

I cannot predict what these techniques will be. For one person it will be to eat slowly, for another it will be to end dichotomous thinking, for another to do aerobic exercise at least four times a week, and for another to keep food out of sight.

These are only examples of the large list of techniques you have learned. Think back over

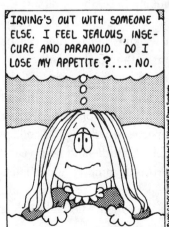
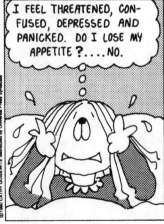
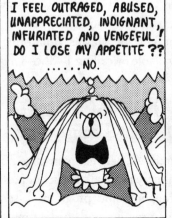
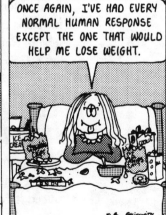

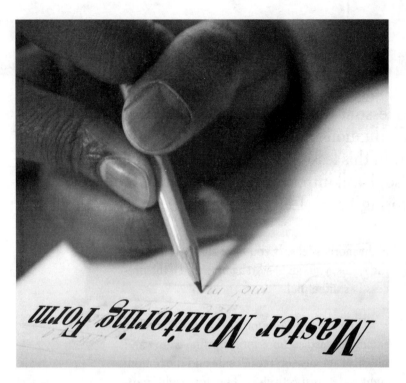

Master Monitoring Form

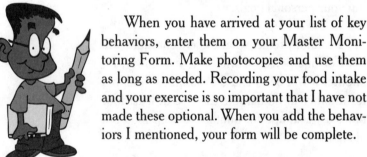

your experiences and decide which techniques are necessary for you. The Master List of Techniques (Appendix A, page 261) described below will be helpful for this task.

When you have arrived at your list of key behaviors, enter them on your Master Monitoring Form. Make photocopies and use them as long as needed. Recording your food intake and your exercise is so important that I have not made these optional. When you add the behaviors I mentioned, your form will be complete.

You are beginning with the Master Monitoring Form in this lesson, so I have the opportunity to discuss your experience with it in the final lesson. Try to start right away, so you will have this experience under your belt for the last lesson. Pocket-sized Master Monitoring Forms are also available by calling 1–888–LEARN–41.

Using the Master List of Techniques

Appendix A, beginning on page 261, contains a summary list of all the techniques I introduced throughout the program. Use this to review your progress and to determine which

techniques were most important to you. Some techniques almost certainly did not apply. If you do no food shopping, the techniques in this area were not relevant. Focus on those most pertinent for you. They may be the techniques you struggled with most, which is one sign that the habits they targeted are difficult to change.

Go through the list in Appendix A and circle the techniques that are most important in your attempts to lose weight. These are not necessarily the behaviors that are easiest for you. They should be the ones that are the keys to your future success. Circle any behavior you feel fits this bill. Think back carefully over your experience with earlier parts of the program and consider programs you have been on in the past. Circle the behaviors that help you control your eating and increase your exercise.

Now that you have circled the important behaviors, it is time to narrow the list. You should end up with 5–10 behaviors that will be the final entries for your Master Monitoring Form. Having too few techniques can make you miss opportunities to change your habits and having too many makes record keeping too complex. It is fine to modify the list as your habits change, but for now, this list should be your marching orders to yourself.

The National Walking Movement

People are walking here, there, almost everywhere. The movement has been bolstered by the discovery that walking can be fun, can be done in the most interesting places, and can be done with a group of similar-minded people. Also, knowledge about the health benefits of walking is increasing. Dr. Ralph Paffenbarger of Stanford University studied 17,000 college alumni as they reached middle and later years. Men who walked briskly nine or more miles each week had 21 percent lower risk of death from heart disease than men who walked less than three miles each week.

The popularity of walking has led Americans to do what they do best, organize. There are walking clubs, walking trails, walking magazines, special walking shoes, and even a clearinghouse for information on walking. Information on these aspects of walking can be a real resource for the person losing or managing their weight. It can help insure that walking is done correctly and that the experience can turn from drudgery to an enriching experience, both socially and physically.

Walking clubs and informal groups have blossomed all over the country. An example is the American Volkssport Association. This group organizes walking events such as a volkswalk, a 6- or 12-mile non-timed walk, where the object is to meet people while enjoying exercise. Another example is Walkabout International, a group that began as a small walking club in San Diego and now publishes a schedule listing more than 90 walks each month. Chapters have now formed in different cities. To find resources in your area, the information in the table below may be helpful. Also, check the weekend section of your newspaper for walking events, which may direct you to local clubs. Finally, many road race events have fun walks attached to them.

"Walking can be fun, can be done in the most interesting places, and can be done with a group of similar-minded people."

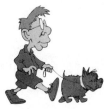

Resources for Walkers

American Volkssport Association
1001 Pat Booker Road, Suite 101
Universal City, Texas 78148
(800) 830–WALK
www.ava.org

Can send you a list of walking clubs in your area. An annual membership ($20 per individual and $25 for families) includes a subscription to *American Wanderer*.

Prevention Walking Club
Rodale Press
33 East Minor
Emmaus, PA 18098
(800) 666-1216
www.healthyideas.com/walking/pvn.walkclub.html

Included as a separate section in *Prevention Magazine* dealing with all aspects of walking. Annual subscription $19.95 plus $1.97 delivery charge.

Walkabout International
835 Fifth Avenue, Room 407
San Diego, CA 92101
(619) 231–7463
www.geocities.com/paris/bristo/2154/walk.htm

Club with chapters in various cities. Organizes and publishes information about walks.

Walking Magazine
P.O. Box 5073
Harlan, IA 51593
(800) 829–5585
www.walkingmagazine.com

Bimonthly commercial magazine about walking. $11.95 per year for subscription.

Walking Handbook
The Cooper Institute for Aerobics Research
12330 Preston Road
Dallas, Texas 75230
(800) 635–7050

Forty-page handbook on all aspects of walking. $7.95 per copy (plus postage).

Revisiting Your Eating and Activity Habits

TAPE 4
SECTION 7

Have you been keeping records of your food intake and physical activity? If so, here's your chance to study your behavior again.

Carefully review your Monitoring Form for the past week and identify your approximate daily calorie intake, your typical times of eating, and any situations that gave you trouble. As I discussed in Lesson Fourteen on page 217, your Monitoring Form is the key to identifying high-risk situations and learning how to prevent them. In addition, be sure to identify situations that you handled well. For example, you may have found new ways to eat out at your favorite restaurant without exceeding your calorie budget. Celebrate these successes. You deserve much credit for them. You also can review your Monitoring Form to determine the composition of your diet in terms of the amounts of carbohydrate, protein, and fat you have eaten.

"Record keeping can be a key in weight control."

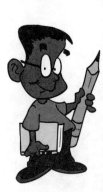

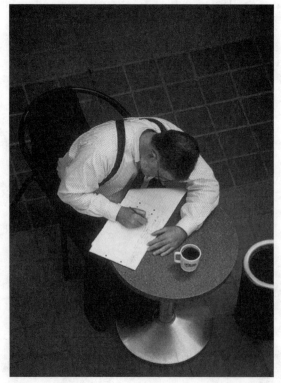

Physical Activity

I hope you are continuing to enjoy your daily activity program. By now, your walking program should feel as familiar to you as your favorite old coat. Hopefully, you have experimented with programmed activity and have found activities that you enjoy doing on a regular basis. Review your Monitoring forms to see how many times you walked or participated in other activities during the past month. You'll probably be amazed at how much you are doing compared to before the program. If you have not been as active as you had planned, what stopped you? Often, it's as simple as getting out of the habit, as a result of a vacation, business travel, or illness. Resolve today to pick up where you left off. Stop feeling guilty and worrying about the fact that you haven't exercised. That's a waste of time and energy. Exercise today, even if only for five minutes. The first step is the hardest. After that, you'll be burning up the sidewalk again!

To Record or Not to Record

You may not be keeping daily records of your food intake or physical activity at this point in the program. This is your decision. Some people find that they are very successful without recording daily; they continue to eat a low-fat diet and walk daily. They occasionally keep a three-day diary to get a snapshot of their eating and activity habits or keep records during the holidays, when everyone struggles to maintain a healthy lifestyle. I think this approach can work. So, if you're happy with your progress and are not keeping daily diaries, the diet police are not going to arrest you! Relax!

I do, however, think that it is important to keep records when you have trouble with your eating and exercise. Your Monitoring Form will serve as a compass or road map by which to get your bearings. In such situations, the sooner you start recording, the sooner you will feel better about your behavior and yourself. Of course, the paradox here is that the times you'll benefit most from keeping a diary (when you're having trouble) are the times you'll least want to. Try it and see if keeping a diary doesn't help relieve "upset" feelings after overeating, gaining a pound, or missing several days of exercise.

A Challenge

If you have not been diligent in keeping your Monitoring Form lately, consider making a strong commitment to yourself to do so over the next week and review it carefully. At the end of the week, ask yourself these questions:

❶ Is my daily calorie intake where it should be?

❷ Is my diet balanced—am I eating the appropriate number of servings from the five food groups of the Food Guide Pyramid?

❸ Is my daily intake of fat less than 30 percent of my total calorie intake?

❹ Are there patterns that may lead me to eat inappropriately?

❺ Are my thoughts about my weight management and health positive?

❻ Am I getting at least 30 minutes of physical activity on most days?

❼ Is there room to increase my physical activity?

❽ Are there other activities I can do to help increase my activity or make it more enjoyable?

Weight Loss

Let's review your Weight Change Record on page 154 of Lesson Nine. Have you been recording you weight changes for weeks 9–16? The first thing you are likely to notice is that your rate of weight loss has slowed substantially since the early part of the program. You may have continued to lose a small amount of weight, or you may have hit a plateau. You may be wondering how I know this. It's because weight loss always slows dramatically after the first three to four months, regardless of the treat-

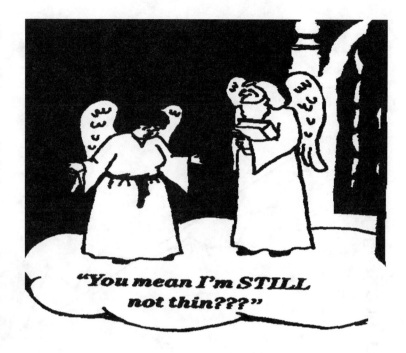

"You mean I'm STILL not thin???"

ment approach used. A slower weight loss after the first three to four months appears to be one of the first laws of nature!

The second law of nature is that this slow-down can be frustrating and perplexing! You may feel that you are working just as hard today as you did the first day of the program. It doesn't seem fair that your efforts are not rewarded accordingly. And, it's not fair.

What can you do about this slower rate of weight loss? Three things:

❶ Understand it

❷ Focus on your accomplishments

❸ Keep up your efforts

Understand it

Your weight loss has slowed, in part, because you are now a smaller person and require fewer calories to maintain basic bodily functions such as your heart rate, breathing, temperature of 98.6 degrees, and so on. These basic functions comprise your resting metabolic rate, which we discussed in Lesson Two on page 34 in the section on "The Benefits of Exercise." As you lose weight, your resting metabolic rate decreases. Smaller bodies generally require

My Weight Change Record

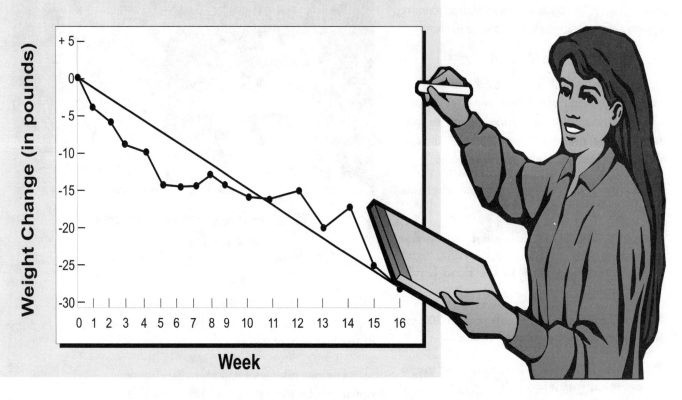

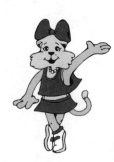

fewer calories than larger ones, just as small cars usually burn less gas than big ones.

Let's say that before the program, your body burned 2000 calories a day. If you consumed 1500 calories a day, you would have a deficit of 500 calories a day or 3500 calories a week (7 x 500 = 3500). Because a pound of fat contains approximately 3500 calories, you would lose about 1 pound a week. Now, after five months, let's say that your body burns only 1750 calories a day because you are a smaller person. If you eat the same 1500-calorie-a-day diet that you did at the start of the program, you will now have a deficit of only 250 calories a day or 1750 a week (250 x 7 = 1750). Do the math and you'll see that you should lose a half pound a week now, rather than a pound.

Your body has a number of other intricate mechanisms that slow the rate of weight loss. These were originally designed to protect us from starvation, a constant threat to our survival until the modern era. Now these same biologi-

cal mechanisms, combined with our more sedentary lifestyle and abundance of food, appear to limit weight loss in some people to about 10 to 15 percent of initial weight.

Focus on Your Accomplishments

This is where I hope that you can change the focus of your efforts from trying to subdue a body (that may be defended like Fort Knox) to recognizing and enjoying all that you have accomplished. Again, see how your quality of life, health, and fitness have improved. Look at all the things that you can do now that you could not five months ago. These are the true measures of success, not some arbitrary number on your bathroom scale or looking like the anorectic teenager who adorns the covers of fashion magazines. If your preoccupation with reaching some "fantasy figure" is preventing you from enjoying and feeling proud of your weight loss, I encourage you to reread the section on body image in Lesson Seven on page 110. Remember, people come in all shapes and sizes; one size does not fit all.

Your ability to celebrate the weight loss that you have achieved is a sign of your self-esteem and self-worth. It is an indication that you know what is truly important—that you have a healthier, fitter, and more active body. Fashions come and go, whether it's skirt lengths, tie widths, or body shapes themselves (remember Twiggy?). Isn't it nice to know that you have taken care of the most important thing—your health and well-being?

The alternative is to remain fixed on reaching a weight that defies your hard work and sincere efforts. A classic recipe for frustration is thinking "If I only work hard enough, I can weigh whatever I want." Unfortunately, your body has not agreed to this deal, any more than it has agreed that you can increase your height by three inches through hard work.

Keep up Your Effort

Focusing on what you have achieved, rather than on what you have not, will keep your spirits and motivation high. Feeling proud that you reached your initial weight loss goal of 10 percent will propel you forward to continue your healthy eating and activity habits. These new habits will help you maintain your improved health.

Does this mean that you will never lose more weight? No, not at all. Many of my clients have gone on to lose more after reducing by approximately 10 percent during the first four to six months and then remaining weight-stable for a while. But I cannot predict whether or when you will lose more, but I hope you enjoy the weight loss you have already achieved. Perhaps the best course is to continue to practice your new eating and activity habits to maintain your improved health and fitness. Over the long term, your body will settle on the appropriate weight.

Quality of Life Self-Assessment

Now we come to the point in the program when it's time to review your quality of life. Use the form on page 248 to check your quality of life. This is the same form you completed on previous occasions. Compare your scores now to those from the survey you completed at the beginning of the program on page 9.

What areas of your life are you most satisfied with now? I would be surprised if you do not have more energy, a more positive mood, greater mobility, and fewer health complications. Think about how remarkable this is. In just four months, you have achieved some impressive benefits. Compare your current responses to those before the program. This comparison will remind you just how much you have changed. Sometimes people lose sight of their accomplishments. I won't let you forget yours!

For those areas in which you are not more satisfied, what can you do to improve things? I suggest that you identify one area and start there. For instance, if you are not satisfied with your leisure and recreational activities, identify a concrete goal that you would like to achieve. It should be something specific such as reading for 30 minutes a day, going for a bike ride with friends on the weekend, or decorating the downstairs bathroom. Make a specific plan concerning what you will do, when, and with whom. That's the best way to get new behaviors going. Use the worksheet on page 249 titled Quality of Life Improvement Worksheet to help you identify specific areas and develop a specific plan of action.

My Salute to You!

If you have been following the LEARN lessons as they were designed, it should now be about four months (or 16 weeks) since you started the program. Let's place this in context. Some people start diets and give up the same day. Others last a few days, perhaps a few weeks, or on rare occasions, a few months. Why?

Many programs are fads, and people find quickly that they are impossible to follow or simply don't work. And let's face it—sticking to

Quality of Life Self-Assessment

Please use the following scale to rate how satisfied you feel now about different aspects of your daily life. Choose any number from this list (1 to 9) and indicate your choice on the questions below.

1 = Extremely Dissatisfied   6 = Somewhat Satisfied

2 = Very Dissatisfied   7 = Moderately Satisfied

3 = Moderately Dissatisfied   8 = Very Satisfied

4 = Somewhat Dissatisfied   9 = Extremely Satisfied

5 = Neutral

1._____ Mood (feelings of sadness, worry, happiness, etc.)

2._____ Self-esteem

3._____ Confidence, self-assurance, and comfort in social situations

4._____ Energy and feeling healthy

5._____ Health problems (diabetes, high blood pressure, etc.)

6._____ General appearance

7._____ Social life

8._____ Leisure and recreational activities

9._____ Physical mobility and physical activity

10._____ Eating habits

11._____ Body image

12._____ Overall quality of life

any program for a long time is difficult. A person in for the long haul encounters many challenges, will feel deprived, will think "it's not fair when other people can eat all they want," and may get frustrated by slow progress. Hence, many people get off the train before it has reached its final destination.

I salute you for staying with the program! It is a REALLY good sign that you have been able to think of your weight management plan as something that requires persistence and flexibility over the long term. It would be nice if there were some easy solution, but when all is said and done, it comes down to personal effort. I am delighted that you have made the effort and hope that the rewards have been and will continue to be substantial. If I could be there with you right now, I'd be giving you a standing ovation!

Rate Your Diet

I promised you at the beginning of the program that I would have you rate your diet three times during the program. It's now time to rate your diet for the third time.

Turn to the Rate Your Diet Quiz—Lesson Sixteen on page 291 in Appendix E. Complete this quiz now, before continuing on. Compare your score on page 294 for this lesson with the total scores on pages 290 (for Lesson Eight) and 286 (Lesson Two). How do your scores compare? Has your diet improved? If so, congratulations! If not, try to decide what has held you back and make corrections.

Quality of Life Improvement Worksheet

Area to Improve	How to Improve	When to Improve
1. _____	_____	_____
2. _____	_____	_____
3. _____	_____	_____
4. _____	_____	_____
5. _____	_____	_____
6. _____	_____	_____

My Personal Goals for This Week

Now is the time to begin keeping the Master Monitoring form. Select the techniques important to you from the Master List of Techniques (Appendix A) and enter them on the form. I will discuss this in the Commencement Lesson, at which time you can develop a permanent version of the Master Monitoring Form.

You have now had four months of experience with setting personal goals. Therefore, you may wish to list goals on the Master Monitoring form that are not listed in Appendix A. This is perfectly fine. It is not important that techniques you employ come from me–just that they work for you. You know best what works for you, and these are what you should enter on the form.

My Self-Assessment

Lesson Sixteen

T (F) 115. Keeping records like the Master Monitoring Form is not of much use after this program.

(T) F 116. Monitoring forms are the key to identifying high-risk situations and learning how to prevent them.

(T) F 117. When weight loss slows, focusing on your accomplishments can help keep you motivated by showing you just how much progress you have made.

(Answers in appendix C, page 271)

Master Monitoring Form

Today's Date: _____

TIME	FOOD AND AMOUNT	CALORIES

TOTAL DAILY CALORIES

PERSONAL GOALS FOR THIS WEEK	MOST OF THE TIME	SOME-TIMES	RARELY
1.			
2.			
3.			
4.			
5. EAT LESS THAN _____ CALORIES PER DAY			
6. EAT LESS THAN _____ GRAMS OF FAT EACH DAY			

FOOD GROUPS FOR TODAY	PHYSICAL ACTIVITY	MINUTES OR STEPS
MILK, YOGURT, AND CHEESE ☐ ☐ ☐	(M)	
MEAT, POULTRY, ETC. ☐ ☐ ☐	(Tu)	
FRUITS ☐ ☐ ☐ ☐	(W)	
VEGETABLES ☐ ☐ ☐ ☐ ☐	(Th)	
BREADS, CEREALS, ETC. ☐ ☐ ☐ ☐ ☐ ☐ ☐ ☐	(F)	
SERVINGS OF WATER (8 OZ) ☐ ☐ ☐ ☐ ☐ ☐ ☐ ☐	(Sa)	
	(Su)	

Here we are, the final lesson of The LEARN Program. I hope you have enjoyed your voyage and have acquired the knowledge and skills to use for permanent weight management. In this lesson, I will discuss a few final steps, but will also look ahead to the future. Let's finish with a flurry of excitement!

Interpreting Your Progress

TAPE 3
SECTION 2

At this stage in the program, individuals have had different experiences and weight losses. Some have done well and attained their goal, and others still have weight to lose. There are those who struggled at times and succeeded at others, and are now on their way to a positive outcome. Others struggled throughout and lost no weight at all. Let's reflect on your progress and use it to forge a picture of the future.

Making the transition from the structure of the program to *free living* can be tricky for some people. If you are fearful of this transition or have had difficulty in the past when ending a program, some work in the "A" (Attitudes) part of the LEARN model might help.

Some people who complete programs have an unfortunate way of not taking credit when credit is due. When they do well on a program they attribute their success to the program, but if they flounder, they blame themselves. I hear people say, "Weight Watchers really helped me lose weight" and later say, "The Weight Watchers program was good, I just couldn't stick with it." This attitude can eventually wear away a person's confidence.

I prefer a different attitude. If you do well on a program, the credit is yours. The program only provides ideas and techniques, but you have the responsibility for implementing them. It is similar to using tools to build a house. Having the right tools can help, but someone has to make the effort to put it all together. Giving the program credit for weight loss is like giving the hammer credit for building the house. When we hear a virtuoso perform a masterpiece on the piano, do we give the piano credit? Whatever you have achieved is yours to boast about. You de-

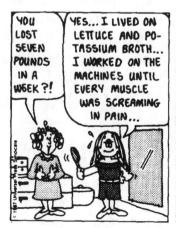

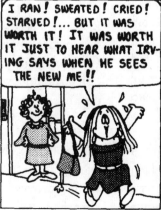

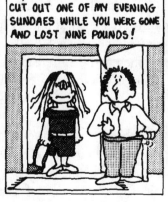

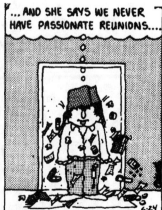

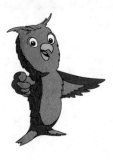

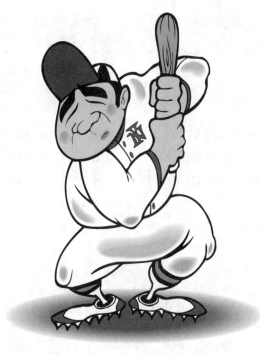

serve to feel good and to remember that your efforts were at work. What does this mean?

If you have been responsible for making progress, the progress can continue. If the program has been responsible, it would be natural for you to fall apart. This is not the case, obviously, but beware of the tendency to give the program credit when the credit is yours.

In the past several paragraphs, I have spoken about the program *ending*. Do you notice the contradiction in this idea and the basic concepts of The LEARN Program? A primary thrust of your effort has been to learn new behaviors and habits that can become permanent. In this sense, the program does not end. The key issue is whether you can take away changes that you will live with. If so, you have accomplished part of your mission. If not, try to identify the lessons in the manual that can best facilitate this notion and then reread the material. The sections on Attitudes are a good place to start.

If you have achieved less than you expected, what can you conclude? Again, the natural tendency is to despair and blame yourself. I do not feel this is fair. Over the course of a lifetime,

overweight individuals go through periods of being very motivated and having the strength to try a program, to periods where nothing seems to work and starting a program is a series of false starts.

There are peaks of success and valleys of disappointment, with lots of terrain in-between. Individuals begin programs at many points in these stages. The ones who do best, of course, are those at the peaks. Those in the valleys have trouble. Others fall somewhere in the middle.

For a person who has not done well, I recommend two approaches. The first is to consider waiting until a peak comes along and then try again. The right timing can be important. The second is to consider trying a different program. This program is not right for everyone, so if something else meets your needs, by all means, try it.

Losing weight is like being a batter on a baseball team. You need not hit a home run on every pitch. Even if you strike out, you will have other chances at bat; even if you go hitless in one game, there will be other games. You just want to avoid a prolonged slump! So, keep a positive attitude and keep trying.

Remember a Reasonable Weight?

TAPE 1
SECTION 6

In the very beginning of this program, I discussed the concept of "reasonable weight." Most people begin programs with expectations of what they will weigh that are based on arbitrary and unrealistic beauty ideals or even on landmarks in their lives (when they got married, finished school, etc.). What should be viewed as terrific progress gets dismissed.

Let me tell you a story about Susan. She began a program at 185 pounds saying she wanted to be 125. Susan weighed 125 when she got married, but she began gaining weight after she had children and had been no less than

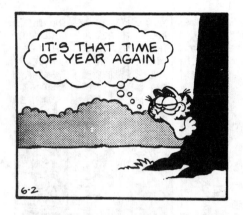

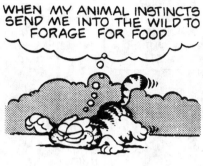

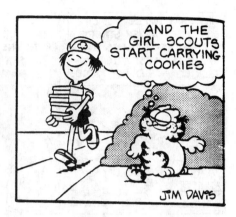

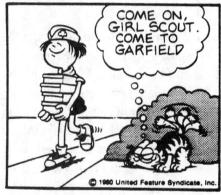

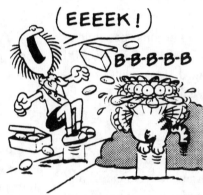

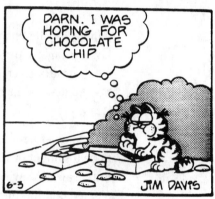

150 most of her adult life. In the 52 weeks on the program, Susan lost 25 pounds and weighed 160. Instead of celebrating the 25 pounds she lost, she focused on the remaining weight. How reasonable is it for her to think that 125 is the only acceptable weight?

You may have lost as much weight as you set out to lose, but if not, which is the case with many people, it is important to view what you have done in a positive context. There is no reason to expect perfection—we do not expect the perfect job, the perfect hair, the perfect eyes, the perfect nose—the perfect life. Why, then, are we only satisfied with total weight loss? The answer is that society teaches us that weight is under total control of the individual, and we have ideals that are highly unrealistic. It would be like saying there is only one acceptable eye color and that people with other colors were imperfect and weren't trying hard enough to change their eye color.

You may be one of the many people who would like to weigh much less but will not or cannot. The choice, then, is whether to wage a wholesale assault on your self-esteem by feeling there is something wrong or to accept what is reasonable and feel good about progress you are able to make. You know which path I favor.

A great deal of research has been done on goal setting. It won't surprise you to hear that people get frustrated, disappointed, and even depressed when they do not reach their goals. Goals, therefore, have to be challenging, but not impossible to reach. By setting realistic goals and rewarding yourself for reaching them, your self-esteem will increase and you will be in a much better position to sustain changes you make.

Making Your Habits Permanent

There are several keys to developing permanent habits. *Practice* is one such key. The lessons in this program may not provide enough time for all your habits to change. Eating habits develop over years and years, so you must be

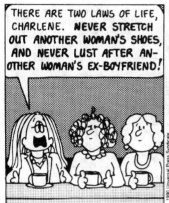
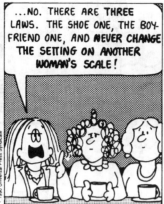
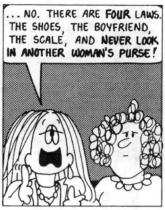
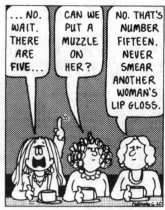

patient for the changes to become permanent. By the time a person is 40, at least 40,000 meals have been consumed. This is lots of practice, so new habits may take time.

Another key is awareness. Try to continue to be a student of your eating and exercise habits. Be aware of what stimulates your eating and of methods for turning the tide. The Master Monitoring Form is designed with this in mind.

Examining Your Master Monitoring Form

I introduced the Master Monitoring Form in the last lesson to give you some experience with it. How did it work for you? This seemingly simple step of getting the form in good order can be quite important. It can help you define which techniques are important for you and provide feedback on how you are doing. Let's review the procedures for making the form work to your advantage.

As I mentioned in Lesson Sixteen, many clients generally list record keeping as one of the most important aspects of the program. You may remember from the early lessons that record keeping has several virtues. It reminds you of the techniques that can help you lose weight and can give you positive feedback about changes you make. It also can help control eating because there is always some accountability when the record is filled out every day.

You can add or delete techniques from the form you completed in Lesson Sixteen. The Master List of Techniques (Appendix A) shows all the techniques used in the program. Pick the ones most likely to help. This is a good time to refer back to the Behavior Chain you completed in Lesson Thirteen on page 206. This showed how trouble can be avoided by interrupting the eating chain at various places. This may give you clues for techniques to add to the Master Monitoring Form.

Don't hesitate to change the Master Monitoring Form in the weeks ahead. A blank form is provided in this lesson. Make as many copies as you need. I recommended in the last lesson that you continue to complete this form for at least eight more weeks. Do it well beyond this point if it will help. I know some people who have kept forms like this for more than 10 years.

Where to Go from Here

TAPE 4
SECTION 9

There are a number of options you might consider for losing more weight, for maintaining what you have lost, or for getting back on the right path if you falter. These are just suggestions—you might have better ideas of your own.

The key is to have a plan, to know what path you will follow, and to know when the plan should be put into action. Here are some of the things to consider.

Use The LEARN Program Again

You might start at the beginning and follow the program through as if you were doing it for the first time. Many people do this. It is not a sign that they failed the first time around. Rather, it shows they know what works for them, and they know when to go back to it. An alternative to starting at the beginning is to use sections in the manual that are most pertinent to you at the time. For example, if holidays are throwing you for a loop, you could pay attention to the sections dealing with this topic.

You may want to pay special attention to the goals you set at the end of each lesson (in the Setting Personal Goals section). The aim of this section was to encourage you to find goals that were particularly important for you. Chances are these goals are still important. Focusing on them is a good way to keep your program moving along as you wish.

Enlist Social Support

If you find your motivation flagging, enlisting a friend or a support partner might be just the thing you need. Two people working together can produce a synergy where each motivates the other and in turn enhances self-motivation. Besides, working with another person on some common goal can really be fun. There is abundant material in this manual on how to identify support people, how to enlist their help, and how to communicate in positive ways to keep the support flowing.

Join a Program

TAPE 4
SECTION 5

Many commercial and self-help programs are available, each offering different approaches. There is no single best approach, but rather best fits between approaches and individuals. Stated another way, some might be better for you and others better for different people.

If you think a program might help, focus on what the most important features of a program are for you. Do you need a structured meal plan, prepared foods, a place to exercise, support from others in the program, a trained counselor, frequent meetings, convenience, low cost, or other factors important to you? Then think about which program does the best job of meeting your needs.

Some people find programs a great help in special times of need. For instance, a person might attend Overeaters Anonymous meetings every few months as a "booster" to their program. This is like getting booster shots to keep immunity high after an initial immunization. Another person might rejoin Weight Watchers at the sign of some crisis (they feel control is slipping, or they have regained some weight).

See a Professional

Professionals offer support and expert advice in a number of areas. By now you should have a good sense of areas where you are strong and other areas where you struggle. Let's take compulsive eating (binge eating) as an example. Many people find that their compulsive eating gets better when following The LEARN Program, but not all. In this case, seeing a psychologist or other health professional to deal with this problem could be a big help. The following is a list of common problems and suggestions for which you may seek professional help.

"How do you feel about your accomplishments in the program?"

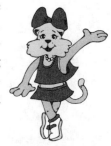

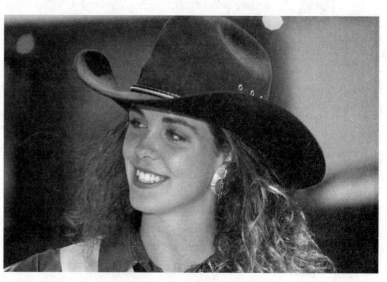

⇨ For nutrition advice—see a Registered Dietitian

⇨ For medical problems—see a Physician

⇨ For medication—see a Physician

⇨ For compulsive eating—see a Specialist in eating disorders (Psychologist, Psychiatrist, or Social Worker)

⇨ For lack of exercise—see a Personal Trainer or Exercise Specialist

⇨ For life stresses—see a Psychologist, Psychiatrist, or Social Worker

⇨ For depression, anxiety—see a Psychologist, Psychiatrist, or Social Worker

⇨ For relationship problems—see a Psychologist, Psychiatrist, or Social Worker

⇨ For weight management—see someone with training in exercise, nutrition, or psychology, or a Certified LifeStyle Counselor® (on the web at www.AALC.org)

Ending Where We Began

TAPE 4
SECTION 9

We can end where we began—with emphasizing the most important principles of all. You may recall that one of the first things I mentioned was a concept called self-efficacy. This concept tells us that the people most likely to make successful, long-term changes are those with the skills and confidence to do so. You have learned many skills—skills to help you confront difficult situations, to handle setbacks, to make changes you can live with, and to enjoy the whole process. You hold your weight management future in your hands. Use the skills and you'll do just fine.

You should be confident in your ability. You should not and could not be confident that you will be perfect, or that you will have an easy path to your goal. But, you can be confident that despite bumps in the road, occasional detours, and perhaps even getting lost on occasion, you can find your way back to the road and continue on your important journey.

Give yourself a pep talk when you need it. If you were your own coach, think about what you would need to hear to be most effective and then inspire yourself in that way. Do whatever you can to be confident that you have the necessary skills, and then use the skills, use the skills, and use them some more. It can work.

A Final Weight Change Record

I leave you with one final Weight Change Record. You will find it on page 257. I have replaced the week numbers at the bottom of the form with blank lines, along with the weight change in pounds. This is so you can start the chart at any point in time. I wish you continued luck with your weight management.

Saying Farewell

TAPE 4
SECTION 10

Let me offer my sincere hope that you enjoyed this program and that you are on your way to accomplishing your weight loss goals. It can be a hard struggle, but with the right attitude and new habits, success can be yours. Keep up the spirit!

Finally, please contact me with your ideas and comments about this program. Success stories are welcome, as are suggestions for improving the program. I pay attention to what I hear and would like to hear from you. Send comments to me at:

American Health Publishing Company
P.O. Box 610430, Dept. 10
Dallas, TX 75261–0430

You may also fax or e-mail your comments to me at the numbers listed in the very beginning of this book.

Good luck!!

Weight Change Record

Week

Weight Change (in pounds)

Master Monitoring Form

*Today's Date:*_____

TIME	FOOD AND AMOUNT	CALORIES

TOTAL DAILY CALORIES

PERSONAL GOALS FOR THIS WEEK	MOST OF THE TIME	SOME-TIMES	RARELY
1.			
2.			
3.			
4.			
5. EAT LESS THAN _____ CALORIES PER DAY			
6. EAT LESS THAN _____ GRAMS OF FAT EACH DAY			

FOOD GROUPS FOR TODAY	PHYSICAL ACTIVITY	MINUTES OR STEPS
MILK, YOGURT, AND CHEESE ☐ ☐ ☐	(M)	
MEAT, POULTRY, ETC. ☐ ☐ ☐	(TU)	
FRUITS ☐ ☐ ☐ ☐	(W)	
VEGETABLES ☐ ☐ ☐ ☐ ☐	(TH)	
BREADS, CEREALS, ETC. ☐ ☐ ☐ ☐ ☐ ☐ ☐ ☐	(F)	
SERVINGS OF WATER (8 OZ) ☐ ☐ ☐ ☐ ☐ ☐ ☐ ☐	(SA)	
	(SU)	

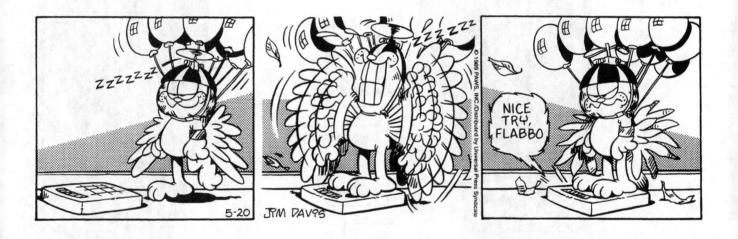

Good Luck!

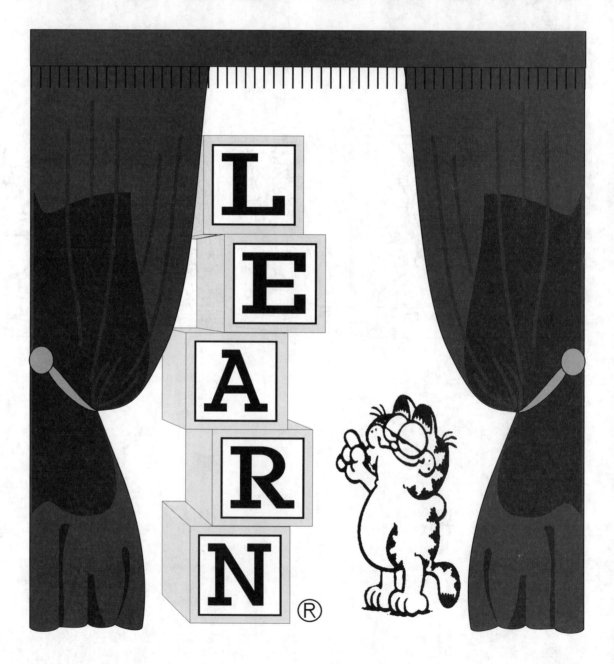

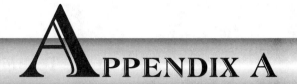

APPENDIX A

Master List of Techniques

Lifestyle Techniques

1. Alter the antecedents to eating (the behavior chain) 58
2. Avoid being a food dispenser 139
3. Be a Forest Ranger and prevent relapses 229
4. Be aware of the toxic environment 209
5. Buy foods that require preparation 102
6. Cope with lapses 227
7. Counter your negative self-talk 95
8. Develop a positive body image 110
9. Distinguish between cravings and hunger.................. 52
10. Do not clean your plate 77
11. Do nothing else while eating.......... 75
12. Eat in one place................... 76
13. Examine patterns in your eating 31, 43
14. Follow an eating schedule........... 76
15. Follow the five-minute rule 139
16. Hide the high-calorie foods.......... 123
17. Identify high-risk situations 217
18. Identify triggers for eating........... 44
19. Identify your behavior chains 202
20. Identify urges.................... 217
21. Interrupt your behavior chains........ 203
22. Keep a food diary 15
23. Keep a weight change record 17
24. Keep problem foods out of sight 124
25. Learn to uncouple stress and eating ... 160
26. Keep healthy foods visible 124
27. Leave the table after eating.......... 138
28. Maximize awareness of eating........ 31
29. Make a list of alternatives to eating 218
30. Pause during your meal 86
31. Plan in advance for high-risk situations . 217
32. Prepare in advance for special events... 231
33. Prevent automatic eating 31
34. Put your fork down between bites 85
35. Remove serving dishes from table 138
36. Serve and eat one portion at a time 138
37. Shop from a list................... 102
38. Shop on a full stomach............. 101
39. Taste every calorie, don't waste any 75
40. Think your way to success 99
41. Use the ABC approach............. 58
42. Use alternatives to eating 218
43. Use the six steps to gain control of lapses 228
44. Use techniques for eating away from home 183
45. Weigh yourself as you see fit......... 48

Exercise Techniques

46. Always warm up and cool down 127
47. Begin with a 15-minute walk 55
48. Choose and use a programmed activity 126
49. Consider a walking partnership........ 58
50. Consider programmed activity. 126
51. Count all activity as exercise 92
52. Counter the exercise threshold concept . 130
53. Do not be embarrassed............. 126
54. Experiment with jogging and running .. 162
55. Experiment with cycling............. 163
56. Experiment with aerobics 173
57. Increase lifestyle activity 91
58. Increase walking 78, 92
59. Keep an exercise diary 93
60. Know the advantages of walking....... 51
61. Know the benefits of exercise 34
62. Know the calorie values of exercise 93
63. Know the new activity formula for Americans.................. 117
64. Maximize pleasure of walking......... 78
65. Perfect your walking. 78
66. Park further away 92
67. Staying motivated to be active........ 56
68. Select something you can do........ 126
69. Select something you would like to do .. 126
70. Select solo or social activities. 126
71. Understand the benefits of exercise 34
72. Use a pedometer to measure your exercise................... 20
73. Use stairs whenever possible.......... 92
74. Use pulse test for positive feedback.... 207
75. Walk in shopping malls 52

Attitude Techniques

76. Ban perfectionist attitudes 99
77. Banish imperatives. 159
78. Be a forest ranger for urges and lapses. . 229
79. Be aware of high-risk situations. . . . 44, 217
80. Beware of attitude
    traps 95, 131, 142, 159, 220
81. Confront or ignore cravings. 60
82. Cope positively with slips and lapses . . . 227
83. Counter food and weight fantasies. 79
84. Counter impossible dream thinking. . . . 142
85. Distinguish hunger from cravings 52
86. Distinguish lapse and relapse 215
87. Focus on behavior rather than weight . . 143
88. Outlast urges to eat 217
89. Realize complex causes of overweight . . . 21
90. Rethink weight loss 12
91. Set flexible goals 143
92. Set realistic goals 7, 61
93. Set short-term goals 143
94. Stop dichotomous thinking. 220
95. Use six steps to gain control
    during lapses 228
96. Use the shaping concept for
    habit change. 60, 62
97. Visualize a reasonable weight change . . . 38

Relationship Techniques

98. Communicate with your family 155
99. Communicate with your partner 90
100. Consider a program partner 80
101. Do shopping with your partner 102
102. Exercise with partner 58
103. Explain your program to friends
     and family 155
104. Have partner do shopping for you. 102
105. Have partner and family read
     this manual. 143, 155
106. Identify and select a support person. 89
107. Make specific and positive requests
     of partner 91
108. Refuse pressures to eat 157
109. Reward your partner 91
110. State your partner requests positively. . . . 91
111. Tell your partner how to help 91
112. Things the family should avoid 156
113. Things the family can do 157
114. Use pleasurable partner activities 174

Nutrition Techniques

115. Be aware of calorie values of foods 183
116. Choose a diet low in fat, saturated
     fat, and cholesterol 64
117. Choose a diet with plenty of vegetables,
     fruits, and grains. 64
118. Consume adequate vitamins 165
119. Count grams of fat 46
120. Deal with pressures to eat. 157
121. Determine your target calorie level 44
122. Drink alcohol in moderation if you drink . 64
123. Eat a balanced diet 63
124. Eat a good breakfast 236
125. Eat a variety of foods 64
126. Eat appropriate servings from
     the five food groups. 64
127. Eating away from home 183
128. Eat great meals 29
129. Follow a balanced diet 63
130. Get adequate carbohydrate in your diet . 165
131. Get adequate protein in diet 148
132. Hide high-calorie foods 123
133. Increase complex carbohydrates 165
134. Increase fiber in diet 176
135. Keep healthy snacks available. 124
136. Know the food guide pyramid. 64
137. Know the importance of carbohydrate . . 165
138. Know the importance of dietary fat 103
139. Know the importance of protein 148
140. Know what makes a pound. 38
141. Learn about calories. 36, 62
142. Learn about portion sizes 86
143. Limit fat to 30 percent of total calories . 104
144. Make low-calorie foods appetizing 107
145. Make small dietary changes you
     can live with 73
146. Plan healthy meals. 107
147. Rate your diet 33
148. Read food labels 145
149. Search for eating patterns 31, 43
150. Select an eating plan 262
151. Set a calorie goal 44, 89
152. Take no more than recommended
     doses of vitamins. 164
153. Understand your triggers for eating. 44
154. Use a calorie guide 17
155. Use salt in moderation 64
156. Use sugars in moderation. 64
157. Use visual guides to control portions . . . 87
158. Watch the calories from alcohol 223

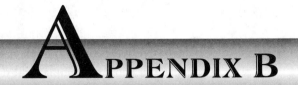

Weight Loss Readiness

Losing weight requires time and effort. This program can help, but the key results will come from your own efforts. Asking yourself if you are ready is an important first step.

For most people who want to lose weight, the main question involves which program to follow. A more fundamental question, however, precedes this issue. The question is whether a person *should* begin a weight loss program. With this is mind, I would like to introduce the issue of weight loss readiness.

Weight loss readiness may seem an unimportant issue at this time, because after all, you're reading this manual. Still, readiness refers to your motivation and commitment not just now, but weeks and months from now. Starting a program when you are truly ready can give you the best chance to succeed over the long run. In addition, if your readiness is low, you can do things to boost it.

What Is Readiness?

People begin weight loss programs for many reasons. Some have made an honest assessment of the effort necessary to stay with a program, while others enter expecting a rapid and simple solution. A health scare prompts some people to lose weight, while family pressure, embarrassment, and feeling uncomfortable may motivate others. Some people may just want to look better. These factors converge to form a person's readiness.

Readiness refers to whether you are truly prepared to begin a weight loss program. Readiness has several components. Among these are how motivated you are, whether the commitment exists to make a sustained effort, whether your life can tolerate the stresses of a program, and whether you can make significant changes in your dietary and activity patterns. Asking yourself the following question is important: Is the time right for me? You may be ready or you may not.

The Consequences of Not Being Ready

Far too often, individuals begin losing weight with a burst of energy that quickly fades. The result is initial weight loss followed by re-

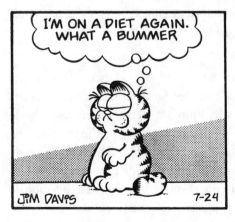
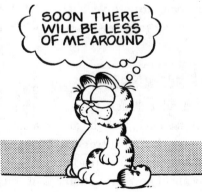
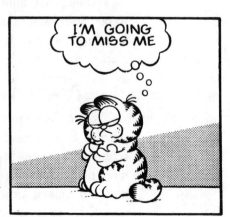

gain. Most overweight people have experienced this and know how unpleasant it can be. Some have referred to this as yo-yo dieting or weight cycling.

The effects of regaining lost weight have not been studied in detail. Professionals must rely, therefore, on experiences with their clients to formulate a picture. This picture is one of discouragement and self-condemnation for failing at yet another attempt to lose weight. This adds to the legacy of failure that plagues so many people.

The failure can be turned inside and affect mood (e.g., depression and anxiety) and wear away at self-esteem. These feelings can be turned outside, into anger at the program and bitterness at having such a difficult problem. Recent research has also raised the possibility that increased weight variability is associated with negative health effects, such as elevated risk for coronary heart disease. Taken together, these consequences argue for being truly ready before beginning a program.

Think ahead to the next few months. Does it look like "all's calm on the horizon" or is "a storm brewing?" Concentrating on weight control can be difficult when you're experiencing major upsets at home or work, when a parent or loved one is seriously ill, or when you have serious financial problems. If you know that such events will be time limited—meaning they will end in the near future—then you may be more likely to succeed if you wait until these stressors pass. Your goal, until that time, is to prevent weight gain rather than trying to lose weight. Let's now look at how you can assess your readiness.

Assessing Readiness

Weight loss can be a difficult and taxing process. Beginning when readiness is high can create an environment in which your success is more likely. Knowing about the idea of readiness and thinking clearly about how this notion applies to you is important.

Assessing readiness can take place in two steps. The first is appreciating the importance of the concept. Recognizing that beginning when the time is right is an important aspect of success. This is a novel idea to many people, so introducing yourself to the notion of readiness is necessary. Readiness is a fluid, changing condition. So, even if you are not ready just now, the right time could arise as time changes. When the conditions are right, this manual can help you.

The second step is in assessing your readiness. For this purpose, I have developed The Weight Loss Readiness Test (see page 267). You can also find The Weight Loss Readiness Test on our website, at www.Learn-Education.com under "Self- Assessments You Can Do."

This readiness test has 23 questions that I have divided into six sections with a scoring key at the end of each section. The sections deal with goals and attitudes, hunger and eating cues, control over eating, binge eating and purging, emotional eating, and exercise patterns and attitudes.

Conveying to you what the test is and what it is not is important. I developed the test to pinpoint the areas you should consider when assessing your readiness. The questions were drawn from my experience with many people and from research on predictors of weight loss. The test is still in its early stages of development, so it must be considered an aid, not a fully developed test.

The test should not be used, therefore, to make specific decisions on starting a program. This is why I did not intend for the test to yield a single summary score for readiness. The test can be used to help you think through the readiness concept and to decide how this notion applies to you. You are in the best position to make a judgment on readiness.

The Weight Loss Readiness Test Categories

As I discussed earlier, questions in The Weight Loss Readiness Test are divided into six sections. The following discussion covers the rationale for each section.

Section 1: Goals and Attitudes

The questions in this section are designed to help you evaluate your motivation. They help you assess how long you anticipate the motivation will last (commitment) and whether you can envision a weight loss program being woven into your lifestyle. In addition, this section deals with setting realistic goals—an important issue. Many people have unrealistic expectations about how quickly they will lose weight and how easy the process will be. When the fantasies fail to become reality, they may feel discouraged and may be more likely to relapse.

Section 2: Hunger and Eating Cues

Common lore suggests that overweight people do not eat in response to physical hunger, but rather, they eat out of habit. Some believe that psychological needs may trigger eating or that eating occurs simply because food is available. This may or may not be true. It is also possible that overweight people experience physical hunger more often, perhaps because internal pressures drive them to have more energy.

Science has shown that many people, regardless of weight, are responsive to external cues to eat. Seeing a dessert cart after a meal may stimulate eating. Driving past a bakery or realizing that it's a regular snack time can make many people want to eat. This section of the test is designed to help you recognize how responsive you are to cues to eat.

Section 3: Control Over Eating

People vary in how much control they feel they have over eating. Some people exert strict control, while others can be thrown off course by seemingly trivial events. The questions in this section deal with whether external pressures to eat threaten your control.

Section 4: Binge Eating and Purging

Binge eating is a common problem in overweight persons. Research on this topic is relatively new. What we do know suggests that weight loss may be especially difficult when binge eating is hard to control. Purging, which involves the use of vomiting, laxatives, or diuretics to rid the body of weight, is less common, but is a serious matter. Individuals who indicate frequent binge eating and purging should be evaluated by an eating disorders specialist to determine whether additional help is necessary.

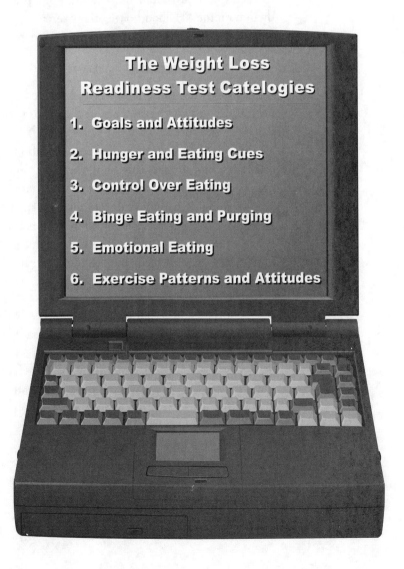

The Weight Loss Readiness Test Catelogies

1. Goals and Attitudes
2. Hunger and Eating Cues
3. Control Over Eating
4. Binge Eating and Purging
5. Emotional Eating
6. Exercise Patterns and Attitudes

Section 5: Emotional Eating

Emotional upheaval can weaken dietary restraint which, in turn, sets the stage for overeating. This can occur when people are depressed, anxious, angry, or lonely. In some cases, even feeling good or relieved about some aspect of life can lead to overeating. This section of the test is designed to help you identify whether eating occurs in response to emotional changes.

Section 6: Exercise Patterns and Attitudes

As I discuss often throughout this manual, exercise is a key component to a comprehensive weight management program. People who exercise are most likely to keep off lost weight. This section contains questions about readiness to exercise. You should think about your prediction on the likelihood of regular exercise because of its central role in weight management.

A Word of Caution

I would like to underscore that the readiness test should not be used as the only basis for deciding whether to begin a program. You should use it to ask yourself questions about readiness, not to make a final decision. As much information as possible should be gathered so that you can think through issues, such as motivation, commitment, and life circumstances. Then you decide on whether the time is right based on your feelings, attitudes, and behaviors.

Please note also that overall readiness may be a less helpful notion than thinking of readiness in different areas. For instance, most people enter a weight loss program expecting to change their diet. They would be in a high state of nutrition readiness. People vary more widely in their readiness to be physically active.

Low scores in one area may be a signal to take action to improve readiness in that specific area. A low physical activity score might be a tip-off to think about obstacles to exercise, either physical or emotional. Try to devise ways to remove the obstacles. Remember that readiness can change—if you take the right steps.

Having you assess your readiness is an interesting process. Even people who are not highly motivated may do an honest self-assessment and then find ways to motivate themselves. Low readiness is not necessarily permanent. It is a snapshot in time to show whether the conditions are right now. Because you may not be ready at this point does not mean that you will not be ready later.

The Weight Loss Readiness Test

Answer the questions below to see how well your attitudes equip you for a weight loss program. For each question, circle the answer that best describes your attitude, then write the number of your answer on the line before each question number. As you complete each of the six sections, add the numbers of your answers and compare them with the scoring guide at the end of each section.

Section 1—Goals and Attitudes

____1. Compared to previous attempts, how motivated are you to lose weight at this time?

   1   Not at all motivated

   2   Slightly motivated

   3   Somewhat motivated

   4   Quite motivated

   5   Extremely motivated

____2. How certain are you that you will stay committed to a weight loss program for the time it will take to reach your goal?

   1   Not at all certain

   2   Slightly certain

   3   Somewhat certain

   4   Quite certain

   5   Extremely certain

____3. Consider all outside factors at this time in your life (the stress you're feeling at work, your family obligations, etc.). To what extent can you tolerate the effort required to stick to a program?

   1   Cannot tolerate

   2   Can tolerate

   3   Uncertain

   4   Can tolerate well

   5   Can tolerate easily

____4. Think honestly about how much weight you hope to lose and how quickly you hope to lose it. Figuring a weight loss of one to two pounds per week, how realistic is your expectation?

   1   Very unrealistic

   2   Somewhat unrealistic

   3   Moderately unrealistic

   4   Somewhat realistic

   5   Very realistic

____5. While losing weight, do you fantasize about eating a lot of your favorite foods?

   1   Always

   2   Frequently

   3   Occasionally

   4   Rarely

   5   Never

____6. While losing weight, do you feel deprived, angry and/or upset?

   1   Always

   2   Frequently

   3   Occasionally

   4   Rarely

   5   Never

_____ **Section 1—TOTAL Score**

If you scored:

6 to 16:   This may not be a good time for you to start a weight loss program. Inadequate motivation and commitment, together with unrealistic goals could block your progress. Think about those things that contribute to this, and consider changing them before undertaking a program.

17 to 23:   You may be close to being ready to begin a program but should think about ways to boost your readiness before you begin.

24 to 30:   The path is clear with respect to goals and attitudes.

Section 2—Hunger and Eating Cues

____7. When food comes up in conversation or in something you read, do you want to eat even if you are not hungry?

   1   Never

   2   Rarely

   3   Occasionally

   4   Frequently

   5   Always

____8. How often do you eat because of physical hunger?

   1   Always

   2   Frequently

   3   Occasionally

   4   Rarely

   5   Never

____9. Do you have trouble controlling your eating when your favorite foods are around the house?

1 Never
2 Rarely
3 Occasionally
4 Frequently
5 Always

_____ **Section 2—TOTAL Score**

If you scored:

3 to 6: You might occasionally eat more than you would like, but it does not appear to be a result of high responsiveness to external cues. Controlling the attitudes that make you eat may be especially helpful.

7 to 9: You may have a moderate tendency to eat just because food is available. Weight loss may be easier for you if you try to resist external cues, and eat only when you are physically hungry.

10 to 15: Some or most of your eating may be in response to thinking about food or exposing yourself to temptations to eat. Think of ways to minimize your exposure to temptations, so that you eat only in response to physical hunger.

Section 3—Control Over Eating

If the following situations occurred while you were on a weight loss program, would you be likely to eat more or less immediately afterward and for the rest of the day?

____10. Although you planned on skipping lunch, a friend talks you into going out for a meal.

1 Would eat much less
2 Would eat somewhat less
3 Would make no difference
4 Would eat somewhat more
5 Would eat much more

____11. You "break" your diet by eating a fattening, "forbidden" food.

1 Would eat much less
2 Would eat somewhat less
3 Would make no difference
4 Would eat somewhat more
5 Would eat much more

____12. You have been following your diet faithfully and decide to test yourself by eating something you consider a treat.

1 Would eat much less
2 Would eat somewhat less
3 Would make no difference
4 Would eat somewhat more
5 Would eat much more

_____ **Section 3—TOTAL Score**

If you scored:

3 to 7: You recover rapidly from mistakes. However, if you frequently alternate between eating out of control and dieting very strictly, you may have a serious eating problem and should get professional help.

8 to 11: You do not seem to let unplanned eating disrupt your program. This is a flexible, balanced approach.

12 to 15: You may be prone to overeat after an event breaks your control or throws you off the track. Your reaction to these eating events can be improved.

Section 4—Binge Eating and Purging

____13. Aside from holiday feasts, have you ever eaten a large amount of food rapidly and felt afterward that this eating incident was excessive and out of control?

2 Yes
0 No

____14. If you answered yes to question 13 above, how often have you engaged in this behavior during the last year?

1 Less than once a month
2 About once a month
3 A few times a month
4 About once a week
5 About three times a week
6 Daily

____15. Have you ever purged (used laxatives, diuretics, or induced vomiting) to control your weight?

5 Yes
0 No

____16. If you answered yes to question 15 above, how often have you engaged in this behavior during the last year?
1   Less than once a month
2   About once a month
3   A few times a month
4   About once a week
5   About three times a week
6   Daily
_____ **Section 4—TOTAL Score**

If you scored:

0 to 1:   It appears that binge eating and purging are problems for you.

2 to 11: Pay attention to these eating patterns. Should they arise more frequently, get professional help.

12 to 19: You show signs of having a potentially serious eating problem. See a counselor experienced in evaluating eating disorders right away.

Section 5—Emotional Eating

____17. Do you eat more than you would like to when you have negative feelings, such as anxiety, depression, anger, or loneliness?
1   Never
2   Rarely
3   Occasionally
4   Frequently
5   Always

____18. Do you have trouble controlling your eating when you have positive feelings—do you celebrate feeling good by eating?
1   Never
2   Rarely
3   Occasionally
4   Frequently
5   Always

____19. When you have unpleasant interactions with others in your life, or after a difficult day at work, do you eat more than you would like?
1   Never
2   Rarely
3   Occasionally
4   Frequently
5   Always
_____ **Section 5—TOTAL Score**

If you scored:

3 to 8:   You do not appear to let your emotions affect your eating.

9 to 11: You sometimes eat in response to emotional highs and lows. Monitor this behavior to learn when and why it occurs, and be prepared to find alternative activities.

12 to 15: Emotional ups and downs can stimulate your eating. Try to deal with the feelings that trigger the eating, and find other ways to express them.

Section 6—Exercise Patterns and Attitudes

____20. How often do you exercise?
1   Never
2   Rarely
3   Occasionally
4   Frequently
5   Always

____21. How confident are you that you can exercise regularly?
1   Not at all confident
2   Slightly confident
3   Somewhat confident
4   Quite confident
5   Extremely confident

____22. When you think about exercise, do you develop a positive or negative picture in your mind?
1   Completely negative
2   Somewhat negative
3   Neutral
4   Somewhat positive
5   Completely positive

____23. How certain are you that you can work regular exercise into your daily schedule?
1   Not at all certain
2   Slightly certain
3   Somewhat certain
4   Quite certain
5   Extremely certain
_____ **Section 6—TOTAL Score**

If you scored:

4 to 10: You are probably not exercising as regularly as you should. Determine whether your attitudes about exercise are blocking your way, then change what you must and put on those walking shoes.

11 to 16: You need to feel more positive about exercise so you can do it more often. Think of ways to be more active that are fun and fit into your lifestyle.

17 to 20: It looks like the path is clear for you to be active. Now think of ways to get motivated.

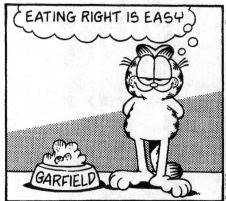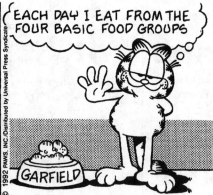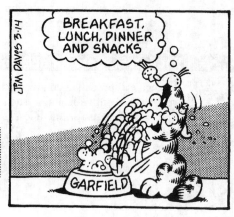

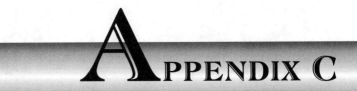

Answers for Self-Assessment Questions

Lesson One

1. **False** Psychological problems are not at the root of all cases of overweight. There is no evidence that uncovering these causes helps with weight loss.

2. **False** People who have been overweight in childhood may have excessive fat cells, but other overweight persons may not. They have fat cells that are too large.

3. **False** There are wide variations in metabolic rate among different people. Some are cursed with a slow metabolism and may be prone to easy weight gains in body weight.

4. **True** One study found that persons losing weight who observed common foods and estimated quantity and calories averaged errors of 60 percent. Therefore, using a calorie guide, measuring tools, and a food scale is important.

5. **True** Persons who have lost weight and maintained their loss often report that record keeping was one key to their success.

6. **False** Activity measuring devices like a pedometer and the LEARN WalkMaster are excellent ways to help you keep up with your daily physical activity. Moreover, these devices can help motivate you by showing you just how much physical activity you are doing each day.

Lesson Two

7. **False** Being on a weight management program does not mean you have to forgo great tasting meals. By learning all about calories, you can enjoy every bit of your food.

8. **True** Many overweight people eat without paying attention to all they consume. They miss the taste in much of what they eat.

9. **True** The Food Diary helps you discover times, foods, feelings, and activities associated with eating. Understanding your eating patterns is a key in changing lifelong habits.

10. **False** Exercise has many benefits aside from the calories you burn. It is one of the most important aspects of weight control.

11. **True** Exercise maximizes the loss of fat and can prevent the loss of muscle. Exercise combined with diet is preferable to diet alone for weight loss.

12. **True** Making the meals that you do eat count. Your meals should be satisfying, good tasting, and nutritious. Otherwise, you'll feel deprived when there is no need to, and your body won't get enough good nutrients.

13. **False** The calorie is a measure of the energy your body gets from a food. Fat supplies some of these calories in some foods, but so do carbohydrate and protein.

14. **False** There are differences in how much weight people lose on the same caloric intake. Some people need to make a greater restriction in caloric intake than others in order to lose weight.

Lesson Three

15. **True** Your food diary will allow you to identify times, places, feelings, activities, and other events which are frequently associated with overeating. Identifying these situations will allow you to intervene appropriately.

16. **False** You decide how frequently you should weigh yourself. Some people benefit from daily weighings, but others do not. It is your call.

17. **True** How far you go is more important than how fast you go, so walking is an ideal exercise. Of course, running will get the job done faster!

18. **False** Expensive exercise clothes contain no special materials and have no advantage over clothes most people have anyway. Their only advantage is cosmetic.

19. **False** Low fat does not mean low calories. Many low-fat foods on the market today have as

many calories as the high-fat foods they replaced.

20. **True** Walking has many advantages for weight management. Moreover, walking is something that just about anyone can do.

21. **False** Overweight people experience physical hunger. However, they often confuse psychological cravings for this hunger and eat when there is no physical need.

Lesson Four

22. **False** The ABC approach stands for Antecedents, Behavior, and Consequences. It shows the importance of what occurs before, during, and after eating.

23. **False** Many people do profit from exercising with a partner, but many enjoy doing their exercise alone. It is a matter of individual preference.

24. **False** Shaping refers to making gradual progress in a step-by-step fashion so that goals are attainable.

25. **False** Different numbers of servings are recommended for each of the five food groups. It is this combination of a different number of servings from each of the five food groups that provides dietary balance.

26. **True** As few as 10 calories make a difference when added up over a year.

27. **True** Many overweight people are embarrassed to exercise, but this is something you need to banish from your mind. Most people give heavy people much credit for increasing their physical activity.

28. **True** Using a pedometer like the LEARN WalkMaster can help you to realize the progress you are making in being more active. Often, you may be more active than you realize. Using a pedometer that tells you that you have been active can be a powerful motivational tool at the end of a long day.

29. **False** No foods are prohibited. You can learn to eat any foods in moderation. Making foods illegal only sets up a person for failure.

30. **True** One size does not fit all. Different approaches to food cravings will help different people.

31. **True** Goals help keep you oriented to the areas of greatest importance, and provide a way for you to reward yourself when you make positive changes.

Lesson Five

32. **False** Only about 22 percent of the American adult population is active enough to realize health benefits. The rest of the population is either totally sedentary or not active enough.

33. **False** This concept of an exercise threshold is a barrier to exercise for many people. Any exercise can help, so do whatever you can.

34. **True** It is wise to break the habit of cleaning the plate so you, and not the server, determine how much you eat. By cleaning the plate, you have no control and eat whatever is in front of you.

35. **False** Eating on a schedule helps define the times you eat so that you minimize the times of the day associated with eating.

36. **False** Many people do benefit from having a weight management partner, but not everyone falls into this category. This decision is best left up to you.

37. **False** Weight loss is one measure of success. Equally, if not more important, are improved health, fitness, and quality of life.

Lesson Six

38. **False** Taste buds catch nothing but a blur if the food shoots past like a rocket. Slowing down can help you enjoy food more.

39. **True** Do not expect your partner to read your mind. Tell your partner exactly what he or she can do to help. Remember, be specific, ask for positive changes, and be nice to your partner in return.

40. **True** Climbing stairs is an excellent way to burn calories. However, most people cannot climb stairs for extended periods of time. Lifestyle activity in which exercise can be added to your daily routine is a much better approach.

41. **False** Pausing gives the body a chance to signal that enough had been eaten so you can be satisfied with less food.

42. **False** Many people underestimate the calories they eat (some, by as much as 60 percent). Part of this error may result from not accurately measuring portion sizes.

43. **True** Relationships are two-way streets. You want your support partner to feel good about helping you, so more help will come your way. Reinforcing him or her for helping is a great way to see that this happens.

Lesson Seven

44. **False** It can be difficult to change thoughts we have had for years, but with repeated practice, old thoughts can give way to new, constructive, and more helpful thoughts.

45. **False** Shopping on an empty stomach is asking for trouble. You will do less impulse buying if you shop after eating.

46. **True** Taking the time to prepare foods will give you a chance to make a determined decision to eat. Many times the food will not be worth the effort, so you can ask yourself how important eating really is.

47. **False** Fat plays an important role in the body and should not be eliminated from your diet. It is important for good health, however, most people eat too much fat.

48. **True** Fat, as a *percentage* of total calories eaten, should be 30 percent or less of your daily diet.

49. **True** One gram of fat contains 9 calories while 1 gram of carbohydrate or protein contain only 4 calories.

50. **False** It is true that saturated fats are generally solid at room temperature, but it is not true that saturated fats are found only in animal products. Coconut and palm oils also contain saturated fats.

51. **False** Yogurt may be used in many creative ways to replace other foods that have calories. However, there is no evidence that eating yogurt everyday helps people lose weight.

52. **True** With the "ideal" being extremely thin, shaped, and sculpted, it is virtually impossible for most people to look like they think they should—no matter how much dieting and exercise they do. People deserve to feel good about their bodies, and the first step is to have a realistic standard.

53. **True** It's not easy, because society places so much importance on being thin. However, many people uncouple weight from their self-esteem and manage to appreciate their personal qualities and to accept their body for the pleasure it can bring them.

Lesson Eight

54. **True** Thirty minutes of incremental physical activity over most days (at least five) is now recommended for people to reach a moderate level of physical fitness.

55. **False** Vitamins, minerals, and water are considered nutrients essential to our bodies, yet, they contain no calories.

56. **True** Remember, the refrigerator battle cry, "Out of Sight, Out of Mouth!"

57. **True** One serving from the milk group is equal to 1 cup or 8 ounces of milk. Remember, drinking skim or low-fat milk will help keep the calories down.

58. **True** The Food Guide Pyramid recommends two to three servings each day from the Milk, Yogurt, and Cheese Group.

59. **True** Each of us holds internal conversations, and many overweight individuals have fat *thoughts*. These thoughts and attitudes can greatly hinder weight loss efforts if they are not countered.

60. **False** The two purposes of stretching and other warm up exercises are to loosen the muscles to avoid strain and to permit the heart and circulatory system to make a gradual transition from rest to hard work. You should warm up and cool down for at least five minutes each time you exercise.

61. **True** These are the three parts of the formula, so if you wish to get a training or aerobic effect, you must do each part in specific amounts.

62. **False** Some people take longer than others to become active because new habits take a while to develop. Also, vigorous activity isn't necessarily the goal. If you do vigorous activity, fine, but anything you do to be more active is helpful.

63. ***True*** A significant number of overweight persons suffer from binge eating. The LEARN Program may help with this problem, as may other resources described in Lesson Eight.

Lesson Nine

64. ***False*** It is best to take one portion at a time because it gives you time to decide whether you need more. It interrupts automatic eating.

65. ***True*** Spot reducing is a myth. Your body adds and removes fat according to genetic and hormonal factors. You can reduce fat in general, but you cannot dictate where it will come off.

66. ***True*** These images and fantasies can distract a person from the day-to-day behaviors needed to lose weight, can lead to serious disappointment when the individual loses weight, and can cause significant life issues.

67. ***False*** The amount of total fat listed under the heading "% Daily Value" of the food label represents the amount of a day's intake in a serving, based on a 2000-calorie diet.

68. ***False*** Protein is important for good health, but too much protein can lead to certain health problems. Most experts agree that between 10 and 15 percent of your total daily calories should come from protein.

69. ***False*** Eating a variety of legumes and grains will also provide high-quality protein.

70. ***True*** Behavior, even helping behavior, fades away if it is not rewarded (people like to be appreciated). So, if a partner helps you, show your appreciation in creative ways—his or her desire to help you will persist.

Lesson Ten

71. ***False*** Families can be a great resource for a person losing weight, but the harmony between the individual and the family requires a special effort.

72. ***True*** These words are a setup for failure because they represent standards that no person can meet.

73. ***True*** Jogging and cycling have both psychological and physical benefits. They are ideal for

many people who are losing and maintaining weight.

74. ***False*** Carbohydrates should make up the largest portion of your daily diet (between 55 and 60 percent of total calories). It is important, however, to watch for *hidden* calories in these foods and limit the *added* calories, such as toppings, butter, and dressings.

75. ***False*** It is nice to be friendly, but it is more important that *you* control what you eat. Be polite, but be firm in not yielding to pressure to eat.

76. ***True*** The Food Guide Pyramid suggests between three and five servings each day from the Vegetable Group.

77. ***False*** There is no weight loss advantage to taking mega doses of any vitamin. Sticking with the Recommended Daily Allowances (RDA) is the best policy. This can usually be done by eating a balanced diet, and at most, can be accomplished with a multiple vitamin.

78. ***False*** It is important to be familiar with the fat content of all foods. Vegetables are usually low in fat; however, nuts are an example of vegetables that are very high in fat.

Lesson Eleven

79. ***False*** Vitamins do not contain energy themselves, but aid in the breakdown of other nutrients into energy that the body can use.

80. ***False*** Small bouts of exercise can help you advance to the moderately-fit category and are likely to have a big impact on health. They will certainly be helpful for weight management.

81. ***False*** Aerobic activities do little for strength. They increase the body's use of oxygen and improve the condition of your heart. They are valuable for both health and weight loss.

82. ***True*** These foods are naturally high in fiber and are good additions to your diet if you wish to increase fiber intake.

83. ***False*** Most Americans do not eat the recommended number of servings of fruit on a daily basis. Hence, most people should increase their intake of fruit.

84. ***True*** With the current state of science, it is not possible to say that increased fiber in the

diet protects against diseases, but there are strong hints that this may be the case.

85. **True**   Most nutritionist suggest that a healthy goal is to aim for an average intake of 25-35 grams of fiber each day.

86. **False**   The great news about exercise is that short bouts of activity, performed at a comfortable level, will improve your health and fitness. Small amounts of activity add up over the coarse of the day.

87. **False**   There are many kinds of exercise that can help with your weight loss. The best kind is the kind you will do—now and in the future. Doing something rigorous is fine, if you keep it up. But low-level activities will be better if you can stick with them over the long term.

88. **False**   Precisely because fiber is indigestible, it facilitates movement of food and waste products through the digestive system. Eating a high-fiber diet may also reduce risk for several chronic diseases.

Lesson Twelve

89. **True**   Alcohol releases inhibitions and weakens dietary restraint. It contains little nutrition and many calories.

90. **True**   Package deals, like getting a hamburger, fries, and cole slaw together more cheaply than separately, deliver more food (and calories) than you may want or need. Only get the package if you are *sure* you want all its components.

91. **True**   Most people have access to stairs, so it is easy to add several flights to your routine.

92. **True**   Foods from this group are very high in complex carbohydrates and most people should increase their intake from this food group. Breads, cakes, cookies, etc., however, have *hidden* calories, and it is important to watch out for these.

93. **True**   Many overweight people avoid eating breakfast because they may not be hungry first thing in the morning or because they hope to save calories by not eating. However, this typically leads to more calories being consumed during the day.

Lesson Thirteen

94. **True**   If you understand the circumstances that prompt you to eat well and be active, and the circumstances that make you eat more and be inactive, you are poised to make positive lifestyle choices.

95. **True**   A Behavior Chain can be broken at any link. Concentrate on the weakest links, where the chain is easiest to break.

96. **False**   People losing weight sometimes feel the chain is out of control, but a chain *can* be broken by using the right techniques at the proper time in a given situation.

97. **False**   It can be difficult to interrupt a chain at one of the final links because the momentum created by the earlier links can be powerful. Consider breaking the links earlier, before the process gets rolling.

98. **False**   As your weight decreases and you become more fit, your resting heart rate will probably decline. This means that your heart can accomplish its work with fewer beats.

99. **False**   Exercise is one predictor of who will keep weight off in the long run.

100. **True**   Just like many people get angry at tobacco companies trying to peddle their toxic products, it can be helpful to think of food advertisements, restaurants that serve enormous portions, and fast-food restaurants with tricks like drive-through windows, package meals, and very large servings of things like french fries as an enemy trying to take your money and make you sick. Resist!!!

101. **True**   Birds differ in the amount of fat they provide. The leanest poultry is turkey. After being skinned and cooked, chicken has double or triple the fat of turkey, and ducks and geese have 50 percent more fat than chicken.

Lesson Fourteen

102. **False**   Some people *think* that a lapse leads to relapse because they feel guilty at any mistake. By using special coping techniques, you can see that a lapse can be a signal to do better, not worse.

103. **True**   Being a good urge surfer involves identifying the urges early in their development and then readying your skills to ride the wave. If you

recognize the wave early, but cannot surf, you will also wipe out.

104. **False** This refers to thinking that you are on or off a program, perfect or terrible with your behavior, and legal or illegal in your eating. This must be replaced with a more rational perspective.

105. **True** Saturated fat can raise your cholesterol level, so it is important to control the intake of foods high in cholesterol *and* foods high in saturated fat.

106. **True** This can provide you with a list of enjoyable activities that can become associated with the signals that are used to stimulate eating.

Lesson Fifteen

107. **False** Different people respond to different techniques. It is best to select a small number of techniques that work for *you* and to focus on them.

108. **False** Anxiety makes it hard to think and weakens restraint that might keep eating in check. It is best to stay calm during a lapse so you can make a rational plan for responding.

109. **True** The longer you wait during a lapse, the more momentum builds for overeating. The best approach is to act swiftly and decisively.

110. **False** Consider yourself a forest ranger. Your task is to prevent fires and to move quickly when a fire breaks out. Occasionally fires do break out, and when they do, take steps immediately to keep the fire from consuming the entire forest.

111. **True** Eating a low-calorie food before you go takes the edge off hunger. This can help you avoid high-calorie foods like chips and nuts, so you can use your calories for special foods you really want.

112. **False** Iron deficiency is not common. Most people obtain adequate iron from normal eating and do not need the popular supplements.

113. **True** Most experts recommend reductions in salt intake. Excess sodium comes from salt in foods naturally and from the salt we add to food.

114. **True** Calcium is needed throughout life to sustain bone strength, but the body needs different amounts at different times of life. The general RDA for calcium is 1 gram per day.

Lesson Sixteen

115. **False** Keeping records is usually rated as one of the most important aspects of the program. Many people continue to keep the records for years. This process helps the new habits become more permanent.

116. **True** This is the main reason for keeping the Monitoring Forms. You should consider keeping Monitoring Forms on a periodic basis (say, one week out of every month) well into the future.

117. **True** Almost everyone experiences a slow down in weight loss after a few months on any program. Turning your attention away from the scale and on all the accomplishments you have made during the program can help you realize just how much you have changed and can provide motivation to continue making positive changes.

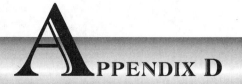

Guidelines for Being a Good Group Member

Many programs deal with participants in groups. This is done for an important reason. Members of the group can provide tremendous help to one another. The help may come in the form of encouraging words, a pat on the back, ideas to solve a specific problem, or just the knowledge that others in similar circumstances care about you.

Importance of the Group

From a problem-solving perspective, a group provides a shared experience that can help you develop an effective program. But beyond providing information, group members can provide support and encouragement. Most people losing weight encounter times when their motivation is high and other times when it is difficult to move in the right direction. When you take a detour from your program, the group can help the motivation return. When you are highly motivated yourself, you can encourage someone else in the group who may have trouble.

Good Chemistry and Teamwork

When a group has the right chemistry, it functions like a well-oiled machine. The meetings are enjoyable, informative, and motivational. Each group member receives as much as he or she gives, and all are better off for the effort.

The analogy of a sports team is especially appropriate. Let's take a basketball team, for example. We all know of teams with great individual players, but the team goes nowhere if the players do not work together. One player may have an opportunity to take a shot, but passing to a teammate who has a better shot will help the team. Teams with far less talent win cham-

pionships by working together and helping one another. This intangible *team spirit* motivates everyone to work harder. Each player receives and gives, and all benefit in the process.

Being a good group member is a **responsibility** of anyone entering a group. But more than duty, it is the best way to lose weight. Entering a group with a spirit of cooperation and the willingness to help others will insure that the help comes back to you. In the long run, you emerge the winner.

To be a good group member means following specific guidelines. There are things to do, things to say, and ways to act. The guidelines that follow can make this happen.

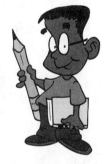

"A good group is like a sports team. Each player receives and gives, and all benefit in the process."

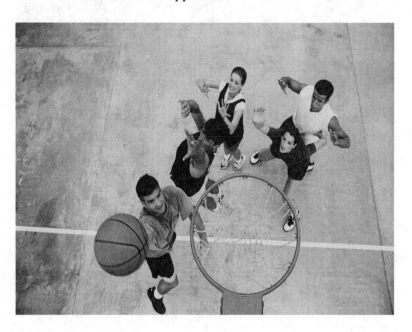

Guidelines and Responsibilities

Attend Meetings and Be Punctual

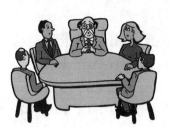

People in a group are responsible for attending meetings, not only for themselves but for others. When a group member misses a meeting, others in the group may worry about the person, may wonder if the absence is a sign of trouble, etc.

There undoubtedly will be times when you question whether you should attend a meeting. You might have overdone it on nacho chips, it may be rainy and miserable outside, or you may have had a difficult time with work or with the kids. These are the times when your program might be most in jeopardy, so it is important to attend the meeting. The group functions best when all attend, so remember that by joining a group you are agreeing to do your level best to make the meetings.

Being on time is another key factor. When you arrive late for a group, you draw attention to yourself, disrupt the proceedings, miss what has happened to that point, and force the group leader to either ignore what you have missed or cover it again. Showing up late, especially if it occurs chronically, is a sign of disrespect for other members of the group.

Sometimes, of course, being late is inevitable. You might have just arrived in town on the flight from Tokyo where you were thinking of acquiring SONY or Toyota. If you live in Arizona, you might have been attacked by the Abominable Cactus. Or you might have some more common reason like a traffic jam, late baby-sitter, or deadlines at the office. These things are fine, but when you are late when you can help it, we start to worry.

Being late can be a sign of many things. Some people are always late because they fall into the Type A behavior pattern. They are always rushing and want to get in every last bit of activity before departing for the group. Such a person would cringe at sitting around for a few minutes with nothing to do. My advice is to go ahead and cringe, but be on time.

Sometimes group members are late because they have done poorly and want to avoid speaking with the group leader. Others might be angry at the group leader or dissatisfied with the program or their progress. These things are usually not done on a conscious level, but if you look closely at your reasons for being late, these things may be the driving factors. If you find yourself being late, or wanting to be late, think about the reasons.

Really Listen

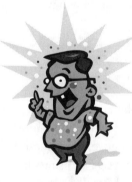

Sure, we all listen in a group, but do we **really** listen? Are you tuned in to what is happening? Do you hear the emotions behind the words of another group member?

It is quite apparent when someone in the group is not listening. Yawning, rolling the eyes, looking out the window, or daydreaming are giveaways. It is easy to get distracted, especially if what is being discussed is not relevant to you, or if something else important is occupying your thoughts. It takes a real effort to listen carefully.

Being a good listener involves watching the person who is speaking. Do they look like they are expressing some strong emotions? Is the topic a sensitive one? Have you experienced a similar situation or feeling? Have you found some approach helpful with the problem? It is fine to ask questions if you don't understand what the person is trying to say, and it is certainly fine to respond with supportive statements or suggestions. It will be nice when others in the group do this for you, so start by really listening.

Be Non-judgmental

This may sound like psychological jargon, but here is what it means to be non-judgmental. Sometimes you might feel that what another group member says or does is wrong, silly, or even stupid. There is a tendency to come down on these people or to point out the folly in their ways. The risk lies in being too negative, which can antagonize the person on the other end and make the remaining group members mad at you for being critical.

This does not mean that you are in a group where *everything is wonderful* and no negative emotions can be expressed. It is important to remember that there are different ways of saying things. What others say can be used as an opportunity for growth or an occasion to create bad feelings. The basic concept is for group members to accept one another. In such a climate, people in the group feel free to say things

they might otherwise hide for fear of being criticized.

The chart provided below gives some examples of judgmental and non-judgmental statements. As you can see, the non-judgmental statements are supportive and understanding, and open the door for further discussion. They show others that you care about them and are willing to help.

Be an Active Participant

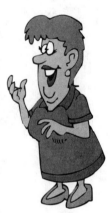

In any group, some people are more active than others. This is fine, and can reflect differences in personalities. Not everyone has to be talkative to benefit from the group. However, opening up to be an active participant can help both you and the other members of the group.

Being silent in a group sometimes reflects being shy or reserved. In other cases, it shows that a person is angry, resentful, or bored. Whatever the reason, try to speak up when you have something worth saying. If you would like to share some of your own experiences, to ask if anyone has a solution to a

"A non-judgmental statements are supportive and understanding and open the door for further discussion."

Being Non-judgmental

One person says	Judgmental Response	Non-judgmental Response
I just couldn't exercise this week.	You must be getting lazy.	It's hard to keep motivated to exercise.
I don't think this group is helping.	You are just making excuses.	Can we do something to help?
Others here don't understand me.	You talk too much.	I would like to. What can I do?

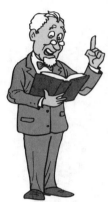

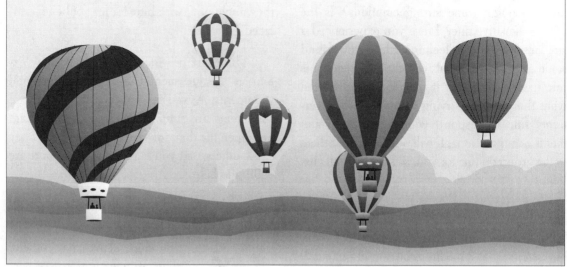

particular problem you face, or provide ideas of your own about an issue, speak up. Many times, what you have to say will be listened to with all the attention given to a group leader, and you might have ideas that the leader or others in the group do not have.

If you are the silent type, don't feel pressured to be exceptionally talkative. Not everyone will participate equally or will speak the same amount. When you do have something to offer, please share it with the others.

Share the Air Space

Think of the air in the group room as the territory around an airport. If too many planes enter the air space, the situation becomes dangerously confusing. If one jet occupies more than its share of the air space, say by circling in an erratic pattern, it would be tough going for the others.

In a group, there is only so much air space. Only so many voices can be heard and so many things said in the course of a group. For members of the group who are particularly verbal, there can be a tendency to monopolize the conversation and to crowd others from the air space.

Again, not everyone speaks the same amount, so if some people are naturally more vocal in the group, there is no need to pull in the reins. But if such a person interrupts or always speaks first, there may be a problem with sharing the air space. If the person takes a long time to make a point or has to say something during every discussion, it may be time to open the air space to others. Look at the way you speak in the group, and see if any of these apply to you. If so, try to pull back and think before speaking. By all means speak up when you have something to say, and say what you feel, but try not to speak just because there is an opportunity.

Be Supportive

One of the fundamental reasons there are groups is for group members to support each other. This can be motivating and encouraging. In fact, sometimes a kind word or a supportive gesture will mean more coming from a fellow group member than the exact same word or gesture coming from the group leader.

Group members should try to be nice, helpful, and understanding. When another group member is troubled by something, do what you can to show that you understand. You can offer moral support by showing that you understand that the person faces a difficult situation. Share similar experiences you might have had, and most of all, give some constructive suggestions if you can think of ways to help.

In Summary

When you enter a group, you enter a situation in which you can reap impressive rewards. You have the opportunity to not only learn the facts and techniques of the program, but to support and be supported, learn and instruct, help and be helped. This does not happen automatically, so people must be serious about their responsibilities as group members. In so doing, they will benefit from you and you will benefit from them. All will be better off, and the long-term result can be permanent weight loss.

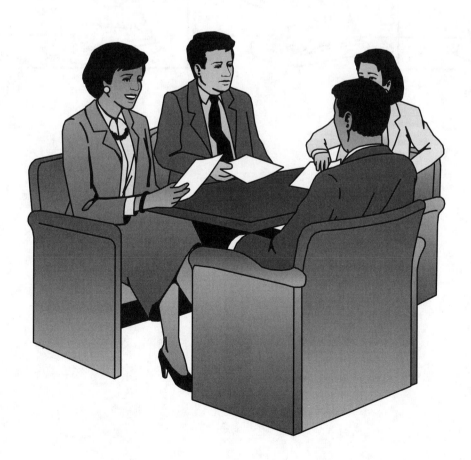

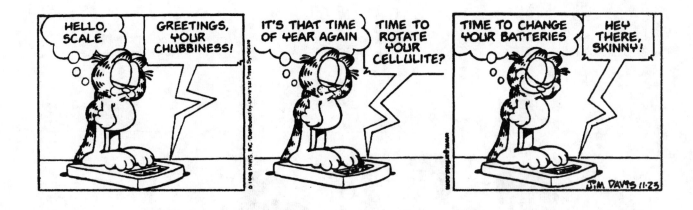

Rate Your Diet Quiz—Lesson Two

The following questions will give you a rough sketch of your typical eating habits. The (+) or (-) number for each answer instantly pats you on the back for good eating habits or alerts you to problems you didn't even know you had. The quiz focuses on fat, saturated fat, cholesterol, sodium, sugar, fiber, and fruits and vegetables. It doesn't attempt to cover everything in your diet. Also, it doesn't try to measure precisely how much of the key nutrients you eat. Next to each answer is a number with a + or - sign in front of it. Circle the number that corresponds to the answer you choose and write that score (e.g., +1) in the space provided in front of each question. That's your score for the question. If two or more answers apply, circle each one. Then average them to get your score for the question.

How to average. In answering question 19, for example, if your sandwich-eating is equally divided among tuna salad (-2), roast beef (+1), and turkey breast (+3), add the three scores (which gives you +2) and then divide by three. That gives you a score of +⅔ for the question. Round it to +1. Pay attention to serving sizes, which are given when needed. For example, a serving of vegetables is ½ cup. If you usually eat one cup of vegetables at a time, count it as two servings. If you're ready, let's start.

Fruits, Vegetables, Grains, and Beans

____ 1. How many servings of fruit or 100% fruit juice do you eat per day? (OMIT fruit snacks like Fruit Roll-Ups and fruit-on-the-bottom yogurt. One serving = one piece or ½ cup of fruit or 6 oz of fruit juice.)

- -3 None
- -2 Less than 1 serving
- 0 1 serving
- +1 2 serving
- +2 3 serving
- +3 4 or more servings

____ 2. How many servings of non-fried vegetables do you eat per day? (One serving = ½ cup. Include potatoes.)

- -3 None
- -2 Less than 1 serving
- 0 1 serving
- +1 2 serving
- +2 3 serving
- +3 4 or more servings

____ 3. How many servings of vitamin-rich vegetables do you eat per week? (One serving = ½ cup. Only count broccoli, Brussels sprouts, carrots, collards, kale, red pepper, spinach, sweet potatoes, or winter squash.)

- -3 None
- +1 1 to 3 servings
- +2 4 to 6 servings
- +3 7 or more servings

____ 4. How many servings of leafy green vegetables do you eat per week? (One serving = ½ cup cooked or 1 cup raw. Only count collards, kale, mustard greens, romaine lettuce, spinach, or Swiss chard.)

- -3 None
- -2 Less than 1 serving
- +1 1 to 2 servings
- +2 3 to 4 servings
- +3 5 or more servings

____ 5. How many times per week does your lunch or dinner contain grains, vegetables, or beans, but little or no meat, poultry, fish, eggs, or cheese?

- -1 None
- +1 1 to 2 times
- +2 3 to 4 times
- +3 5 or more times

____ 6. How many times per week do you eat beans, split peas, or lentils? (Omit green beans.)

- -3 None
- -1 Less than 1 time
- 0 1 times
- +1 2 times
- +2 3 times
- +3 4 or more times

____ 7. How many servings of grains do you eat per day? (One serving = 1 slice of bread, 1 oz of crackers, 1 large pancake, 1 cup pasta or cold cereal, or ½ cup granola, cooked cereal, rice, or bulgur. Omit heavily sweetened cold cereals.)

- -3 None
- 0 1 to 2 servings
- +1 3 to 4 servings
- +2 5 to 7 servings
- +3 8 or more servings

____ 8. What type of bread, rolls, etc., do you eat?

- +3 100% whole wheat as the only flour
- +2 Whole-wheat flour as 1st or 2nd flour
- +1 Rye, pumpernickel, or oatmeal
- 0 White, French, or Italian

____ 9. What kind of breakfast do you eat?

- +3 Whole-grain (like oatmeal or Wheaties)
- 0 Low-fiber (like Cream of Wheat or Corn Flakes)
- -1 Sugary low-fiber (like Frosted Flakes or low-fat granola)
- -2 Regular granola

Meat, Poultry, and Seafood

____ 10. How many times per week do you eat high-fat red meats (*hamburgers, pork chops, ribs, hot dogs, pot roast, sausage, bologna, steaks other than round steak, etc.*)?

+3   None
+2   Less than 1 time
-1   1 time
-2   2 times
-3   3 times
-4   4 times

____ 11. How many times per week do you eat lean red meats (*hot dogs or luncheon meats with no more than 2 grams of fat per serving, round steak, or pork tenderloin*)?

+3   None
+1   Less than 1 time
0   1 time
-1   2 to 3 times
-2   4 to 5 times
-3   6 or more times

____ 12. After cooking, how large is the serving of red meat you eat? (*To convert from raw to cooked, reduce by 25 percent. For example, 4 oz of raw meat shrinks to 3 oz after cooking. There are 16 oz in a pound*).

-3   6 oz or more
-2   4 to 5 oz
0   3 oz or less
+3   Don't eat red meat

____ 13. If you eat red meat, do you trim the visible fat when you cook or eat it?

+1   Yes
-3   No

____ 14. What kind of ground meat or poultry do you eat?

-4   Regular ground beef
-3   Ground beef that's 11 to 25% fat
-2   Ground chicken or 10% fat ground beef
-1   Ground turkey
+3   Ground turkey breast
+3   Don't eat ground meat or poultry

____ 15. What chicken parts do you eat?

+3   Breast
+1   Drumstick
-1   Thigh
-2   Wing
+3   Don't eat poultry

____ 16. If you eat poultry, do you remove the skin before eating?

+2   Yes
-3   No

____ 17. If you eat seafood, how many times per week? (*Omit deep-fried foods, tuna packed in oil, and mayonnaise-laden tuna salad—low-fat mayo is okay.*)

0   Less than 1 time
+1   1 time
+2   2 times
+3   3 or more times

Mixed Foods

____ 18. What is your most typical breakfast? (*Subtract an extra 3 points if you also eat sausage.*)

-4   Biscuit sandwich or croissant sandwich
-3   Croissant, Danish, or doughnut
-3   Eggs
-1   Pancakes, French toast, or waffles
+3   Cereal, toast, or bagel (no cream cheese)
+3   Low-fat yogurt or low-fat cottage cheese
0   Don't eat breakfast

____ 19. What sandwich fillings do you eat?

-3   Regular luncheon meat, cheese, or egg salad
-2   Tuna or chicken salad or ham
0   Peanut butter
+1   Roast beef
+1   Low-fat luncheon meat
+3   Tuna or chicken salad made with fat-free mayo
+3   Turkey breast or humus

____ 20. What do you order on your pizza? (*Subtract 1 point if you order extra cheese, cheese-filled crust, or more than one meat topping*).

+3   No cheese with at least one vegetable topping
-1   Cheese with at least one vegetable topping
-2   Cheese
-3   Cheese with one meat topping
+3   Don't eat pizza

____ 21. What do you put on your pasta? (*Add one point if you also add sautéed vegetables.*)

+3   Tomato sauce or red clam sauce
-1   Meat sauce or meat balls
-3   Pesto or another oily sauce
-4   Alfredo or another creamy sauce

22. How many times per week do you eat deep-fried foods (*fish, chicken, French fries, potato chips, etc.)*?

+3 None
0 1 time
-1 2 times
-2 3 times
-3 4 or more times

23. At a salad bar, what do you choose?

+3 Nothing, lemon, or vinegar
+2 Fat-free dressing
+1 Low- or reduced-calorie dressing
-1 Oil and vinegar
-2 Regular dressing
-2 Cole slaw, pasta salad, or potato salad
-3 Cheese or eggs

24. How many times per week do you eat canned or dried soups or frozen dinners? *(Omit lower-sodium, low-fat ones.)*

+3 None
0 1 time
-1 2 times
-2 3 to 4 times
-3 5 or more times

25. How many servings of low-fat calcium-rich foods do you eat per day? *(One serving = ⅔ cup low-fat or nonfat milk or yogurt, 1 oz low-fat cheese, 1½ oz sardines, 3½ oz canned salmon with bones, 1 oz tofu made with calcium sulfate, 1 cup collards or kale, or 200 mg of a calcium supplement.)*

-3 None
-1 Less than 1 serving
+1 1 serving
+2 2 servings
+3 3 or more servings

26. How many times per week do you eat cheese? *(Include pizza, cheeseburgers, lasagna, tacos or nachos with cheese, etc. Omit foods made with low-fat cheese.)*

+3 None
+1 1 time
-1 2 times
-2 3 times
-3 4 or more times

27. How many egg yolks do you eat per week? *(Add 1 yolk for every slice of quiche you eat.)*

+3 None
+1 1 yolk
0 2 yolks
-1 3 yolks
-2 4 yolks
-3 5 or more yolks

Fats & Oils

28. What do you put on your bread, toast, bagel, or English muffin?

-4 Stick butter or cream cheese
-3 Stick margarine or whipped butter
-2 Regular tub margarine
-1 Light tub margarine or whipped light butter
0 Jam, fat-free margarine, or fat-free cream cheese
+3 Nothing

29. What do you spread on your sandwiches?

-2 Mayonnaise
-1 Light mayonnaise
+1 Catsup, mustard, or fat-free mayonnaise
+2 Nothing

30. With what do you make tuna salad, pasta salad, chicken salad, etc.?

-2 Mayonnaise
-1 Light mayonnaise
0 Fat-free mayonnaise
+2 Nothing

31. What do you use to sauté vegetables or other food? *(Vegetable oil includes safflower, corn, sunflower, and soybean.)*

-3 Butter or lard
-2 Margarine
-1 Vegetable oil or light margarine
+1 Olive or canola oil
+2 Broth
+3 Cooking spray

Beverages

32. What do you drink on a typical day?

+3 Water or club soda
0 Caffeine-free coffee or tea
-1 Diet soda
-1 Coffee or tea (up to 4 a day)
-2 Regular soda (up to 2 a day)
-3 Regular soda (3 or more a day)
-3 Coffee or tea (5 or more a day)

____ 33. What kind of "fruit" beverage do you drink?

+3 Orange, grapefruit, prune, or pineapple juice

+1 Apple, grape, or pear juice

0   Cranberry juice blend or cocktail

-3 Fruit "drink," "ade," or "punch"

____ 34. What kind of milk do you drink?

-3 Whole

-1 2% fat

+2 1% low-fat

+3 skim

____ 35. What do you eat as a snack?

+3 Fruits or vegetables

+2 Low-fat yogurt

+1 Low-fat crackers

-2 Cookies or fried chips

-2 Nuts or granola bar

-3 Candy bar or pastry

____ 36. Which of the following "salty" snacks do you eat?

-3 Potato chips, corn chips, or popcorn

-2 Tortilla chips

-1 Salted pretzels or light microwave popcorn

+2 Unsalted pretzels

+3 Baked tortilla or potato chips or homemade air-popped popcorn

+3 Don't eat salty snacks

____ 37. What kind of cookies do you eat?

+2 Fat-free cookies

+1 Graham crackers or reduced-fat cookies

-1 Oatmeal cookies

-2 Sandwich cookies (like Oreos)

-3 Chocolate coated, chocolate chip, or peanut butter cookies

+3 Don't eat cookies

____ 38. What kind of cake or pastry do you eat?

-4 Cheesecake

-3 Pie or doughnuts

-2 Cake with frosting

-1 Cake without frosting

0   Muffins

+1 Angle food, fat-free cake, or fat-free pastry

+3 Don't eat cakes or pastries

____ 39. What kind of frozen dessert do you eat? (*Subtract 1 point for each of the following toppings: hot fudge, nuts, or chocolate candy bars or pieces.*)

-4 Gourmet ice cream

-3 Regular ice cream

-1 Frozen yogurt or light ice cream

-1 Sorbet, sherbet, or ices

+1 Nonfat frozen yogurt or fat-free ice cream

+3 Don't eat frozen desserts

____ **Total Score**

Add up your score for each question and write it in the "total score" line above. **If your score is:**

1 to 29   Don't be discouraged. Eating healthy is tough, but you can learn to eat healthier.

30 to 59   Congratulations. Your are doing just fine. Pin your Quiz to the nearest wall.

60 or above Excellent. You're a nutrition superstar. Give yourself a big pat on the back.

Source: Adapted with permission from *Nutrition Action Healthletter*, May 1996, V23/N4. (*Nutrition Action Healthletter*, 1875 Connecticut Ave., N.W., Suite 300, Washington DC 20009-5728. $24 for 10 issues.)

Rate Your Diet Quiz—Lesson Eight

The following questions will give you a rough sketch of your typical eating habits. The (+) or (-) number for each answer instantly pats you on the back for good eating habits or alerts you to problems you didn't even know you had. The quiz focuses on fat, saturated fat, cholesterol, sodium, sugar, fiber, and fruits and vegetables. It doesn't attempt to cover everything in your diet. Also, it doesn't try to measure precisely how much of the key nutrients you eat. Next to each answer is a number with a + or - sign in front of it. Circle the number that corresponds to the answer you choose and write that score (e.g., +1) in the space provided in front of each question. That's your score for the question. If two or more answers apply, circle each one. Then average them to get your score for the question.

How to average. In answering question 19, for example, if your sandwich-eating is equally divided among tuna salad (-2), roast beef (+1), and turkey breast (+3), add the three scores (which gives you +2) and then divide by three. That gives you a score of +⅔ for the question. Round it to +1. Pay attention to serving sizes, which are given when needed. For example, a serving of vegetables is ½ cup. If you usually eat one cup of vegetables at a time, count it as two servings. If you're ready, let's start.

Fruits, Vegetables, Grains, and Beans

____ 1. How many servings of fruit or 100% fruit juice do you eat per day? (*OMIT fruit snacks like Fruit Roll-Ups and fruit-on-the-bottom yogurt. One serving = one piece or ½ cup of fruit or 6 oz of fruit juice.*)

-3 None
-2 Less than 1 serving
0 1 serving
+1 2 serving
+2 3 serving
+3 4 or more servings

____ 2. How many servings of non-fried vegetables do you eat per day? (*One serving = ½ cup. Include potatoes.*)

-3 None
-2 Less than 1 serving
0 1 serving
+1 2 serving
+2 3 serving
+3 4 or more servings

____ 3. How many servings of vitamin-rich vegetables do you eat per week? (*One serving = ½ cup. Only count broccoli, Brussels sprouts, carrots, collards, kale, red pepper, spinach, sweet potatoes, or winter squash.*)

-3 None
+1 1 to 3 servings
+2 4 to 6 servings
+3 7 or more servings

____ 4. How many servings of leafy green vegetables do you eat per week? (*One serving = ½ cup cooked or 1 cup raw. Only count collards, kale, mustard greens, romaine lettuce, spinach, or Swiss chard.*)

-3 None
-2 Less than 1 serving
+1 1 to 2 servings
+2 3 to 4 servings
+3 5 or more servings

____ 5. How many times per week does your lunch or dinner contain grains, vegetables, or beans, but little or no meat, poultry, fish, eggs, or cheese?

-1 None
+1 1 to 2 times
+2 3 to 4 times
+3 5 or more times

____ 6. How many times per week do you eat beans, split peas, or lentils? (*Omit green beans.*)

-3 None
-1 Less than 1 time
0 1 times
+1 2 times
+2 3 times
+3 4 or more times

____ 7. How many servings of grains do you eat per day? (*One serving = 1 slice of bread, 1 oz of crackers, 1 large pancake, 1 cup pasta or cold cereal, or ½ cup granola, cooked cereal, rice, or bulgur. Omit heavily sweetened cold cereals.*)

-3 None
0 1 to 2 servings
+1 3 to 4 servings
+2 5 to 7 servings
+3 8 or more servings

____ 8. What type of bread, rolls, etc., do you eat?

+3 100% whole wheat as the only flour
+2 Whole-wheat flour as 1st or 2nd flour
+1 Rye, pumpernickel, or oatmeal
0 White, French, or Italian

____ 9. What kind of breakfast do you eat?

+3 Whole-grain (like oatmeal or Wheaties)
0 Low-fiber (like Cream of Wheat or Corn Flakes)
-1 Sugary low-fiber (like Frosted Flakes or low-fat granola)
-2 Regular granola

Meat, Poultry, and Seafood

____ 10. How many times per week do you eat high-fat red meats (*hamburgers, pork chops, ribs, hot dogs, pot roast, sausage, bologna, steaks other than round steak, etc.*)?

+3 None
+2 Less than 1 time
-1 1 time
-2 2 times
-3 3 times
-4 4 times

____ 11. How many times per week do you eat lean red meats (*hot dogs or luncheon meats with no more than 2 grams of fat per serving, round steak, or pork tenderloin*)?

+3 None
+1 Less than 1 time
0 1 time
-1 2 to 3 times
-2 4 to 5 times
-3 6 or more times

____ 12. After cooking, how large is the serving of red meat you eat? (*To convert from raw to cooked, reduce by 25 percent. For example, 4 oz of raw meat shrinks to 3 oz after cooking. There are 16 oz in a pound*).

-3 6 oz or more
-2 4 to 5 oz
0 3 oz or less
+3 Don't eat red meat

____ 13. If you eat red meat, do you trim the visible fat when you cook or eat it?

+1 Yes
-3 No

____ 14. What kind of ground meat or poultry do you eat?

-4 Regular ground beef
-3 Ground beef that's 11 to 25% fat
-2 Ground chicken or 10% fat ground beef
-1 Ground turkey
+3 Ground turkey breast
+3 Don't eat ground meat or poultry

____ 15. What chicken parts do you eat?

+3 Breast
+1 Drumstick
-1 Thigh
-2 Wing
+3 Don't eat poultry

____ 16. If you eat poultry, do you remove the skin before eating?

+2 Yes
-3 No

____ 17. If you eat seafood, how many times per week? (*Omit deep-fried foods, tuna packed in oil, and mayonnaise-laden tuna salad—low-fat mayo is okay.*)

0 Less than 1 time
+1 1 time
+2 2 times
+3 3 or more times

Mixed Foods

____ 18. What is your most typical breakfast? (*Subtract an extra 3 points if you also eat sausage.*)

-4 Biscuit sandwich or croissant sandwich
-3 Croissant, Danish, or doughnut
-3 Eggs
-1 Pancakes, French toast, or waffles
+3 Cereal, toast, or bagel (no cream cheese)
+3 Low-fat yogurt or low-fat cottage cheese
0 Don't eat breakfast

____ 19. What sandwich fillings do you eat?

-3 Regular luncheon meat, cheese, or egg salad
-2 Tuna or chicken salad or ham
0 Peanut butter
+1 Roast beef
+1 Low-fat luncheon meat
+3 Tuna or chicken salad made with fat-free mayo
+3 Turkey breast or humus

____ 20. What do you order on your pizza? (*Subtract 1 point if you order extra cheese, cheese-filled crust, or more than one meat topping*).

+3 No cheese with at least one vegetable topping
-1 Cheese with at least one vegetable topping
-2 Cheese
-3 Cheese with one meat topping
+3 Don't eat pizza

____ 21. What do you put on your pasta? (*Add one point if you also add sautéed vegetables.*)

+3 Tomato sauce or red clam sauce
-1 Meat sauce or meat balls
-3 Pesto or another oily sauce
-4 Alfredo or another creamy sauce

22. How many times per week do you eat deep-fried foods (*fish, chicken, French fries, potato chips, etc.*)?

+3 None
0 1 time
-1 2 times
-2 3 times
-3 4 or more times

23. At a salad bar, what do you choose?

+3 Nothing, lemon, or vinegar
+2 Fat-free dressing
+1 Low- or reduced-calorie dressing
-1 Oil and vinegar
-2 Regular dressing
-2 Cole slaw, pasta salad, or potato salad
-3 Cheese or eggs

24. How many times per week do you eat canned or dried soups or frozen dinners? (*Omit lower-sodium, low-fat ones.*)

+3 None
0 1 time
-1 2 times
-2 3 to 4 times
-3 5 or more times

25. How many servings of low-fat calcium-rich foods do you eat per day? (*One serving = ⅔ cup low-fat or nonfat milk or yogurt, 1 oz low-fat cheese, 1½ oz sardines, 3½ oz canned salmon with bones, 1 oz tofu made with calcium sulfate, 1 cup collards or kale, or 200 mg of a calcium supplement.*)

-3 None
-1 Less than 1 serving
+1 1 serving
+2 2 servings
+3 3 or more servings

26. How many times per week do you eat cheese? (*Include pizza, cheeseburgers, lasagna, tacos or nachos with cheese, etc. Omit foods made with low-fat cheese.*)

+3 None
+1 1 time
-1 2 times
-2 3 times
-3 4 or more times

27. How many egg yolks do you eat per week? (*Add 1 yolk for every slice of quiche you eat.*)

+3 None
+1 1 yolk
0 2 yolks
-1 3 yolks
-2 4 yolks
-3 5 or more yolks

Fats & Oils

28. What do you put on your bread, toast, bagel, or English muffin?

-4 Stick butter or cream cheese
-3 Stick margarine or whipped butter
-2 Regular tub margarine
-1 Light tub margarine or whipped light butter
0 Jam, fat-free margarine, or fat-free cream cheese
+3 Nothing

29. What do you spread on your sandwiches?

-2 Mayonnaise
-1 Light mayonnaise
+1 Catsup, mustard, or fat-free mayonnaise
+2 Nothing

30. With what do you make tuna salad, pasta salad, chicken salad, etc.?

-2 Mayonnaise
-1 Light mayonnaise
0 Fat-free mayonnaise
+2 Nothing

31. What do you use to sauté vegetables or other food? (*Vegetable oil includes safflower, corn, sunflower, and soybean.*)

-3 Butter or lard
-2 Margarine
-1 Vegetable oil or light margarine
+1 Olive or canola oil
+2 Broth
+3 Cooking spray

Beverages

32. What do you drink on a typical day?

+3 Water or club soda
0 Caffeine-free coffee or tea
-1 Diet soda
-1 Coffee or tea (up to 4 a day)
-2 Regular soda (up to 2 a day)
-3 Regular soda (3 or more a day)
-3 Coffee or tea (5 or more a day)

_____ 33. What kind of "fruit" beverage do you drink?

+3   Orange, grapefruit, prune, or
      pineapple juice

+1   Apple, grape, or pear juice

0   Cranberry juice blend or cocktail

-3   Fruit "drink," "ade," or "punch"

_____ 34. What kind of milk do you drink?

-3   Whole

-1   2% fat

+2   1% low-fat

+3   skim

_____ 35. What do you eat as a snack?

+3   Fruits or vegetables

+2   Low-fat yogurt

+1   Low-fat crackers

-2   Cookies or fried chips

-2   Nuts or granola bar

-3   Candy bar or pastry

_____ 36. Which of the following "salty" snacks do you
      eat?

-3   Potato chips, corn chips, or popcorn

-2   Tortilla chips

-1   Salted pretzels or light microwave
      popcorn

+2   Unsalted pretzels

+3   Baked tortilla or potato chips or
      homemade air-popped popcorn

+3   Don't eat salty snacks

_____ 37. What kind of cookies do you eat?

+2   Fat-free cookies

+1   Graham crackers or reduced-fat
      cookies

-1   Oatmeal cookies

-2   Sandwich cookies (like Oreos)

-3   Chocolate coated, chocolate chip,
      or peanut butter cookies

+3   Don't eat cookies

_____ 38. What kind of cake or pastry do you eat?

-4   Cheesecake

-3   Pie or doughnuts

-2   Cake with frosting

-1   Cake without frosting

0   Muffins

+1   Angle food, fat-free cake, or
      fat-free pastry

+3   Don't eat cakes or pastries

_____ 39. What kind of frozen dessert do you eat? (Sub-
      *tract 1 point for each of the following toppings:
      hot fudge, nuts, or chocolate candy bars or
      pieces.)*

-4   Gourmet ice cream

-3   Regular ice cream

-1   Frozen yogurt or light ice cream

-1   Sorbet, sherbet, or ices

+1   Nonfat frozen yogurt or fat-free
      ice cream

+3   Don't eat frozen desserts

_____   **Total Score**

Add up your score for each question and write it in the "total score" line above. **If your score is:**

1 to 29   Don't be discouraged. Eating healthy is
            tough, but you can learn to eat healthier.

30 to 59   Congratulations. Your are doing just fine.
            Pin your Quiz to the nearest wall.

60 or above Excellent. You're a nutrition superstar.
            Give yourself a big pat on the back.

Source: Adapted with permission from *Nutrition Action Healthletter,* May 1996, V23/N4. (*Nutrition Action Healthletter,* 1875 Connecticut Ave., N.W., Suite 300, Washington DC 20009-5728. $24 for 10 issues.)

Rate Your Diet Quiz—Lesson Sixteen

The following questions will give you a rough sketch of your typical eating habits. The (+) or (-) number for each answer instantly pats you on the back for good eating habits or alerts you to problems you didn't even know you had. The quiz focuses on fat, saturated fat, cholesterol, sodium, sugar, fiber, and fruits and vegetables. It doesn't attempt to cover everything in your diet. Also, it doesn't try to measure precisely how much of the key nutrients you eat. Next to each answer is a number with a + or - sign in front of it. Circle the number that corresponds to the answer you choose and write that score (e.g., +1) in the space provided in front of each question. That's your score for the question. If two or more answers apply, circle each one. Then average them to get your score for the question.

How to average. In answering question 19, for example, if your sandwich-eating is equally divided among tuna salad (-2), roast beef (+1), and turkey breast (+3), add the three scores (which gives you +2) and then divide by three. That gives you a score of +⅔ for the question. Round it to +1. Pay attention to serving sizes, which are given when needed. For example, a serving of vegetables is ½ cup. If you usually eat one cup of vegetables at a time, count it as two servings. If you're ready, let's start.

Fruits, Vegetables, Grains, and Beans

1. How many servings of fruit or 100% fruit juice do you eat per day? (*OMIT fruit snacks like Fruit Roll-Ups and fruit-on-the-bottom yogurt. One serving = one piece or ½ cup of fruit or 6 oz of fruit juice.*)

-3	None
-2	Less than 1 serving
0	1 serving
+1	2 serving
+2	3 serving
+3	4 or more servings

2. How many servings of non-fried vegetables do you eat per day? (*One serving = ½ cup. Include potatoes.*)

-3	None
-2	Less than 1 serving
0	1 serving
+1	2 serving
+2	3 serving
+3	4 or more servings

3. How many servings of vitamin-rich vegetables do you eat per week? (*One serving = ½ cup. Only count broccoli, Brussels sprouts, carrots, collards, kale, red pepper, spinach, sweet potatoes, or winter squash.*)

-3	None
+1	1 to 3 servings
+2	4 to 6 servings
+3	7 or more servings

4. How many servings of leafy green vegetables do you eat per week? (*One serving = ½ cup cooked or 1 cup raw. Only count collards, kale, mustard greens, romaine lettuce, spinach, or Swiss chard.*)

-3	None
-2	Less than 1 serving
+1	1 to 2 servings
+2	3 to 4 servings
+3	5 or more servings

5. How many times per week does your lunch or dinner contain grains, vegetables, or beans, but little or no meat, poultry, fish, eggs, or cheese?

-1	None
+1	1 to 2 times
+2	3 to 4 times
+3	5 or more times

6. How many times per week do you eat beans, split peas, or lentils? (*Omit green beans.*)

-3	None
-1	Less than 1 time
0	1 times
+1	2 times
+2	3 times
+3	4 or more times

7. How many servings of grains do you eat per day? (*One serving = 1 slice of bread, 1 oz of crackers, 1 large pancake, 1 cup pasta or cold cereal, or ½ cup granola, cooked cereal, rice, or bulgur. Omit heavily sweetened cold cereals.*)

-3	None
0	1 to 2 servings
+1	3 to 4 servings
+2	5 to 7 servings
+3	8 or more servings

8. What type of bread, rolls, etc., do you eat?

+3	100% whole wheat as the only flour
+2	Whole-wheat flour as 1st or 2nd flour
+1	Rye, pumpernickel, or oatmeal
0	White, French, or Italian

9. What kind of breakfast do you eat?

+3	Whole-grain (like oatmeal or Wheaties)
0	Low-fiber (like Cream of Wheat or Corn Flakes)
-1	Sugary low-fiber (like Frosted Flakes or low-fat granola)
-2	Regular granola

Meat, Poultry, and Seafood

____ 10. How many times per week do you eat high-fat red meats *(hamburgers, pork chops, ribs, hot dogs, pot roast, sausage, bologna, steaks other than round steak, etc.)*?

+3	None
+2	Less than 1 time
-1	1 time
-2	2 times
-3	3 times
-4	4 times

____ 11. How many times per week do you eat lean red meats *(hot dogs or luncheon meats with no more than 2 grams of fat per serving, round steak, or pork tenderloin)*?

+3	None
+1	Less than 1 time
0	1 time
-1	2 to 3 times
-2	4 to 5 times
-3	6 or more times

____ 12. After cooking, how large is the serving of red meat you eat? *(To convert from raw to cooked, reduce by 25 percent. For example, 4 oz of raw meat shrinks to 3 oz after cooking. There are 16 oz in a pound)*.

-3	6 oz or more
-2	4 to 5 oz
0	3 oz or less
+3	Don't eat red meat

____ 13. If you eat red meat, do you trim the visible fat when you cook or eat it?

+1	Yes
-3	No

____ 14. What kind of ground meat or poultry do you eat?

-4	Regular ground beef
-3	Ground beef that's 11 to 25% fat
-2	Ground chicken or 10% fat ground beef
-1	Ground turkey
+3	Ground turkey breast
+3	Don't eat ground meat or poultry

____ 15. What chicken parts do you eat?

+3	Breast
+1	Drumstick
-1	Thigh
-2	Wing
+3	Don't eat poultry

____ 16. If you eat poultry, do you remove the skin before eating?

+2	Yes
-3	No

____ 17. If you eat seafood, how many times per week? *(Omit deep-fried foods, tuna packed in oil, and mayonnaise-laden tuna salad—low-fat mayo is okay.)*

0	Less than 1 time
+1	1 time
+2	2 times
+3	3 or more times

Mixed Foods

____ 18. What is your most typical breakfast? *(Subtract an extra 3 points if you also eat sausage.)*

-4	Biscuit sandwich or croissant sandwich
-3	Croissant, Danish, or doughnut
-3	Eggs
-1	Pancakes, French toast, or waffles
+3	Cereal, toast, or bagel (no cream cheese)
+3	Low-fat yogurt or low-fat cottage cheese
0	Don't eat breakfast

____ 19. What sandwich fillings do you eat?

-3	Regular luncheon meat, cheese, or egg salad
-2	Tuna or chicken salad or ham
0	Peanut butter
+1	Roast beef
+1	Low-fat luncheon meat
+3	Tuna or chicken salad made with fat-free mayo
+3	Turkey breast or humus

____ 20. What do you order on your pizza? *(Subtract 1 point if you order extra cheese, cheese-filled crust, or more than one meat topping)*.

+3	No cheese with at least one vegetable topping
-1	Cheese with at least one vegetable topping
-2	Cheese
-3	Cheese with one meat topping
+3	Don't eat pizza

____ 21. What do you put on your pasta? *(Add one point if you also add sautéed vegetables.)*

+3	Tomato sauce or red clam sauce
-1	Meat sauce or meat balls
-3	Pesto or another oily sauce
-4	Alfredo or another creamy sauce

22. How many times per week do you eat deep-fried foods (*fish, chicken, French fries, potato chips, etc.*)?

+3 None
0 1 time
-1 2 times
-2 3 times
-3 4 or more times

23. At a salad bar, what do you choose?

+3 Nothing, lemon, or vinegar
+2 Fat-free dressing
+1 Low- or reduced-calorie dressing
-1 Oil and vinegar
-2 Regular dressing
-2 Cole slaw, pasta salad, or potato salad
-3 Cheese or eggs

24. How many times per week do you eat canned or dried soups or frozen dinners? (*Omit lower-sodium, low-fat ones.*)

+3 None
0 1 time
-1 2 times
-2 3 to 4 times
-3 5 or more times

25. How many servings of low-fat calcium-rich foods do you eat per day? (*One serving = ⅔ cup low-fat or nonfat milk or yogurt, 1 oz low-fat cheese, 1½ oz sardines, 3½ oz canned salmon with bones, 1 oz tofu made with calcium sulfate, 1 cup collards or kale, or 200 mg of a calcium supplement.*)

-3 None
-1 Less than 1 serving
+1 1 serving
+2 2 servings
+3 3 or more servings

26. How many times per week do you eat cheese? (*Include pizza, cheeseburgers, lasagna, tacos or nachos with cheese, etc. Omit foods made with low-fat cheese.*)

+3 None
+1 1 time
-1 2 times
-2 3 times
-3 4 or more times

27. How many egg yolks do you eat per week? (*Add 1 yolk for every slice of quiche you eat.*)

+3 None
+1 1 yolk
0 2 yolks
-1 3 yolks
-2 4 yolks
-3 5 or more yolks

Fats & Oils

28. What do you put on your bread, toast, bagel, or English muffin?

-4 Stick butter or cream cheese
-3 Stick margarine or whipped butter
-2 Regular tub margarine
-1 Light tub margarine or whipped light butter
0 Jam, fat-free margarine, or fat-free cream cheese
+3 Nothing

29. What do you spread on your sandwiches?

-2 Mayonnaise
-1 Light mayonnaise
+1 Catsup, mustard, or fat-free mayonnaise
+2 Nothing

30. With what do you make tuna salad, pasta salad, chicken salad, etc.?

-2 Mayonnaise
-1 Light mayonnaise
0 Fat-free mayonnaise
+2 Nothing

31. What do you use to sauté vegetables or other food? (*Vegetable oil includes safflower, corn, sunflower, and soybean.*)

-3 Butter or lard
-2 Margarine
-1 Vegetable oil or light margarine
+1 Olive or canola oil
+2 Broth
+3 Cooking spray

Beverages

32. What do you drink on a typical day?

+3 Water or club soda
0 Caffeine-free coffee or tea
-1 Diet soda
-1 Coffee or tea (up to 4 a day)
-2 Regular soda (up to 2 a day)
-3 Regular soda (3 or more a day)
-3 Coffee or tea (5 or more a day)

_____ 33. What kind of "fruit" beverage do you drink?

+3   Orange, grapefruit, prune, or pineapple juice

+1   Apple, grape, or pear juice

0   Cranberry juice blend or cocktail

-3   Fruit "drink," "ade," or "punch"

_____ 34. What kind of milk do you drink?

-3   Whole

-1   2% fat

+2   1% low-fat

+3   skim

_____ 35. What do you eat as a snack?

+3   Fruits or vegetables

+2   Low-fat yogurt

+1   Low-fat crackers

-2   Cookies or fried chips

-2   Nuts or granola bar

-3   Candy bar or pastry

_____ 36. Which of the following "salty" snacks do you eat?

-3   Potato chips, corn chips, or popcorn

-2   Tortilla chips

-1   Salted pretzels or light microwave popcorn

+2   Unsalted pretzels

+3   Baked tortilla or potato chips or homemade air-popped popcorn

+3   Don't eat salty snacks

_____ 37. What kind of cookies do you eat?

+2   Fat-free cookies

+1   Graham crackers or reduced-fat cookies

-1   Oatmeal cookies

-2   Sandwich cookies (like Oreos)

-3   Chocolate coated, chocolate chip, or peanut butter cookies

+3   Don't eat cookies

_____ 38. What kind of cake or pastry do you eat?

-4   Cheesecake

-3   Pie or doughnuts

-2   Cake with frosting

-1   Cake without frosting

0   Muffins

+1   Angle food, fat-free cake, or fat-free pastry

+3   Don't eat cakes or pastries

_____ 39. What kind of frozen dessert do you eat? (*Subtract 1 point for each of the following toppings: hot fudge, nuts, or chocolate candy bars or pieces.*)

-4   Gourmet ice cream

-3   Regular ice cream

-1   Frozen yogurt or light ice cream

-1   Sorbet, sherbet, or ices

+1   Nonfat frozen yogurt or fat-free ice cream

+3   Don't eat frozen desserts

_____ **Total Score**

Add up your score for each question and write it in the "total score" line above. **If your score is:**

1 to 29   Don't be discouraged. Eating healthy is tough, but you can learn to eat healthier.

30 to 59   Congratulations. Your are doing just fine. Pin your Quiz to the nearest wall.

60 or above   Excellent. You're a nutrition superstar. Give yourself a big pat on the back.

Source: Adapted with permission from *Nutrition Action Healthletter*, May 1996, V23/N4. (*Nutrition Action Healthletter*, 1875 Connecticut Ave., N.W., Suite 300, Washington DC 20009-5728. $24 for 10 issues.)

INDEX

A

ABC's of Behavior, 58, 197
   Antecedents, 58, 124, 198
     Behavior, 58, 198
     Consequences, 59
Achievements
   See reviewing your progress
Activity
   See physical activity
Aerobics, 128, 173
   See also physical activity
Alcohol, 185, 223
   Calories in, 223
     Making you vulnerable to eat more, 223
American Association of LifeStyle Counselors, 304
American College of Sports Medicine, 118
American Dietetic Association, 66
Amino acids, 148
   Essential, 148
   Nonessential, 148
Antecedents, 58
   See also ABC's of Behavior
Appetite
   The effects of exercise on, 34
Arsenic, 120
Attitude traps
   Dichotomous (light bulb) thinking, 220
   Imperatives, 159
   Impossible dream thinking, 142
   Internal, 131
     Countering, 131
   Negative self-talk, 95
Attitudes
   Shaping, 60

B

Baked Italian chicken dinner, 30
B-complex vitamins
   See vitamins
Behavior chain
   Analyzing, 207
   Interrupting, 203
   My, 206
   Sample, 204
Binge eating
   See eating
   Overcoming Binge Eating, 125
Binge Eating Disorder, 124
Body image

Challenging faulty assumptions, 112
Confront what is realistic, 112
Effect on self-esteem, 110
Getting accustomed to seeing your body, 112
Improving, 111
The Body Image Workbook, 111
Uncoupling from self-esteem, 112
Your body as a gift, 112
Boron, 120
Breakfast, 236
   Importance of, 236
   Strategies for eating, 237
Breast cancer, 103
Brownell, Kelly D.
   About the author, 311
Burger King, 209
Butter, 104

C

Calcium, 120, 121, 234
Calisthenics, 173
Calorie
   Burning through physical activity, 34
   Definition, 36
   Empty, 185
   Hidden, 185
   How many make a pound, 38
   The mighty, 62
   Where you can get just 10, 62
Calorie guide
   How to get one, 16
   Using, 17
Calorie levels
   Determining your target, 44
   Of fat, 104
   Setting your target, 88
     Not all people are created equal, 37
Carbohydrate, 119
   Calories per gram, 166
   Complex, 166
   Definition of, 166
   Extra calorie burning, 166
   In your diet, 165
   Recommended amount in diet, 166
   Simple, 166
   Starch, 166
Cardiorespiratory fitness, 129
Cardiovascular conditioning, 173

Cardiovascular training
   See physical activity
Cellulose, 176
Cereal, 192
Charts
   See tables and charts, 128
Chlorine, 120
Cholesterol, 12, 151, 189, 221
   Blood, 223
   Content of common foods, 222
   Definition, 221
   HDL, 221
   Recommended blood levels, 221
Chromium, 120
Chutes and Ladders, 230
Cobalamin
   See vitamin B_{12}
Cobalt, 120, 233
Collapse
   See relapse
Colon cancer, 103
Communicating with your partner, 90
Complex sugars (carbohydrate)
   See carbohydrate
Compulsive eating
   See eating
Confidence
   Building, 13
   Effects of exercise on, 34
   See also skills
Consequences, 59
Controlling eating
   Calories should be tasted, not wasted, 75
   Do not clean your plate, 77
   Do nothing else while eating, 75
   Eat in one place, 76
   Follow an eating schedule, 76
   Slowing your eating rate, 85
     Techniques for, 85
   Strategies for, 76
Cooking tips to reduce fat, 107
Cooper Institute for Aerobics Research, 172
Copper, 120
Cravings
   Conquering, 60
     Confrontation, 60
     Distraction, 60
   See also hunger

Vs. hunger quiz, 53
Vs. hunger, 52

D

Daily Reference Value, 147

Dessert, 185
    Dietary fat in, 107
Diabetes, 12

Dichotomous (light bulb) thinking
    See attitude traps,
Diet
    Following a balanced, 63
    Making small changes in, 73
    Rate your diet quizzes, 283, 287, 291
    Rating your diet, 33
    Vs. lifestyle change, 12
Dietary balance, 63

Dietary fat
    Calculating daily calorie goal, 106
    Calorie content of, 104
    Chart of common foods with, 105
    Cooking tips to reduce, 107
    See also fat
    From the Bread, Cereal, Rice, & Pasta
        Group, 107
    From the Meat, Poultry, Fish, Dry
        Beans, Eggs, & Nuts Group, 107
    From the Milk, Yogurt, & Cheese
        Group, 106
    From the Vegetable and Fruit Groups,
        107
    How much to eat, 104
    Importance of, 103
    In snacks and desserts, 107
    Monounsaturated, 103
    Polyunsaturated, 103, 223
    Reduced-fat foods, 47
    Reducing the amount in your diet, 106
    Saturated, 103, 189, 223
    Sources of, 106
    The role of, 102
Dietary fiber
    See fiber
Dietary guidelines for Americans, 64

Dietary Reference Intakes, 147

DNA, 148

E

Eating
    Away from home, 183
    Binge, 124
    Compulsive, 124
    Dealing with pressures to eat, 157
    Dessert, 185
    Effect of alcohol on, 223
    Great meals, 29

Habits, 136
    Revisiting, 244
    Making a list of alternatives to, 218
    Restaurants, 183
    Sensible meals, 29
    See also stress
    Triggers for, 44
        See also controlling eating
        See also high-risk situations
    Using alternative activities, 218
Eating disorders
    See also Binge Eating Disorder
    See also eating
    Support groups, 125
Eating patterns
    Amount of food, 31
    Foods you eat, 32
    My eating patterns worksheet, lesson
        three, 45
    My eating patterns worksheet, lesson two,
        32
    Places you eat, 32
    Times that you eat, 31
Eating plan
    Calorie counting, 66
    Exchange plan, 66
    Selecting, 66
Emotional response, 186

Empty calories, 223

Enzymes, 148

Essential fatty acids, 103

Exercise
    A new view, 34
    Benefits of, 34
    Is it safe, 49
    See also physical activity
    The role of, 33
Expanded Food Diary
    See food diary

F

Family
    For them to read, 155
    Things they can do, 157
    Things they should avoid, 156
Family upbringing, 22

Fast food, 189

Fast-food restaurants, 209

Fat
    See dietary fat
    Vegetable, 103
Fat cells, 22

Fat grams
    Counting, 46

Fiber
    Description of, 176
    Facts and fantasies, 176
    Foods containing, 177
    In fast foods, 189
    Recommended daily intake of, 177
    Sources of, 176
Fluorine, 120

Folacin, 120, 167

Food
    Hiding the high-calorie, 123
    Importance of, 119
    Serving and dispensing, 137
        Avoid being a food dispenser, 139
        Follow the five-minute rule, 139
        Leave the table after eating, 138
        Remove dishes from the table, 138
        Serve and eat one portion at a time,
            138
    See also shopping for food
    Storing out of sight, 123
Food and weight fantasies, 79

Food diary
    Expanded food diary, 32
        Analyzing your, 43
        Lesson two sample, 40
        Lesson two, 41
    Lesson one, 27
    See also monitoring forms
    Purpose of, 15
    See also record keeping
    Reviewing, 30
    Sample, lesson one, 26
    Searching for patterns, 31
        Activity, 44
        Amount, 31
        Feelings, 43
        Foods, 32, 44
        Places, 32
        Time, 31, 43
Food Guide Pyramid
    A graphic illustration, 65
    Bread, Cereal, Rice, & Pasta Group,
        107, 190
    Description of, 64
    Dietary fat from, 105
    Fats, Oils, & Sweets, 106
    Fruit Group, 107, 178
    History of, 64
    Meat, Poultry, Fish, Dry Beans, Eggs,
        & Nuts Group, 107, 150
    Milk, Yogurt, & Cheese Group, 106,
        121
    Servings and calorie guide, 88
    Servings from the five food groups, 82

The importance of the five food groups, 87
Vegetable Group, 107, 167
Food labels
Daily Reference Value, 147
Daily values, 146
Dietary Reference Intakes, 147
Ingredients list, 147
Nutrition facts panel, 146
Nutrition Labeling and Education Act of 1990 (NLEA), 146
Purpose, 146
Reading, 145
Reference Daily Intakes, 147
Food portions
Food portion quiz, 87
Measuring, 86
The importance of knowing, 86
Visual guides, 87
Foods
Keeping healthy snacks, 124
Reduced-fat, 47
Forms
See worksheets and forms
Fructose, 166

Fruit
See also Food Guide Pyramid
In your diet, 178
Increasing dietary intake of, 178

G

Genetics, 21

Glands, 21

Goals
Automatic setting, 99
Setting out of reach, 100
The process of setting, 100
Goals and expectations
Setting program goals, 61
Setting realistic goals, 7, 99
Your goals and expectations, 6
Your vision of reasonable weight change, 38
Groups
Being a good group member, 36
Guidelines and responsibilities, 278
Guidelines for being a good member, 277
Importance of, 277
Responsibilities of members, 277

H

Habits
Making them permanent, 253
HDL
See cholesterol
Heart rate, 208

Height-weight tables, 12

Helpful resources
Certified LifeStyle Counselor, 304
LEARN Healthy Eating and Calorie Guide, 9, 304
LEARN Program Cassettes 2000, 8
LEARN Program Monitoring Forms, 304
LEARN WalkMaster, 9, 304
Living with Exercise 2000, 35, 304
Mastering Stress 2000—A LifeStyle Approach, 162, 304
Overcoming Binge Eating, 125, 304
The Body Image Workbook, 111, 304
Weight Control Digest, 304
Hemicellulose, 176

Hemoglobin, 148

High blood pressure, 12
See also hypertension

High density lipoprotein (HDL)
See cholesterol
High-risk situations
Identifying, 217
Triggers for eating, 44
Holidays, parties, and special events, 79, 231

Hunger
See also cravings
Cravings vs. quiz, 53
Cravings vs., 52
Hypertension, 235
See also blood pressure

I

Impossible Dream Thinking
See attitude traps
Insulin, 148

Internal attitude traps
See attitude traps
Iodine, 120

Iron, 120, 167, 236
Suggested intake of, 236

K

Kentucky Fried Chicken, 209

Kilocalories, 37

L

Lactose, 166

Lapse
See relapse
LDL
See cholesterol
LEARN Education Center, 303

LEARN Healthy Eating and Calorie Guide

Daily calorie requirements, 45
Description, 9
How to order, 304
LEARN Institute for LifeStyle Management, 303, 304

LEARN Program
A two month review, 135
Approach of, 11, 12
Description, 3, 11
Format of, 4
How the program is used, 12
Long-term results, 6
What it is all about, 2
LEARN Program Cassettes 2000
Description, 8, 304
How to use with The LEARN Program, 2, 11
LEARN Program Monitoring Forms, 304

LEARN WalkMaster
An impressive study, 20
Description, 9
Getting feedback and staying motivated to be active, 56
Measuring physical activity with, 20
See also physical activity
Light bulb thinking
See also attitude traps
Lignin, 176

Lipoproteins, 221

Living with Exercise 2000, 35, 304

Low density lipoprotein (LDL)
See cholesterol

M

Macronutrients
See minerals
Magnesium, 120, 167

Maintenance
See weight loss
Manganese, 120

Margarine, 104

Master List of Techniques, 242

Master Monitoring Form, 241
Examining, 254
Mastering Stress 2000—A LifeStyle Approach, 162, 304

McDonald's, 209

Metabolism, 21
Effects of exercise on, 34
Micronutrients
See minerals
Milk, yogurt, and cheese food group
See Food Guide Pyramid
In your diet, 121
Recommended servings from, 122

Serving sizes, 122
Sample foods from, 122
Minerals, 119, 233
Functions of, 120
Macronutrients, 119
Micronutrients, 119
See also under individual names
Molybdenum, 120

Monitoring form
See also food diary
See also record keeping
Recording your physical activity on, 93
See worksheets and forms
Monounsaturated fats
See dietary fat
Mood
How your thoughts effect, 99
Multiple vitamins
See vitamins
Muscle, 148

My Self-Assessment
See self assessments

N

National Cholesterol Education Program, 221

Niacin, 120, 164, 165

Nickel, 120

Non-judgmental
Being, 279
Nutrients with energy, 119

Nutrients without energy, 119

Nutrition
Importance of, 233
Nutrition facts panel, 146

Nutrition Labeling and Education Act of 1990 (NLEA), 146

O

Oil
Coconut, 103
Corn, 103
Cotton Seed, 103
Fish, 103
Palm kernel, 103
Palm, 103
Safflower, 103
Soybean, 103
Sunflower, 103
Ordering information, 303

Osteoporosis, 234

Overcoming Binge Eating, 125, 304

Overweight
Reasons for, 21

Why losing weight is difficult, 35

P

Partnership
A shopping, 102
A walking, 58
Eating out with, 186
Something for your partner to read, 143
Pectin, 176

Phosphorus, 120

Physical activity
A new formula for Americans, 117
A walking partnership, 58
Aerobics, 173
Barriers to, 55
Benefits of exercise, 34
Benefits of, 172, 198
Calorie values for 10 minutes of, 94
Calorie values of, 93
Cardiovascular training, 128
Clothes, shoes, and weather, 51
Count all activity as exercise, 92
Cycling, 163
Advantages of, 163
Effect of technology on, 117
Effect on learning ability, 109
Effect on weight maintenance, 108
Effects on stress, 172
Environmental effects on, 118
See also exercise
Exercise threshold, 130
F.I.T. approach, 129
Duration, 129
Frequency, 129
Intensity, 129
Resistance training, 129
Type of activity, 129
Getting feedback and staying motivated, 56
Getting started, 19
Habits, 136
Importance of being active, 33
Is exercise safe for you, 49
Jogging and running, 162
Benefits of, 163
Labor-saving devices, effect on, 117
Levels in America, 117
Lifestyle activity, 92
Developing permanent habits, 110
Reviewing your progress, 110
Techniques for, 92
Making it count, 91
Matching to your goals, 139
Measuring
The LEARN WalkMaster, 20

Using a pedometer, 20
Misconceptions about, 118
Myth of spot reducing, 141
New guidelines for, 118
Predictor of long-term success, 198
Presidential Sports Award, 57
Programmed, 126
Choosing, 126
Pulse test, 207
Reasons people resist, 139
Reasons to be active, 108, 188
Revisiting, 244
Stairs, 187
Stretching exercises
Arm circles, 128
Sit-and-reach, 128
Toe touches, 128
Trunk twists, 128
The 15-minute prescription, 55
The LEARN concept of, 49
Tracking your progress, 93
See also walking
Warming up and cooling down, 127
Work at the office, 211
Physical Activity Readiness Questionnaire (PAR-Q), 49, 50

Planning healthy meals, 107

Pleasurable partner activities, 174

Polyunsaturated fat
See dietary fat
Potassium, 120, 233, 235

Poultry, 210

President's Council on Physical Fitness and Sports, 118

Presidential Sports Award, 57
Requirements for fitness walking award, 57
Requirements for tennis award, 57
Pressures to eat
See eating
Principle of Shaping, 62

Program partnerships, 80
See also partnership
Progress
See reviewing your progress,
Reviewing your, 251
Taking credit for your, 251
Protein, 119
Definition, 148
High-quality, 148
Importance of, 148
Low-quality, 148
Recommended intake, 150
Sources of, 148
Soy, 148

Prothrombin, 174

Psychological factors, 22

Pulse test, 207
  Steps for taking, 208
Pyridoxine
  See vitamin B6

Q

Quality of life
  Assessing, 68
  Weight loss, 74
  Your health, 73
Quality of Life Self-Assessment
  Introduction and orientation lesson, 9
  Lesson eight, 133
  Lesson four, 69
  Lesson sixteen, 247, 248
  Lesson twelve, 194
  Review of
  See worksheets and forms

R

Readiness
  See Weight loss readiness
Reasonable weight loss, 74
  Your vision of, 38
    See also goals and expectations
Reasonable weight, 252

Recommended Daily Allowance, 120

Record keeping
  A challenge, 245
  Purpose and importance, 14, 244
    See also food diary
    See also monitoring forms
Reference Daily Intakes, 147

Relapse
  Collapse,
    Definition, 216
  Definition, 216
  Distinguishing between lapse, relapse,
    and collapse, 216
  Lapse,
    Coping with, 227
    Definition, 216
  Preventing, 215, 227
  Six steps to gaining control, 228
  Slip, 215
Relationships
  See also partnership
Restaurants
  See eating
Reviewing your progress, 197
  Attitude achievements, 199
  Exercise achievements, 198
  Lifestyle achievements, 197
  Nutrition achievements, 201

Relationship achievements, 200
Riboflavin, 120, 164, 165

S

Salt, 234
  See also sodium
Saturated fat
  See dietary fat
Selecting an Eating Plan, 66

Selenium, 120

Self assessment
  Purpose of, 23
Self-Assessments
  Lesson eight, 133
  Lesson eleven, 181
  Lesson fifteen, 238
  Lesson five, 83
  Lesson four, 70
  Lesson fourteen, 224
  Lesson nine, 152
  Lesson one, 24
  Lesson seven, 114
  Lesson six, 97
  Lesson sixteen, 249
  Lesson ten, 169
  Lesson thirteen, 212
  Lesson three, 53
  Lesson twelve, 195
  Lesson two, 39
Self-esteem
  See also body image
  Your body and, 110
Semi-essential fatty acid, 103

Serving and dispensing food, 137
  See also food
Shaping
  Principles of, 62
Shaping the Right Attitudes, 60

Shopping for food
  Foods requiring preparation, 102
  On a full stomach, 101
  Using a list, 102
  With a partner, 102
Silicon, 120

Simple sugars (carbohydrate)
  See carbohydrate
Skills
  Building, 13
  See also confidence
Sleep disturbances, 12

Slimnastics, 173

Slip
  See relapse
Snacks
  Dietary fat in, 107
  Healthful, 124
Social changers, 80

Social support
  Choosing a support person, 89
    A quiz for, 89
  Enlisting, 255
  Its importance, 81
  See also partnership
  Support partner quiz, 90
Sodium, 120, 189, 233, 234
  Suggested daily intake, 234
Solo changers, 80

Spot reducing
  The myth of, 141
Starches
  See carbohydrate,
Storing foods, 123

Stress
  And eating, 160
    Questions to ask yourself, 161
  Effects of exercise on, 172
  How to overcome, 161
  Relationship between body, mind, and
    environment, 161
Stroke, 221

Sucrose, 166

Sulfur, 120

T

Tables and charts
  A dozen other reasons to exercise, 188
  Alternatives incompatible with eating,
    219
  Benefits of various exercises, 140
  Breaking the links in Laura's behavior
    chain, 205
  Calorie values for 10 minutes of activity,
    94
  Calories and fat in poultry, 210
  Cholesterol content of common foods,
    222
  Fat from the different food group choices,
    105
  Foods from the Bread, Cereal, Rice, &
    Pasta Group, 191
  Foods from the Fruit Group, 179
  Foods from the Meat, Poultry, Fish, Dry
    Beans, Eggs, & Nuts Group, 149
  Foods from the Milk, Yogurt, & Cheese
    Group, 122
  Foods from the Vegetable Group, 168
  High-fiber fruits, vegetables, and cereals,
    177
  Imperative and counter statements, 160
  Minerals, 120
  Office calories (burning), 211
  Pulse test, 208
  Resources for walkers, 243
  Six classifications of nutrients, 120
  Sodium content of foods, 235

Support organizations for eating disorders, 125
Vitamins, 120
Taking control of your eating, 75

Technology
Effect on physical activity, 117
The Body Image Workbook, 304

The LifeStyle Company
Address, 10
E-mail address, 10
Ordering information, 303
To order from, 10
Thiamine, 120, 164

Thoughts
Determining how you feel, 99
Effect on mood, 99
Emotional responses to, 100
How they can help you succeed, 99
Your thinking process, 99
Toxic environment, 209
Bracing against, 209
Triggers
See eating

U

U.S. Centers for Disease Control and Prevention, 118

Urges
Being an urge surfer, 217
Identifying, 217
Outlasting, 217
Using alternative activities, 218
Using the stairs
See physical activity

V

Vanadium, 120

Vegetables
See also Food Guide Pyramid
In your diet, 167
Vegetarian diets, 148

Very-low-calorie diet (VLCD), 46

Vigorous activity, 130

Vitamin A, 120, 121, 145, 167, 174, 189

Vitamin B$_1$
See thiamine
Vitamin B$_{12}$, 120, 164, 165

Vitamin B$_2$
See riboflavin
Vitamin B$_3$
See niacin
Vitamin B$_6$, 120, 164, 165

Vitamin C, 120, 145, 164, 165, 167

Vitamin D, 120, 121, 145, 174, 189

Vitamin E, 120, 145, 174

Vitamin K, 120, 145, 174

Vitamins, 103, 119, 144
B-complex, 145, 164, 165
Effect on weight loss, 144
Fat soluble, 120, 174
Multiple, 165
See under individual names
Water soluble, 120, 164

W

Walking
A partnership, 58
Advantages of, 51
Clothing, 51
Continuing, 110
Increasing, 78
Lifestyle activity, 110
Mall, 52
Maximizing the pleasure of, 78
Not overdoing, 78
Paying attention while, 78
Perfecting, 78
Resources for walkers, 243
Reviewing your progress, 110
Starting your program, 51
Taking a gradual approach, 78
Using entertainment, 78
Weather, 51
Water, 119, 121

Weekly personal goals
Lesson eight, 132
Lesson eleven, 180
Lesson fifteen, 237
Lesson five, 82
Lesson four, 69
Lesson fourteen, 223
Lesson nine, 152
Lesson one, 23
Lesson seven, 113
Lesson six, 97
Lesson ten, 168
Lesson thirteen, 211
Lesson three, 52
Lesson twelve, 194
Lesson two, 39
Weighing yourself
How often, 48
Weight Change Record
Description, 17
Sample, lesson one, 19
See also worksheets and forms
Weight Control Digest, 304
Description, 10
How to order, 304
Weight loss

A revolution in thinking, 12
A two month review, 137
Calorie intake, 74
Maintenance, 6, 108, 201, 215
Why losing weight is difficult, 35
Your vision of reasonable weight changes, 38
Weight loss benefits
What it can mean in your life, 3
Weight loss readiness
About, 264
Benefits and sacrifices, 5
Consequences of not being ready, 263
Discussion of, 263
Is the time right for you, 4
Test categories, 265
Test, 267
What is readiness, 263
Weight Loss Readiness Test, 267

Weight management
Like life on Chutes and Ladders, 230
Wendy's, 209

Wine, 185

Worksheets and forms
Calculating my daily fat intake, 104
Countering Dichotomous (Light Bulb) Thinking, 220
Cravings vs. hunger quiz, lesson three, 53
Expanded food diary—lesson three, 54
Expanded food diary—lesson two, 41
Food diary—lesson one, 27
Master Monitoring Form, commencement lesson, 258
Master Monitoring Form, lesson sixteen, 250
Monitoring form, lesson eight, 134
Monitoring form, lesson eleven, 182
Monitoring form, lesson fifteen, 239
Monitoring form, lesson five, 84
Monitoring form, lesson four sample, 71
Monitoring form, lesson four, 72
Monitoring form, lesson fourteen, 225
Monitoring form, lesson nine, 153
Monitoring form, lesson seven, 115
Monitoring form, lesson six, 98, 153
Monitoring form, lesson ten, 170
Monitoring form, lesson thirteen, 213
Monitoring form, lesson twelve, 196
My alternatives to Eating, 219
My eating patterns worksheet, lesson three, 45
My eating patterns worksheet, lesson two, 32
My eating schedule, 76
My goals for this program, 61
My plans for dining out, 186

My reasonable weight loss, lesson two, 42

My Weight Change Record (weeks 1–8), 25

My Weight Change Record (weeks 9–16), 154

Physical Activity Readiness Questionnaire (PAR-Q), 50

Progress in my program, lesson six, 96

Quality of Life Self-Assessment, introduction and orientation lesson, 9

Quality of Life Self-Assessment, lesson eight, 133

Quality of Life Self-Assessment, lesson four, 69

Quality of Life Self-Assessment, lesson sixteen, 248

Quality of Life Self-Assessment, lesson twelve, 194

Quality of Life Improvement Worksheet, 249

Rate your diet quiz
    Lesson eight, 287
    Lesson sixteen, 291
    Lesson two, 283

Review of Quality of Life
    Self-Assessment, lesson four 70
    Self-Assessments, lesson nine, 136
    Self-Assessment, lesson twelve, 195

Support partner quiz, 90

Your calorie target, lesson three, 46

Z

Zinc, 120

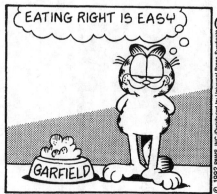
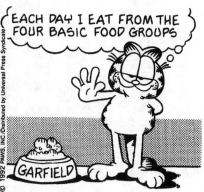
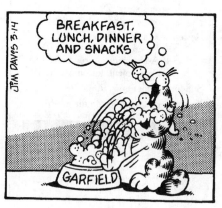

SUPPLEMENTAL RESOURCES AND ORDERING INFORMATION

This manual and the other materials distributed through The Life-Style Company are not available in bookstores. You may write, call, or visit us on the Internet to obtain current pricing and shipping charges. Discounts are available for bulk orders. Below are other materials and services also available.

The LifeStyle Company

The LifeStyle Company, a division of The LEARN Education Center, was established to respond to the increasing demand for scientifically sound, state-of-the-art publications, training courses, and services. The LifeStyle Company is dedicated to the development of health and wellness materials, including audio tapes, newsletters, professional training guides, leadership training programs, and professional counseling services.

For your ordering convenience, a toll free telephone number is available and may be called 24 hours a day. In addition, you can order via our Internet address at www.TheLifeStyleCompany.com. Payments can be made with a major credit card, check, or money order.

All orders are shipped with 24 hours of receipt, and next day and second day delivery service is available. As you use our publications, we sincerely welcome any comments you may have to improve these materials, and we encourage you to tell us how we are doing.

For ordering or general information, please write or call us at:

The LifeStyle Company
P.O. Box 610430, Dept. 70
Dallas, Texas 75261–0430

Telephone (In the U.S.)	**1-888–LEARN–41**
Telephone (Outside the U.S.)	**817–545–4500**
Fax	**817–545–2211**

E-mail address:

LEARN@TheLifeStyleCompany.com

Internet address:

www.TheLifeStyleCompany.com

The LEARN Institute for LifeStyle Management

The LEARN Institute was established to provide state-of-the-art training programs to health professionals working with overweight clients. The LEARN Institute is the first to offer specific training and certification in the field of weight control. The LifeStyle Counselor Certification Program has been developed to provide a comprehensive cross-disciplinary training program to health professionals working in the field of weight and stress management.

Two certifications are currently offered and training is provided in various cities throughout the United States. Certifications currently being offered include:

Certification in Weight Control
Certification in Stress Management

For more detailed information on The LifeStyle Counselor Certification Program or a free brochure call or write to:

**The LEARN Institute for
  LifeStyle Management**
P.O. Box 610430, Dept. 50
Dallas, Texas 75261–04308
Telephone (In the U.S.)   1-888–LEARN–50
Telephone (Outside the U.S.)   817–545–4500
Fax   817–545–2211

E-mail address:
          TheInstitute@LearnEducation.com
Internet address:
          www.LearnEducation.com

The American Association of LifeStyle Counselors

The American Association of LifeStyle Counselors is a nonprofit corporation dedicated to providing its members and the public with the most current, safe, and sound lifestyle-management programs and services. Individuals who complete the LifeStyle Counselor Certification Program become eligible for membership in the American Association of LifeStyle Counselors (AALC). Only members of the AALC can use the title of Certified LifeStyle Counselor®. If you would like to locate a Certified LifeStyle Counselor in your area you may write, call, or visit the AALC's Internet site as follows:

**The American Association
  of LifeStyle Counselors**

P.O. Box 610410, Dept. 55
Dallas, Texas 76261–0410

Telephone   817–545–3220
Fax   817–545–2211

E-mail address   AALC@AALC.org
Internet address   www.AALC.org

Other Materials

Publications currently available from The LEARN Education Center are as follows:

Weight Management

The LEARN Program Cassettes 2000, by Kelly D. Brownell, Ph.D.

The LEARN Program for Weight Management 2000, by Kelly D. Brownell, Ph.D.

The LEARN Program for Weight Management—Meal Replacement Edition, by Kelly D. Brownell, Ph.D.—Available in 2000.

The LEARN Program for Weight Control—Special Medication Edition, by Kelly D. Brownell, Ph.D. and Thomas A. Wadden, Ph.D.

The LEARN Program Monitoring Forms

The LifeStyle Counselor's Guide for Weight Control, by Brenda L. Wolfe, Ph.D., et al.

The Weight Control Digest—annual subscription.

Diet and Nutrition

Health Ways to Manage Your Weight, by Kelly D. Brownell, Ph.D.—Available in 2000.

The LEARN Healthy Eating and Calorie Guide.

Eating Disorders

Overcoming Binge Eating, by Christopher Fairburn, M.D.

Physical Activity

Living with Exercise 2000, by Steven N. Blair, P.E.D.—Available in 2000.

Stress Management

Mastering Stress 2000—A LifeStyle Approach, by David H. Barlow, Ph.D., Leslie Reisner, Ph.D., Ronald M. Rapee, Ph.D.—Available in 2000.

Mind Over Mood, by Dennis Greenberger, Ph.D. and Christine A. Padesky, Ph.D.

Other Materials

The Body Image Workbook, by Thomas F. Cash, Ph.D.

Motivational Interviewing, by William R. Miller and Stephen Rollnick.

The LEARN WalkMaster.

Notes

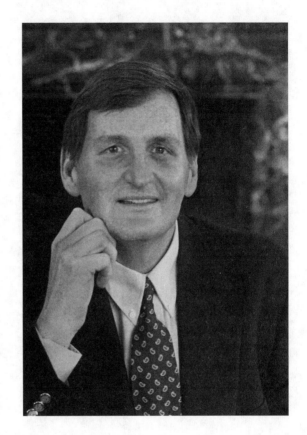

Kelly D. Brownell, Ph.D., is an internationally known expert on weight management. He received training at Purdue University, Rutgers University, and Brown University. After serving on the faculty of the University of Pennsylvania School of Medicine for 13 years, he joined the faculty at Yale University, where he is Professor of Psychology, Professor of Epidemiology and Public Health, Director of the Yale Center for Eating and Weight Disorders, and Master of Silliman College. He has written 12 books and more than 200 research papers and book chapters, and holds appointments on 10 editorial boards.

TAPE 1
SECTION 3

Dr. Brownell has received awards from the American Psychological Association and the New York Academy of Sciences, and has been awarded research grants from the National Institutes of Health, the MacArthur Foundation, and the National Institute of Mental Health. He has been the President of the Society of Behavioral Medicine, the Division of Health Psychology of the American Psychological Association, and the Association for the Advancement of Behavior Therapy. He has been an advisor to the U.S. Navy, American Airlines, Johnson & Johnson and other organizations.

He has appeared on the *Today Show*, *Good Morning America*, *Nova* and *20/20*, and his work has been featured in the *New York Times, Washington Post, Glamour, Redbook, Family Circle, Vogue*, and other publications.